Advanced Concepts and Strategies in Central Nervous System Tumors

Edited by Frances Chow
and Lindsay Hwang

Published in London, United Kingdom

Advanced Concepts, Strategies in Central Nervous System Tumors
http://dx.doi.org/10.5772/intechopen.1003586
Edited by Frances Chow, Lindsay Hwang

Contributors
Abdullah Alobaid, Alejandro González, Alma Ortiz-Plata, Andres F. Cardona, Antonina S. Rait, Arianna Casciati, Caterina Merla, Christopher Hancock, Ciltlaltepetl Salinas-Lara, Conrado Martínez-Cadenas, Cristiano Palego, Daniel Hieber, Daniel Rembao-Bojórquez, Diana Chavez-Muñoz, Diego Pineda, Diocelina Navarro-Bastida, Dongjiang Chen, Elena Rampazzo, Elvira M. Carbonell-Martínez, Esther H. Chang, Felix Holl, Frances Chow, Friederike Liesche-Starnecker, Ivan Pašalić, Iván Bobadilla, Javier A. Jacobo, Jenny Christine Kienzler, Jie Huang, Joe B. Harford, Johannes Schobel, Johnny Odeh, Jorge H. Aristizabal, Juan L. Gómez-Amador, Julia L. Gutiérrez-Arroyo, Kathleen F. Pirollo, Kyle Conway, Lesly Portocarrero-Ortiz, Lindsay Hwang, Luca Persano, Lucas Santana-Santos, Luis G. González-Bonet, Madina Sukhanova, Maria Angeles Marqués-Torrejón, Mariateresa Mancuso, Martha Tena-Suck, Matthew McCord, Miguel A. Ramos-Peek, Mirella Tanori, Miroslav Vukić, Natalia Villa-Corral, Nicolle Wagner-Gutiérrez, Noemi Gelista-Herrera, Oscar Arrieta, Pia Gallego-Porcar, Ping Shi, Pouya Jamshidi, Pramath Kakodkar, Qian Dai, Razan Almufarriji, Ricardo Gómez-Rivera, Rudolph Castellani, Samuel Guzman, Sang-Soo Kim, Santiago Vallejo, Sarah Binabdulqader, Sergio Zavala-Vega, Tadej Strojnik, Vera Nickl, Xuan Zhai, Yazeed Alotaibi

First published in London, United Kingdom, 2025 by IntechOpen
IntechOpen is the global imprint of INTECHOPEN LIMITED, registered in England, Wales, registration number: 11086078, 167-169 Great Portland Street, London, W1W 5PF, United Kingdom

For EU product safety concerns: IN TECH d.o.o., Prolaz Marije Krucifikse Kozulić 3, 51000 Rijeka, Croatia, info@intechopen.com or visit our website at intechopen.com.

British Library Cataloguing-in-Publication Data
A catalogue record for this book is available from the British Library

Advanced Concepts, Strategies in Central Nervous System Tumors
Edited by Frances Chow, Lindsay Hwang
p. cm.

This title is part of the Oncology Book Series, Volume 2
Series Editor: Thomas J. FitzGerald

Print ISBN 978-0-85014-808-4
Online ISBN 978-0-85014-807-7
eBook (PDF) ISBN 978-0-85014-809-1
ISSN 3049-8864

IntechOpen Book Series
Oncology
Volume 2

Aims and Scope of the Series

The field of oncology has undergone extraordinary change and progress over the past several decades. Today, information is evolving at a rapid rate, with standards of management far different than standards of care applied during the training of most practicing oncologists. Oncology practitioners in all disciplines must remain current to optimize patient care. Basic and translational science remain critical in developing process improvements for patient care. The closer we understand the mechanism, the more we can improve targeted therapies and apply them to patient care. The pace of information is moving faster than at any previous time in history, and all oncology disciplines must remain current to provide excellent service to patients. The modern oncologist must be fluent in using big data and the volume of information generated in clinical trials. As we move closer to personalized patient care based on genomics and molecular biomarkers, the modern oncologist has to be nimble in assessing all available information and how this would be applied to each patient, balanced by the clinical status and medical co-morbidities of each patient. Targeted therapies can bring new and different sequelae, and oncology teams need to remain fluent in managing the consequences of therapy and primary management. In this book series, we will present how modern care has progressed in multiple disease areas and how modern oncology teams need to adapt in order to manage the cancer patients of today successfully. Surgery, radiation therapy, and medical oncology are practiced today with the support of exceptional modern technology, and in this series, we will review how these improvements are applied to each disease site to maintain excellence in patient care.

Meet the Series Editor

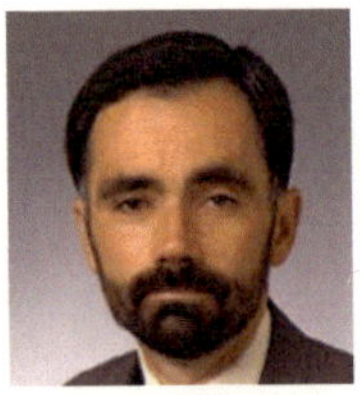

Dr. FitzGerald is the professor and chair of the Department of Radiation Oncology at UMass Chan Medical School in the USA. He serves as one of the principal investigators of the Imaging and Radiation Oncology Core (IROC) service for the National Cancer Institute clinical trials program and is directly involved in the quality assurance of clinical trials in the National Clinical Trials Network (NCTN). Dr. Fitzgerald manages NCTN clinical trials with a real-time pre-therapy review of imaging and radiation therapy treatment objects to ensure the care plan complies with study objectives and the patient stage has been assigned to the correct study. His basic science interest is in hematopoietic stem cell biology and cellular adhesion molecules as they pertain to therapeutic resistance and mitigation of injury from therapy.

Meet the Volume Editor

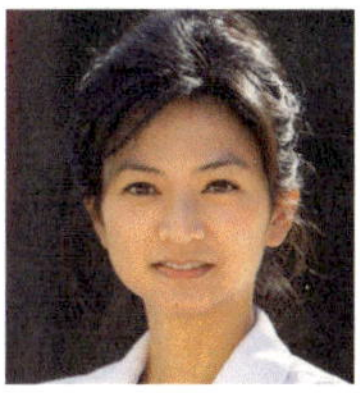

Frances Chow, MD, is an Assistant Professor of Neurological Surgery and Neurology at the Keck School of Medicine at the University of Southern California in the USA. She specializes in neuro-oncology and the management of central nervous system tumors. As a National Institutes of Health-supported scientist and National Cancer Institute Cancer Therapy Evaluation Program principal investigator, Dr. Chow's research focuses on the tumor microenvironment and systemic effects of immunotherapy, biomarker development, and clinical trials for central nervous system tumors. Dr. Chow was inducted into the Society for Immunotherapy of Cancer Women in Immunotherapy Leadership Institute and the Society for Neuro-Oncology Future Leaders Development Program. She has been named a Top Doctor by Los Angeles Magazine.

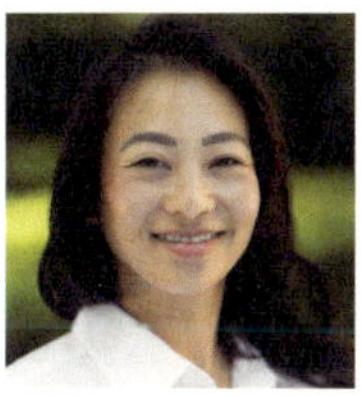

Lindsay Hwang, MD, is a Clinical Assistant Professor of Radiation Oncology (LAGMC) at the Keck School of Medicine at the University of Southern California and Los Angeles General Medical Center. She specializes in radiation treatment of benign and malignant central nervous system tumors and radiosurgical techniques. Dr. Hwang is the associate program director of the radiation oncology residency training program and has been awarded the Association of Residents in Radiation Oncology Educator of the Year Award.

Contents

Preface

The central nervous system (CNS) has been regarded as a sacred frontier in medicine. Despite valiant efforts, managing primary tumors of the central nervous system has been relatively unchanged in the past decades, with incremental improvements in outcomes. Modern scientific and technological advancements have spurred new explorations and resulted in numerous exciting preclinical and clinical trials that may bring us to the next era in diagnosing and treating tumors of the central nervous system.

In this edition, we will begin by exploring the molecular classification of CNS tumors and reviewing advances in imaging-based pathologic diagnosis. Next, we present several chapters covering recent learnings on the etiology and biology of glioblastoma and other CNS tumors including pediatric tumors associated with neurofibromatosis. Finally, we offer a selection of chapters on novel therapeutics in managing benign and malignant brain tumors, ranging from electrical tumor treatment fields, encapsulated chemotherapeutic techniques, immunotherapeutic advances, and therapeutic stem cells.

Frances Chow, MD
Departments of Neurological Surgery and Neurology,
University of Southern California,
Los Angeles, USA

Lindsay Hwang, MD
Department of Radiation Oncology,
Los Angeles General Medical Center,
Los Angeles, USA

Section 1

Introduction

Chapter 1

Introductory Chapter: Mind and Matter – Applications of Artificial Intelligence in CNS Tumors

Lindsay Hwang and Frances Chow

1. Introduction

The term artificial intelligence (AI) was first coined by John McCarthy during the Dartmouth Conference in 1955 [1]. Since then, its application in medicine has steadily increased with wide *applications* in data management and analytics, diagnostic tools, surgical robotic systems, and even decision-making. Modern medicine harnesses the pattern-recognition power of computers and artificial intelligence to aid scientists and physicians in making advances in the detection and treatment of a wide range of diseases. In the management of brain tumors, specifically, artificial intelligence has led to advancements in diagnosis and prognostication.

We discuss how artificial intelligence assists radiology and pathology-based tumor segmentation and ways in which artificial intelligence-based approaches are advancing drug discovery in brain tumors.

2. Deep learning in radiology

Applications of AI radiomics include novel methods of classification, guidance of radiation treatment volumes, early recognition of tumor progression versus necrosis, and prediction of therapeutic response. An increasing number of studies employ deep learning features to improve the accuracy, sensitivity and specificity of imaging modalities (such as MRI, positron emission tomography (PET), and spectroscopy) and to link an array of imaging features to prognostic outcomes in gliomas [2].

While individual cohorts are instrumental in the initial development of AI systems, there remain challenges in validation. Therefore, larger multi-institutional cohorts through international collaborative efforts are helping to streamline AI-driven advances in radiology. The Brain Tumor Segmentation (BraTS) challenge—launched in 2012 through the collective efforts of the Radiological Society of North America (RSNA), the American Society of Neuroradiology (ASNR), and the Medical Image Computing and Computer-Assisted Interventions (MICCAI) Society—releases annual themed challenges to focus on state-of-the-art methods to segment, classify, and predict outcomes for publicly available datasets. The libraries compiled by BraTS facilitate the development of deep-learning models for CNS tumors including glioblastoma, diffuse midline glioma, and low-grade glioma. Global efforts such as BraTS in data-sharing and collaboration are critical in the advancement of AI radiomics for rare conditions like primary CNS tumors.

3. Pathology-based tumor segmentation

The pace of diagnostic and therapeutic advancements for brain tumors continues to rapidly accelerate. The major updates of the 2021 WHO Classification of CNS Tumors reflect the incorporation of histologic, genomic, transcriptomic, and methylomic data into the diagnosis and prognosis of tumors [3]. Additional computational approaches to integrate and analyze invasive pathological data with non-invasive imaging include the evolution of prediction algorithms to classify tumor subtypes rather than histological grade, IDH mutation status, 1p/19q codeletion status, MGMT promoter methylation, and prognostic markers that integrate clinical features. Some strategies in progress include using radiomics-based machine learning classifiers to differentiate between enhancing intracranial lesions (brain metastasis versus glioma versus lymphoma) or to determine vasogenic edema from non-contrast-enhancing tumors [4–6]. These potential tools can not only minimize invasive procedures such as biopsies, but they can also help to better define treatment volumes in the planning of radiation therapy.

In recognition of the significant and potential role of AI-based biomarkers, the Artificial Intelligence for Response Assessment in Neuro Oncology (AI-RANO) international working group recently proposed a set of recommendations to offer policy and guidance to this rapidly developing field [7, 8]. In addition to summarizing strides made in the last decade, the recommendations highlight the potential role of adapting AI in neuro-oncology clinical trials and the importance of trustworthiness and centralized efforts.

4. *In silico* prediction of novel drugs

Drug discovery is a field enriched by rapidly growing tools to more efficiently identify and develop candidate therapies. The computational technique of molecular docking can predict the affinity of ligands to receptors in a virtual, simulation-based *in silico* platform. This novel strategy can screen large libraries to identify candidate molecules based on drug-likeness or binding affinity *in silico*, to then be evaluated *in vitro*, thus facilitating drug design and development [9]. Molecular docking is playing an expanding role in precision medicine by speeding the rate of discovery while reducing the cost of expensive experiments and trials.

5. Social implications: Diversity and inclusion

The quality of data fed into AI drives the quality of its results. A concerted effort to include diverse demographics and historically underrepresented populations is critical as AI continues to integrate into the future of neuro-oncology. Women and minorities remain significantly under-accrued in neuro-oncology clinical trials, representing only 1.5% (Asians), 1.7% (Hispanics), and 2.6% (Blacks) of trial participants [10]. As therapeutics evolve with a greater emphasis on targeted therapies and personalized medicine, a diverse representation in clinical trials and tissue repository datasets will be necessary to ensure the validity and generalizability of results.

6. Conclusion and future directions

Thus far, the use of AI models in clinical practice has been limited by poor generalizability and external validity. As we develop meticulously annotated public and collaborative radiology, pathology, and clinical databases, it is critical to promote reference standards and employ widespread use of standardized imaging protocols and metadata libraries across institutions and diagnoses. Furthermore, the implications of inclusion and ethical considerations of data privacy are imperative in the collaboration, storage, and sharing of data. AI serves as a transformative tool in the advancement of concepts and strategies for central nervous system tumors.

Author details

Lindsay Hwang and Frances Chow*
University of Southern California, United States of America

*Address all correspondence to: frances.chow@med.usc.edu

References

[1] McCarthy J. What Is Artificial Intelligence? Stanford: Stanford University; 2007. Available from: https://www-formal.stanford.edu/jmc/whatisai.pdf

[2] Luo J, Pan M, Mo K, Mao Y, Zou D. Emerging role of artificial intelligence in diagnosis, classification and clinical management of glioma. Seminars in Cancer Biology. 2023;**91**:110-123. DOI: 10.1016/j.semcancer.2023.03.006

[3] Central Nervous System Tumours. WHO Classification of Tumours. 5th ed. Vol. 6. Lyon: International Agency for Research on Cancer; 2021

[4] Alcaide-Leon P, Dufort P, Geraldo AF, Alshafai L, Maralani PF, Spears J, et al. Differentiation of enhancing glioma and primary central nervous system lymphoma by texture-based machine learning. AJNR. American Journal of Neuroradiology. 2017;**38**(6):1145-1150

[5] Qian Z, Li Y, Wang Y, et al. Differentiation of glioblastoma from solitary brain metastases using radiomic machine-learning classifiers. Cancer Letters. 2019;**451**:128-135. DOI: 10.1016/j.canlet.2019.02.054

[6] Sengupta A, Agarwal S, Gupta PK, et al. On differentiation between vasogenic edema and non-enhancing tumor in high-grade glioma patients using support vector machine classifier based upon pre- and post-surgery MRI images. European Journal of Radiology. 2018;**106**:199-208. DOI: 10.1016/j.ejrad.2018.07.018

[7] Villanueva-Meyer JE, Bakas S, Tiwari P, Lupo JM, Calabrese E, Davatzikos C, et al. Galldiks N; response assessment in neuro oncology (RANO) group. Artificial intelligence for response assessment in neuro oncology (AI-RANO), part 1: Review of current advancements. The Lancet Oncology. 2024;**25**(11):e581-e588

[8] Bakas S, Vollmuth P, Galldikis N, Booth TC, HJWL A, Bi WL, et al. Artificial intelligence for response assessment in neuro oncology (AI-RANO), part 2: Recommendations for standardisation, validation, and good clinical practice. The Lancet Oncology. 2024;**25**(11):e589-e601

[9] Gentile F, Yaacoub JC, Gleave J, et al. Artificial intelligence–enabled virtual screening of ultra-large chemical libraries with deep docking. Nature Protocols. 2022;**17**:672-697

[10] Reihl SJ, Patil N, Morshed RA, Mehari M, Aabedi A, Chukwueke UN, et al. A population study of clinical trial accrual for women and minorities in neuro-oncology following the NIH revitalization act. Neuro-Oncology. 2022;**24**(8):1341-1349

Section 2

Classification

Chapter 2

DNA Methylation-Based Classification of the Central Nervous System Tumors, Achievements, and Challenges

Pramath Kakodkar, Kyle Conway, Lucas Santana-Santos, Matthew McCord, Madina Sukhanova, Rudolph Castellani and Pouya Jamshidi

Abstract

The classification, grading, and risk stratification of central nervous system (CNS) tumors have rapidly evolved with the advent of integrative advanced molecular testing. Here, we review the advances and challenges associated with DNA methylation-based classification of central nervous system (CNS) tumors. Specifically, we will review the brief background information about the role of epigenetic signatures, including DNA methylation status of CpG islands, in identifying the cell of origin, bioinformatic methods, and products of DNA methylation profiling, namely t-distributed stochastic neighbor embedding (t-SNE) plot vs. uniform manifold approximation and projection (UMAP), CNS tumor classifications, methylguanine methyltransferase (MGMT), and chromosomal copy number variations. We will follow with the diagnostic utility, accuracy, and impact on clinical outcomes. We will conclude the chapter by highlighting the limitations of DNA methylation, bioethical issues, and the future directions for this diagnostic tool.

Keywords: whole-genome DNA methylation, CpG islands, t-SNE plot, UMAP, CNS tumors, molecular, bioethics

1. Introduction

Advances in molecular diagnostics have enhanced our understanding of central nervous system (CNS) tumors from morphologically defined to biologically defined entities. Historically, morphology has been the mainstay of CNS tumor pathology assessment despite interobserver variability and subjectivity inherent in pathological interpretation. Since 2016, each edition of the World Health Organization (WHO) CNS tumor classification system has been progressively incorporating cytogenetics and integrative molecular diagnosis attributed to key genetic alterations (i.e., *IDH1*, *ATRX*, *TP53*, *TERT* promoter, *BRAF*, *H3F3A*, *CTTNB1*) [1].

These advances in integrated molecular diagnosis in CNS tumors have now leveraged a relatively novel technology called whole-genome DNA methylation profiling that classifies tumors based on epigenomic lineage signatures. Whole-genome DNA methylation profiling can distinguish tumor types and subtypes, identify new tumor types, and help in the prognosis and risk stratification of tumors [2–5]. It is important to note that DNA methylation-based tumor subclassifications remain consistent with immunohistochemistry identified (ependymoma with ZFTA1 and YAP1 fusions) as well as transcriptomics verified tumor entities such as WNT-activated medulloblastoma [6, 7]. Moreover, whole-genome DNA methylation-based profiling has been utilized to assess prognosis and offer an objective method of risk stratification in several tumor types such as chordomas, meningiomas, atypical teratoid/rhabdoid tumors, and ependymal tumors [5, 8–10].

The whole-genome DNA methylation profiling technology relies on its comparison against a reference tumor methylation library and utilizes a machine learning classifier. This technology was first pioneered by the German Cancer Research Network (Deutsches Krebsforschungszentrum: DKFZ) and the University Hospital Heidelberg [2, 11]. In a landmark study, Capper *et al.* utilized the methylome analysis *via* a random forest algorithm with multinomial logistic regression on the CNS tumor methylation data. While this methylome classifier has not been validated for clinical use, it remains available as an open-source online tool for research (https://www.molecularneuropathology.org/mnp/classifiers, last accessed Oct 29, 2024). In this chapter, we will introduce the common cytosine-guanine (CpG) methylation array-based platforms, and briefly review the bioinformatic analysis regarding the t-distributed Stochastic Neighbor Embedding (t-SNE), Uniform Manifold Approximation and Projection (UMAP) plot, chromosome copy number variation (CNV), and O-6-methylguanine-DNA methyltransferase (MGMT) methylation status. Lastly, as methylation-based profiling gains more widespread use for diagnosis, we overview the potential ethical issues associated with this novel diagnostic tool.

2. Epigenetic signatures

CNS neoplasms have epigenetic determinants that modulate gene transcription, distinct from classical gene sequence alterations [11]. The epigenetic profile of these neoplastic cells can therefore dictate aberrant cell cycle signaling and phenotypic expression. Epigenetic modulation can be achieved with DNA methylation, histone modifications, and microRNAs [12]. It is important to note that DNA methylation remains the well-characterized among the above modalities.

DNA methylation is mediated by DNA methyltransferase (DNMT), which deploys a methyl moiety *via* covalent transfer onto the fifth carbon position of cytosine within the CpG sites subjacent to gene promoters called CpG islands (CGI) [13]. As part of normal development, a cell-type-specific lineage is established by methylation or unmethylation of certain CpG islands. These established DNA methylation patterns remain stable throughout subsequent cell divisions *via* DNMT and can therefore be utilized as a proxy for delineating the cell origin [14]. During tumorigenesis, the mutational burden acquired aims to mitigate apoptosis and promote survival signaling without altering the core epigenetic signatures [12]. Therefore, lineage-defining epigenetic modification evades selective pressure since any alteration in these CpGs will not confer a survival advantage.

In tumors of the central nervous system, there is a global reduction in methylated CGIs coupled with hypermethylation in CGIs pertaining to tumor suppressor genes [13]. Furthermore, cell lineage-specific CpG methylation patterns are retained as the tumor acquires mutational burden [2, 13, 15]. The combination of these features portends the utility of DNA methylation profiling in classification of CNS tumors.

DNA modifications can happen at any of the DNA bases which span from N6-methyladenine (6-mA), N4-methylcytosine (4-mC), 5-methylcytosine (5-mC), 5-hydroxymethylcytosine (5-hmC), 5-formylcytosine (5-fC), or 5-carboxylcytosine (5-caC). These modifications can modulate genomic imprinting, chromatin reorganization, transposon activity, cell differentiation, and gene silencing [16].

The presence of CpG is inferred by bisulfite sequencing of genomic DNA [17]. Unmethylated cytosine is modified to uracil when treated with sodium bisulfite (**Figure 1A**) [17]. In contrast, epigenetic modification with 5′ methylated cytosine (5-mC) or 5′ hydroxymethylated cytosine (5-hmC) remains unaltered after sodium bisulfite treatment (**Figure 1B**) [14]. Therefore, whole-genome bisulfite sequencing (WGBS) can yield a single base-level resolution for nearly 29 million CpG within the human CGI [14]. This high-level resolution paired with the computational complexity and expense makes WGBS a less practical option for high-volume implementation.

A practical solution to WGBS is pairing bisulfite-transformed DNA with CGI microarrays. Commercially available assays such as Illumina Infinium genotyping assay amplify the fragments of the bisulfite-converted DNA and utilize hybridization technology with beads that bind to oligonucleotide probes complementary to specific CpG sites of interest. There have been many iterations of these microarray assays leading to increasing CGI coverage such as the HumanMethylation450 (>450,000 CpGs) and HumanMethylationEPIC (>850,000 CpGs) [18]. These microarray assays

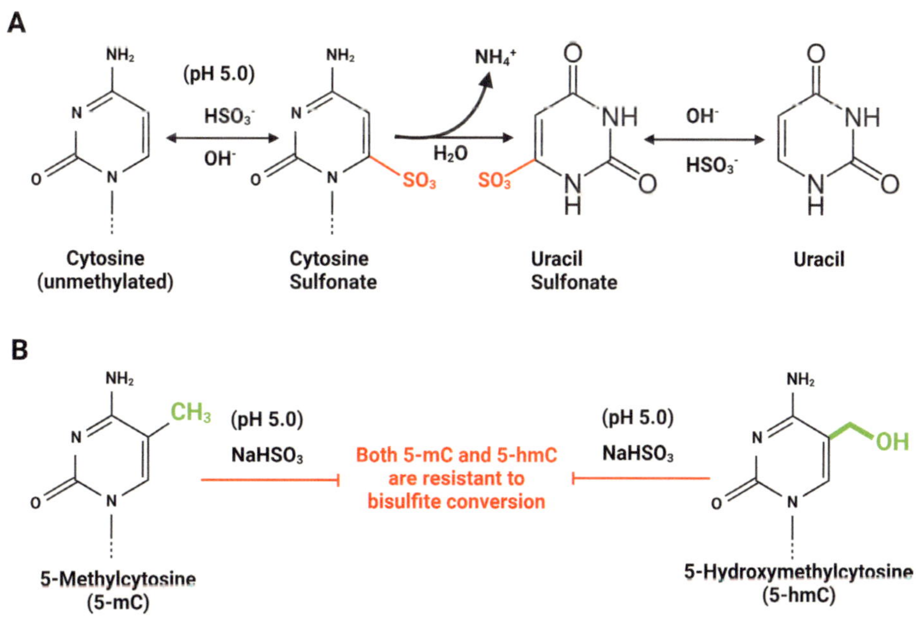

Figure 1.
(A) Unmethylated cytosine is modified to uracil when treated with sodium bisulfite as the initial step in bisulfite sequencing. (B) Epigenetic modification with 5′ methylated cytosine (5-mC) or 5′ hydroxymethylated cytosine (5-hmC) remains unaltered after sodium bisulfite treatment.

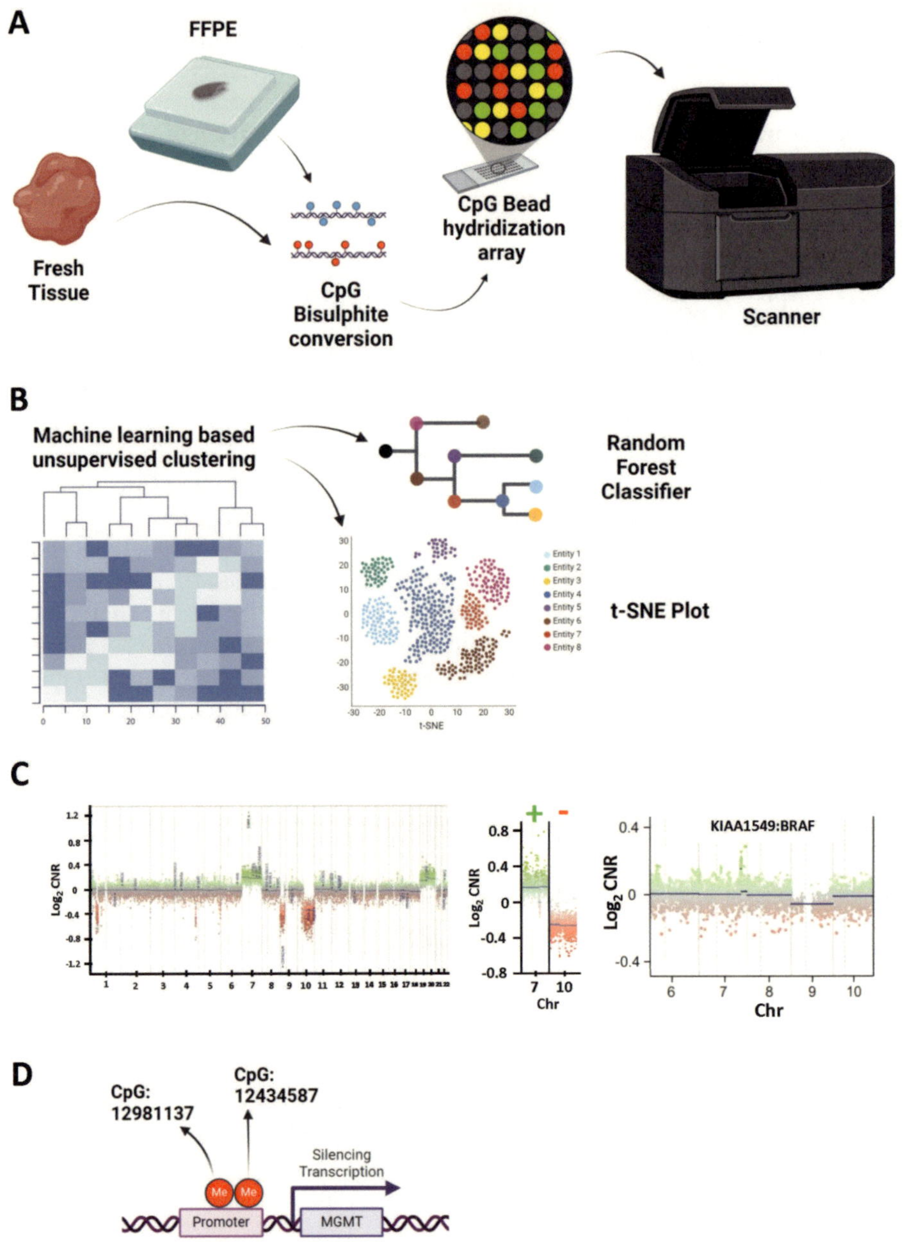

Figure 2.
DNA methylation profiling workflow in surgical neuropathology service. (A) DNA is extracted from both fresh tissue and Formalin-Fixed Paraffin-Embedded (FFPE), which is then bisulfite converted and hybridized to CpG Bead hybridization chip. The chip is scanned, and the resultant methylated and unmethylated fluorescent signals require processing. (B) The DNA methylation data is processed and represented as hierarchical clustering with t-Distributed Stochastic Neighbor Embedding (t-SNE) via *unsupervised machine learning algorithms or as supervised random forest classifiers. (C) The ratio of methylated and unmethylated signal intensities can be utilized to assess copy number alterations. DNA methylation profiling can identify chromosome 7 gain and chromosome 10 loss in glioblastoma as well as copy number breakpoints which can detect BRAF fusions in pilocytic astrocytomas. (D) DNA methylation profiling can be used to assess the methylation status of O-6-methylguanine-DNA methyltransferase (MGMT) promoter in glioblastoma.*

offer lower cost, provide comprehensive CGI coverage, and can use formalin-fixed paraffin-embedded (FFPE) tissue as DNA input. **Figure 2** provides a schematic showing the diagnostic flow of DNA methylation profiling and its role in neuropathology service.

The third-generation sequencing (long read-sequencing) is another modality that can profile CpG methylation. The commercially available Oxford Nanopore MinION sequencer uses sequencing-by-synthesis to detect 5-mC, which produces a subtle but unique ionic signal as the single-stranded DNA passes through the voltage-biased nanopore sensor [19]. Due to the subtlety of the ionic current signal, a statistical model called the modified hidden Markov model (HMM) is implemented, which can distinguish cytosine from 5-mC within the CGI with 95% accuracy [20]. The low-pass whole-genome sequencing *via* nanopore was able to predict the DNA methylation profile in primary brain tumors (n = 15 patients) within a rapid median turn-around time (TAT) of 21 hours [21]. These alternatives to bisulfite-based DNA methylation profiling present an optimistic goal shortening the TAT with each iteration eventually resulting in intraoperative tumor classification.

3. Bioinformatic approach

Once the robust methylation array data is obtained, various analytical and computation transformations are required to interpret this complex output. The output from Illumina Infinium assays contains raw fluorescence signal intensities indicating the methylation status of CGI encoded in their proprietary ".IDAT" format. These are processed *via* the R Studio graphical user interface with packages such as "Minfi," which can normalize these raw signal intensities, ensure data reliability, and calculate the beta value to quantify DNA methylation at each CPG site [22]. Feature selection is undertaken as the predominant informative CpG probes are chosen for subsequent analysis.

After processing, the methylation dataset remains high dimensional. Therefore, it requires dimensionality reduction *via* real-time unsupervised algorithms. The popular methodologies utilized in bioinformatics for this purpose of dimensionality reduction are the t-distributed Stochastic Neighbor Embedding (t-SNE) and the Uniform Manifold Approximation and Projection (UMAP) techniques [23, 24]. The t-SNE creates visualizing clusters and patterns facilitate distinguishing tumor subtypes with similar DNA methylation profiles. This nonlinear dimensionality reduction technique groups samples with similar methylation patterns at specific CpG sites together, which preserves the local dataset structure (**Figure 3A**). Conversely, another nonlinear dimensionality reduction technique called UMAP preserves both the global and local dataset structures that represent the complex relationships (**Figure 3B**). Global dataset structure might show the overarching distinction between samples such as normal brain tissue compared to neoplastic tissue or pediatric versus adult samples. Furthermore, UMAP categorizes these groups with higher computational speeds and presents stable interpretable data compared to t-SNE.

In both t-SNE and UMAP plots, the distance between different clusters indicates how similar or distinct the methylation patterns are between those clusters. Conversely, tight clusters indicate a well-defined cell of origin or a degree of biological uniformity within the cluster.

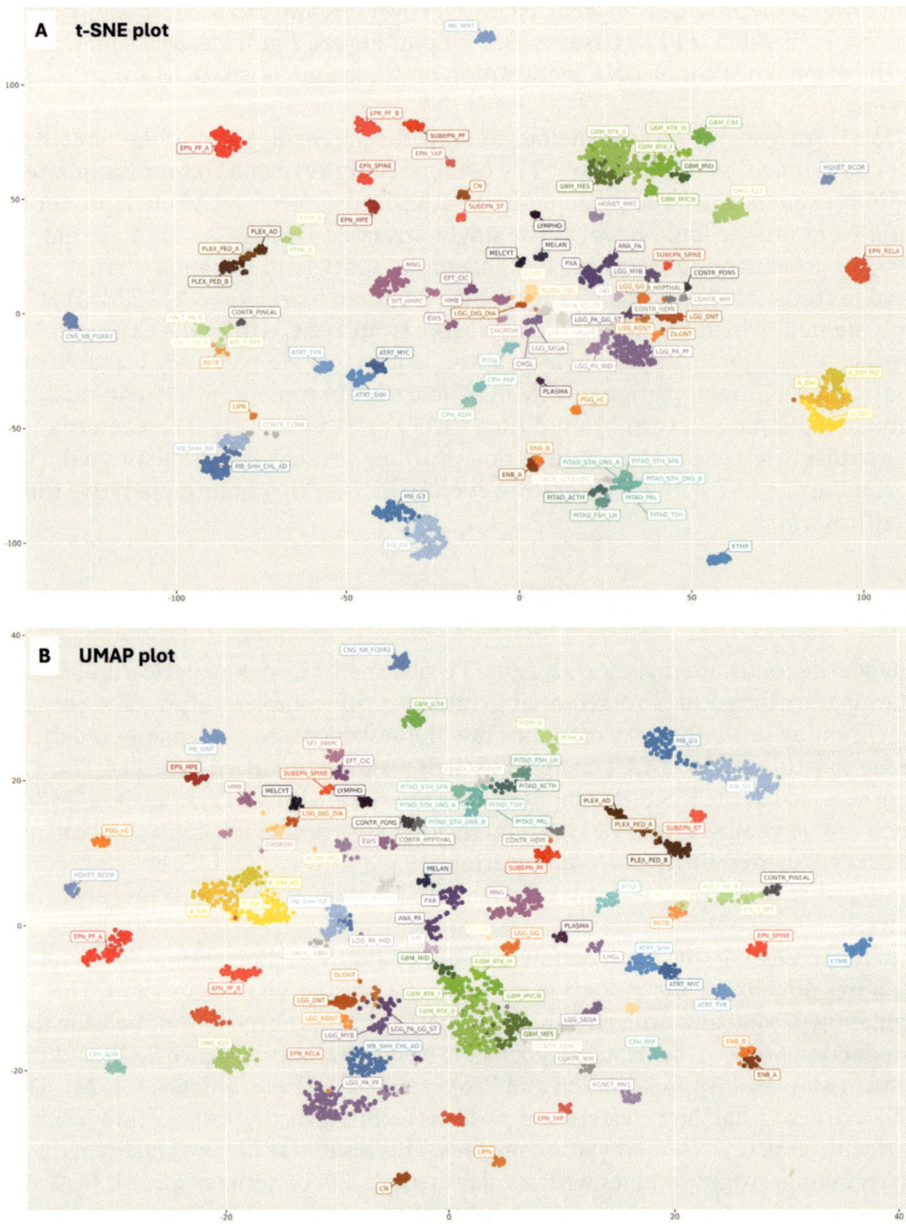

Figure 3.
Clustering of 2801 reference central nervous system (CNS) tumors based on methylation profiles. The top 32,000 most variable probes across samples were utilized. The methylation class labels correspond to the group centroid coordinates. These methylation classes are color-coded based on histology. (A) t-Distributed Stochastic Neighbor Embedding (t-SNE) dimensionality reduction. (B) Uniform Manifold Approximation and Projection (UMAP) dimensionality reduction.

4. Genome-wide copy number variations (CNVs) inference

The differential probes with distinct fluorescent labeling dyes can distinguish the signal intensities between the methylated and unmethylated CpG sites. The sum of these signal intensities is proportion to the quantity of hybridized DNA which can be utilized to infer the copy number variation. A copy number gain or loss can be inferred from the higher-than-normal or lower-than-normal intensity, respectively. Observing the consistent gains or losses across chromosomes (Chr) can help identify clinically significant cytogenetic aberrations such as Chr7+ and Chr10– seen in IDH-wildtype glioblastoma [25]. A similar computational strategy can be implemented at a chromosomal arm level to detect important alterations such as 1p/19q codeletion seen in oligodendrogliomas (**Figure 4**) [25]. Furthermore, signal intensity changes can be monitored at a gene level to identify prognostically significant genetic alterations such as EGFR amplification or homozygous loss of CDKN2A/B. Interestingly, abrupt alteration in signal intensities aligning at fusion gene locations such as KIAA1549:BRAF can be indicated by these copy number breakpoints [11]. Although CNV is generated by DNA-methylation based microarray, it is important to note that for each chromosome the coverage of CpG sites is insufficient to detect nuanced chromosomal copy number alterations [26]. The probes in the assays such as HumanMethylation450 span both intergenic and intragenic regions but often concentrate at the intragenic promoter regions [26]. Due to this distribution in the probe coverage, the CNV calls derived from these methylation arrays vary in sensitivity [26]. One study compared the reliability of the CMV calls obtained from the HumanMethylation450 and HumanMethylationEPIC arrays that were then analyzed by computational pipelines such as ChAMP, conumee, and cnAnalysis450k [27]. The conumee pipeline provided the highest reliability (57.6%) for the sample run on the HumanMethylationEPIC array and the cnAnalysis450k pipeline provided the highest reliability (43.0%) for the sample run on the HumanMethylation450 array [27]. This study showed that all three pipelines had low reliability despite the type of array used, which highlights the need for further refinement. Currently, it does not meet the current threshold for clinical validation.

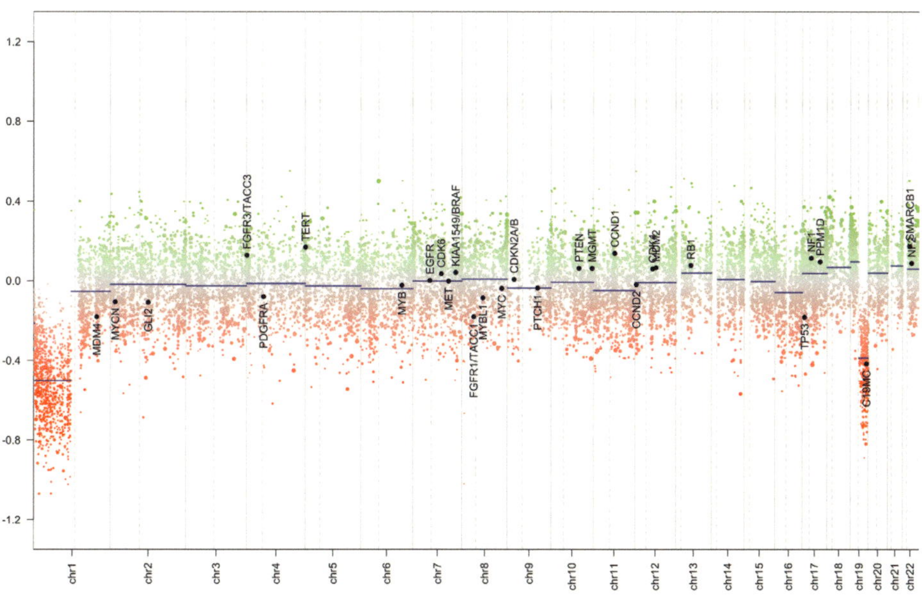

Figure 4.
CNV generated by DNA methylation-based microarray for IDH mutant subclass 1p/19q codeleted oligodendroglioma.

5. MGMT promoter methylation

The DNA methylation arrays can also identify the methylation status of the promoter of the repair gene O-6-methylguanine-DNA methyltransferase (MGMT). Methylation of the MGMT promoter is a known predictor of response to alkylation agents such as temozolomide in patients with glioblastoma [28]. The best model based on the HumanMethylation27K array identified the two CpG sites (probes: cg1243587 and cg12981137) to reliably classify the methylation status of the MGMT promoter [29]. MGMT-STP27 logistical regression model was validated (n = 50; kappa = 0.88; outcome, log-rank $p < 0.001$) for predicting the MGMT promoter methylation status on data obtained from the HumanMethylation450 platform for patients with IDH-wildtype glioblastoma [29]. The clinical validation of MGMT promoter methylation prediction by DNA methylation has shown high concordance with the conventional pyrosequencing method [29, 30].

It is important to note that the MGMT-STP27 logistical regression model was validated on cases of isocitrate dehydrogenase 1 and 2 (IDH)-wildtype glioblastomas, but its predictive value has been extrapolated for use in IDH-mutant astrocytomas [31]. Another limitation in detecting MGMT methylation status with DNA methylation arrays such as HumanMethylation450 and EPIC platforms is their incomplete coverage of all critical CpG sites within the MGMT promoter region [29]. Furthermore, CNV at the MGMT gene locus at 10q26 confounds the interpretation of the methylation status [31]. Tumor heterogeneity in the input samples also poses another challenge, as these methylation arrays cannot distinguish the methylation status of neoplastic and non-neoplastic cells mixed in the input sample [32]. Lastly, these DNA methylation assays can only detect the presence or absence of methylation at select MGMT promoter CpG sites, but it does not detect the transcriptional silencing of the MGMT gene [31].

6. Diagnostic and prognostic utility

DNA methylation profiling is emerging as a beneficial ancillary molecular tool in supplementing the clinical diagnosis of CNS tumors. The landmark study by Capper *et al.* showed that DNA methylation profiling on a larger patient cohort (n = 2801) resulted in the development of 91 unique methylation classes [2]. High concordance was achieved between DNA methylation profiling and routine diagnostic work-up in most of the cases (n = 838, 76%) [2]. This study showed that clinically significant reclassification resulted in the upgrade (n = 53, 4.8%) and downgrade (n = 39, 3.5%) of routinely diagnosed entities [2]. Most upgraded cases were initially diagnosed as IDH-wildtype astrocytomas and anaplastic astrocytomas which were then reclassified by DNA methylation as IDH-wildtype glioblastoma [2]. Conversely, IDH-wildtype glioblastomas were often downgraded by DNA methylation to pleomorphic xanthoastrocytoma, ependymoma, and pilocytic astrocytoma [2].

In another large prospective study of primary CNS tumors (n = 1921), Galbraith *et al.* highlighted how whole-genome DNA methylation profiling confirmed the classification, diagnostic revision, and discovery of novel entities [33]. High concordance was achieved between DNA methylation profiling and routine diagnostic work-up (histology, immunohistochemistry (IHC), and ancillary molecular) in most of the cases (n = 1189, 74%) [33]. DNA methylation profiling was also able to provide additional prognostic information by refining it into subclassifications for already concordant entities (n = 110, 7%) [33]. This above study showed that the pediatric medulloblastoma cases were concordant with the routine diagnostic workup and were accurately classified into their corresponding four prognostic subgroups (94%, n = 110) [33]. Furthermore, this study was also able to appropriately upgrade IDH-mutant Astrocytoma (WHO grade 2) to high-grade IDH-mutant Astrocytoma (13%) as well as downgrade IDH-mutated Astrocytoma (WHO grades 3 and 4) to high-grade IDH-mutant Astrocytoma in 43% and 28% of these cases, respectively [33]. Additionally, the ependymoma cases (n = 75) benefited from the prognostic subgroup classification. DNA methylation has now been incorporated into the WHO 5th edition to facilitate the distinction between ependymoma Posterior Fossa A and Posterior Fossa B [33]. Similarly, Zuccato *et al.* stratified chordomas based on their DNA methylome into the immune-infiltrated subtype associated with poorer disease-specific survival and the cellular subtype that is associated with better disease-specific survival [8]. Analogous work was done in meningioma DNA methylome studies that have stratified them into Merlin-intact (favorable clinical course), immune-enriched (favorable-intermediate clinical course), hypermetabolic (intermediate-poor clinical course), and proliferative type (poorest clinical course) [34, 35].

Machine learning integration into the DNA methylation profile classifier is a powerful tool for evaluating prospective tumor samples. Many subsequent large prospective studies have continued to bolster similar diagnostic utility for DNA methylation profiling in both adult and pediatric CNS tumors. One such study called the AIM BRAIN (AB) project (Access to Innovative Molecular Diagnostic Profiling in Brain Tumors) tested the Illumina EPIC arrays on pediatric CNS tumors (n = 269) [36]. In this clinical trial, they utilized the DKFZ's classifier versions 11b4 and 12.5. Consistent with all the previous studies the reliability of the tumor designation was based on the probability score > 0.90 (67%, n = 176) [36]. Additionally, for any tumors with <0.90 probability the closest tumor designation was still reported with a disclaimer indicating the level of reliability was less than the assigned benchmark. Among those tumors with >0.90 probability score on the classifier, the majority (92%, n = 162) showed concordance with routine diagnostic work-up (histology, IHC, and ancillary molecular) [36]. Only 4% (n = 7) of the tumors with >0.90 probability score showed discordance. These discordant tumors were identified based on routine diagnostic work-up as anaplastic ependymoma, pleomorphic xanthoastrocytoma, ependymoma, neurofibroma, pilocytic astrocytoma, ganglioglioma, and embryonal tumors that were then reclassified on the DNA methylation classifier as glioblastoma, ependymoma, pineal papillary tumor, schwannoma, dysembryoplastic neuroepithelial tumor, pilocytic astrocytoma, and CIC altered sarcoma, respectively [36]. Lastly, some cases attained a probability score ranging from 0.89 to 0.30 (24.1%, n = 64) and > 0.30 (9.4%, n = 25) [36]. Interestingly, even in these lower probability score cohorts, there was consensus with histologic diagnosis in some cases (n = 36). These cohorts predominantly consisted of low-grade gliomas (n = 25), tumor content less than 50% or unknown (n = 11), non-neoplastic control samples (n = 7), and no match (n = 14) [36].

Capper *et al.* provided the foundation for the methylome classifier [2]. Subsequent studies by Galbraith *et al.* [33] and White *et al.* [36] highlighted the significance of DNA methylation profiling in primary CNS tumor diagnosis. Galbraith *et al.* [33] suggested a clinical framework for the indications for the use of DNA methylation profiling in adult and pediatric CNS tumor cases. In contrast, White *et al.* [36] highlighted the practical advantages and challenges of implementing DNA methylation on clinical service for pediatric CNS tumors. All three of these studies provided insights into the diagnostic utility and considerations for implementing DNA methylation profiling into the neuropathology tumor service.

7. Clinical integration

It has been established that DNA methylation profiling is instrumental in refining tumor classifications, but the question still remains as to what are the appropriate criteria for integrating this technology into the current workflow of neuropathology tumor service. A suggested three-tiered system was created by Galbraith et al. [33] based on the outcomes of their large prospective study which divided the clinical indication for DNA methylation profiling into high-, intermediate-, and low-yield categories. The high-yield cohort consists of tumors reported out with descriptive diagnoses, entities with low concordance on histology and IHC alone, entities with inconclusive IHC or molecular results, and tumors with the established prognostic subcategories [33]. The 2021 WHO classification has recognized entities that are exclusively defined by DNA methylation profiling such as high-grade astrocytoma with piloid features (HGAP) and diffuse glioneuronal tumors with oligodendroglioma-like features and nuclear clusters (DGONC) [1]. Interestingly, no data is available to assess whether this level of tumor "subclassification" is clinically meaningful or not [37]. The intermediate-yield cohort consists of tumors wherein DNA methylation could facilitate ancillary molecular testing, entities with a medium level of diagnostic error rate devoid of ancillary molecular testing, or in cases that require expedited results instead of large IHC and molecular panel testing, or when routine diagnostic workup is insufficient for diagnosis [33]. This category underscores the importance of cost efficiency and tissue preservation. Lastly, the low-yield cohort consists of tumors where this technology will provide minimal diagnostic utility, cases with minimal diagnostic error rate, or entities wherein routine diagnostic testing has established the designation and DNA methylation profiling can provide no additional prognostic information [33].

8. Technical limitations

A notable preanalytical limitation of performing DNA methylation profiling with assays such as the Infinium BeadChip is their minimum input DNA requirement of 250 ng. Our institutional validation study has seen good results with DNA as low as 50 ng [30].

On the neuropathology service, we often receive small biopsy specimens that are suboptimal for extensive IHC and molecular workup. Furthermore, these biopsies may be mixed with adjacent non-neoplastic tissue, inflammatory cells, blood clots, or necrotic tissue. The analysis of the DNA methylation profile of the tumoral content can be obscured or attenuated by the amount of these non-neoplastic contents. We have shown that a tumor cellularity of 62–64% is needed for a successful DNA methylation classification in adult-type diffuse gliomas [38]. To optimize the outcome, laboratory techniques such as microdissection, laser capture, or punching FFPE blocks may be employed to enrich the tumoral cellularity.

There are instances where the DNA methylation classifier provides a non-contributory probability score or presents an entity that is incongruent with one obtained by a routine diagnostic workup. In these cases, it may be helpful to visualize the unsupervised t-SNE or UMAP plots to glean information about the clustering and similarity to other tumors, having said that the utility of these classifiers is dependent on the library size, an up-to-date database, and a sample representative of the population.

In a scenario where these plots display clusters that do not align with the suggested diagnosis in the setting of a probability score < 0.85, it may be prudent to only report a descriptive diagnosis instead of a definitive one. All discordances associated with the primary classifier or complementary classification methods such as UMAP or t-SNE plots must be considered only after appropriate bioinformatic quality control measures are met.

Another limitation of DNA methylation profiling is that it does not provide predictions for response to therapies or actionable insights. Therefore, there is still a reliance on DNA and RNA NGS panels to find targetable drivers to guide therapy.

9. Future directions

Future directions for this technology include exploring the implementation of DNA methylation in a reverse diagnostic algorithm wherein early utility of this technology can decrease the overall financial cost and significantly limit the tissue usage for ancillary studies. The initial results from DNA methylation profiling can point us toward the most appropriate molecular test (PCR, RNA fusion NGS panel, or FISH testing) to rapidly confirm the final integrative diagnosis. This Pan-CNS tumor diagnostic assay is superior as it has a shorter turnaround time, lower overall cost than the large DNA and RNA NGS panels, and lower diagnostic error rate. A comprehensive cost-effectiveness study comparing this reverse diagnostic algorithm to routine diagnostic workup is necessary to determine the financial impact.

A novel utilization of a deep learning model is called Deep lEarning from histoPathoLOgy and methYlation (DEPLOY) and integrating it with DNA methylation profiling. DEPLOY can directly classify CNS tumors based on analysis of histopathological images [39]. It can also indirectly predict the DNA methylation beta values to quantify DNA methylation at each CpG site which can then be processed for further classification *via* the classifiers [39]. Lastly, DEPLOY incorporates the patient demographics into its tumor classification prediction [39]. Once this technology is validated and widely adapted, it can facilitate utilization of DNA methylation profiling in regions where there is inaccessibility to the upstream molecular technologies.

DNA methylation profiling has also found a niche in bone and soft tissue tumor diagnostics [40]. Due to the objective unbiased functionality of the DNA methylation profiling tool, it can be utilized in vetting the inclusion criteria for the enrollment of patients into clinical trials for primary CNS as well as bone and soft tissue neoplasms.

There is a constant drive to expand and refine the existing methylation classifiers. Brain metastases make up a significant percentage of cases on the neuropathology services. Multiple studies are validating their DNA methylation classifiers to include tumors involved in brain metastases [41, 42]. Similarly, a random forest machine learning classifier has now been created for the identification of tumors of unknown origin in metastatic cases [43]. These advances reflect the transformative role of DNA methylation profiling in supplementing tumor diagnostics and insights into tumor biology.

10. Bioethical considerations

Bioethical principles are relevant to all aspects of DNA methylation profiling, from ordering the test to interpreting and integrating results. While this technology enhances CNS tumor classification, it raises unique concerns about patient autonomy, potential harm, and distributive justice [44]. Unlike other genetic tests, DNA methylation profiling is often ordered by pathologists rather than clinicians with direct patient contact, creating challenges in ensuring informed consent [45]. Patients may lack awareness of the risks, benefits, and implications of the test, including the potential use of their data for classifier training. Pathologists play a critical role in supporting treating physicians to ensure patients understand the purpose of the test, its limitations, and how their tissue data may be used.

The utility of DNA methylation profiling in tumor diagnostics raises concerns about health equity and distributive justice. While it is a required or supportive criterion for many CNS tumors under WHO guidelines, access to this technology is limited to a few laboratories, primarily in North America and Western Europe, exacerbating global health disparities. Additionally, biases in machine-learning classifiers can arise from training datasets that lack appropriate diagnostic parameters or fail to represent the disease distribution in diverse populations [46].

Many new tumor entities are defined by a unique DNA methylation profile, with histology and other molecular features retrospectively characterized. The extensive granularity with which tumors are now classified offers the benefit of better understanding of tumor biology. But this paradigm may result in additional expensive testing for limited clinical benefit, particularly where the biologic behavior of new entities is not well understood. Additionally, it remains only an assumption that a DNA methylation profile is a gold standard definition of a tumor type; therefore, many tumors defined by unique DNA methylation profiles may in fact be unusual presentations of defined tumor types. As classification of these tumors is limited to classification schema widely available only *via* a small number of classifiers, these results are not readily independently reproducible by separate laboratories as may be done with traditional molecular testing.

Multiple ethical considerations arise regarding the interpretation and reporting of DNA methylation results. Although many tumors show high confidence matches and good concordance across classifiers, challenges arise in ambiguous cases, cases with low tumor cellularity, and entities not included in existing classifiers. It is common for results to suggest an entity without meeting the threshold for a defined match, analogous to interpreting variants of uncertain significance (VUS) in molecular pathology. Despite existing VUS guidelines, no clear framework exists for addressing ambiguous methylation results, particularly in cases with discrepant methylome, routine diagnostic workup, or conflicting classifications [47]. Rigorous validation and standardized reporting are critical in such cases.

Interpretive challenges arise when histology-based classifier nomenclature generates seemingly inaccurate results, such as high-grade gliomas with FGFR3::TACC3 fusions aligning with ganglioglioma in certain versions of the DKFZ classifier [48]. Clear communication with clinical teams is essential to avoid misinterpreting methylation results as definitive diagnoses. Additionally, the vast amount of data generated by DNA methylation arrays raises ethical concerns about storage, sharing, and re-evaluation. Unlike clinical genetics, no guidelines exist for re-reviewing methylation data, making it unclear when unmatched cases should be reassessed with updated classifiers. Regular re-review is impractical for most molecular pathology labs and typically occurs only upon clinical request, often benefiting patients with higher access to specialized care [47].

The possible dangers from exposure of protected patient genetic data are yet another unknown. Some tumor DNA methylation profiles are associated with certain germline variants and may carry implications for patients and families. Additionally, non-neoplastic elements are invariably sampled together with the tumor or, in certain cases, the entire sample. Powerful information can be obtained from these data, such as predicting susceptibility to breast cancer or even predicting a patient's age [49, 50]. Currently, various algorithms exist to perform de-convolutional analysis capable of separating certain non-neoplastic cell types from tumors. How extensive the data obtained from a non-neoplastic methylome can be remains to be seen, but this capability poses potential risks for how this genetic data may be shared and highlights the importance that patients have a clear understanding of what data are being interpreted and shared.

11. Conclusion

In this chapter, we discussed the basics of DNA methylation as a stable epigenetic marker that is resistant to tumor mutational burden and indicates cell lineage. We discussed the bioinformatics strategies used to process the methylation datasets and construct t-SNE and UMAPs to help interpret the robust methylation data. We highlight the diagnostic utility and accuracy of DNA methylation profiling of primary CNS tumors in three large prospective studies. DNA methylation profiling can detect novel entities and appropriately upgrade and downgrade diagnostic classifications resulting in change in clinical intervention and follow-up. The final section of the chapter highlighted the suggested clinical indications for utilizing DNA methylation profiling. We also discussed the limitations and bioethical considerations of this technology and the future directions for this powerful diagnostic tool.

Conflict of interest

The authors declare no conflict of interest.

Author details

Pramath Kakodkar[1], Kyle Conway[2], Lucas Santana-Santos[3], Matthew McCord[4], Madina Sukhanova[3], Rudolph Castellani[3] and Pouya Jamshidi[3*]

1 University of Saskatchewan, Saskatoon, Canada

2 University of Michigan, Ann Harbor, Michigan, USA

3 Feinberg School of Medicine, Northwestern University, Chicago, IL, USA

4 University of Virginia School of Medicine, Charlottesville, VA, USA

*Address all correspondence to: pouya.jamshidi@northwestern.edu

References

[1] Louis DN et al. The 2021 WHO classification of tumors of the central nervous system: A summary. Neuro-Oncology. 2021;**23**(8):1231-1251

[2] Capper D et al. DNA methylation-based classification of central nervous system tumours. Nature. 2018;**555**(7697):469-474

[3] Jaunmuktane Z et al. Methylation array profiling of adult brain tumours: Diagnostic outcomes in a large, single Centre. Acta Neuropathologica Communications. 2019;**7**(1):24

[4] Sturm D et al. New brain tumor entities emerge from molecular classification of CNS-PNETs. Cell. 2016;**164**(5):1060-1072

[5] Sahm F et al. DNA methylation-based classification and grading system for meningioma: A multicentre, retrospective analysis. The Lancet Oncology. 2017;**18**(5):682-694

[6] Ellison DW et al. cIMPACT-NOW update 7: Advancing the molecular classification of ependymal tumors. Brain Pathology. 2020;**30**(5):863-866

[7] Korshunov A et al. DNA methylation profiling is a method of choice for molecular verification of pediatric WNT-activated medulloblastomas. Neuro-Oncology. 2019;**21**(2):214-221

[8] Zuccato JA et al. DNA methylation-based prognostic subtypes of chordoma tumors in tissue and plasma. Neuro-Oncology. 2022;**24**(3):442-454

[9] Johann PD et al. Atypical teratoid/rhabdoid tumors are comprised of three epigenetic subgroups with distinct enhancer landscapes. Cancer Cell. 2016;**29**(3):379-393

[10] Pajtler KW et al. Molecular classification of ependymal tumors across all CNS compartments, histopathological grades, and age groups. Cancer Cell. 2015;**27**(5):728-743

[11] Capper D et al. Practical implementation of DNA methylation and copy-number-based CNS tumor diagnostics: The Heidelberg experience. Acta Neuropathologica. 2018;**136**(2):181-210

[12] Baylin SB, Jones PA. Epigenetic determinants of cancer. Cold Spring Harbor Perspectives in Biology. 2016;**8**(9):a019505

[13] Li S, Tollefsbol TO. DNA methylation methods: Global DNA methylation and methylomic analyses. Methods. 2021;**187**:28-43

[14] Lister R et al. Human DNA methylomes at base resolution show widespread epigenomic differences. Nature. 2009;**462**(7271):315-322

[15] Klughammer J et al. The DNA methylation landscape of glioblastoma disease progression shows extensive heterogeneity in time and space. Nature Medicine. 2018;**24**(10):1611-1624

[16] Lv H et al. Advances in mapping the epigenetic modifications of 5-methylcytosine (5mC), N6-methyladenine (6mA), and N4-methylcytosine (4mC). Biotechnology and Bioengineering. 2021;**118**(11):4204-4216

[17] Frommer M et al. A genomic sequencing protocol that yields a positive display of 5-methylcytosine residues in individual DNA strands. Proceedings of the National Academy of Sciences

of the United States of America. 1992;**89**(5):1827-1831

[18] Bibikova M et al. High density DNA methylation array with single CpG site resolution. Genomics. 2011;**98**(4):288-295

[19] Wang Y et al. Nanopore sequencing technology, bioinformatics and applications. Nature Biotechnology. 2021;**39**(11):1348-1365

[20] Simpson JT et al. Detecting DNA cytosine methylation using nanopore sequencing. Nature Methods. 2017;**14**(4):407-410

[21] Kuschel LP et al. Robust methylation-based classification of brain tumours using nanopore sequencing. Neuropathology and Applied Neurobiology. 2023;**49**(1):e12856

[22] Aryee MJ et al. Minfi: A flexible and comprehensive Bioconductor package for the analysis of Infinium DNA methylation microarrays. Bioinformatics. 2014;**30**(10):1363-1369

[23] van der Maaten L, Hinton G. Viualizing data using t-SNE. Journal of Machine Learning Research. 2008;**9**:2579-2605

[24] McInnes L, Healy J. UMAP: Uniform manifold approximation and projection for dimension reduction. Journal of Open Source Software. 2018;**3**:861

[25] Feber A et al. Using high-density DNA methylation arrays to profile copy number alterations. Genome Biology. 2014;**15**(2):R30

[26] Cho S et al. Measuring DNA copy number variation using high-density methylation microarrays. Journal of Computational Biology. 2019;**26**(4):295-304

[27] Kilaru V et al. Critical evaluation of copy number variant calling methods using DNA methylation. Genetic Epidemiology. 2020;**44**(2):148-158

[28] Gilbert MR et al. Dose-dense temozolomide for newly diagnosed glioblastoma: a randomized phase III clinical trial. Journal of Clinical Oncology. 2013;**31**(32):4085-4091

[29] Bady P et al. MGMT methylation analysis of glioblastoma on the Infinium methylation BeadChip identifies two distinct CpG regions associated with gene silencing and outcome, yielding a prediction model for comparisons across datasets, tumor grades, and CIMP-status. Acta Neuropathologica. 2012;**124**(4):547-560

[30] Santana-Santos L et al. Validation of whole genome methylation profiling classifier for central nervous system tumors. The Journal of Molecular Diagnostics. 2022;**24**(8):924-934

[31] Tesileanu CMS et al. MGMT promoter methylation determined by the MGMT-STP27 algorithm is not predictive for outcome to temozolomide in IDH-mutant anaplastic astrocytomas. Neuro-Oncology. 2022;**24**(4):665-667

[32] Pratt D, Sahm F, Aldape K. DNA methylation profiling as a model for discovery and precision diagnostics in neuro-oncology. Neuro-Oncology. 2021;**23**(23 Suppl 5):S16-s29

[33] Galbraith K et al. Clinical utility of whole-genome DNA methylation profiling as a primary molecular diagnostic assay for central nervous system tumors-a prospective study and guidelines for clinical testing. Neuro-Oncology Advances. 2023;**5**(1):vdad076

[34] Choudhury A et al. Meningioma DNA methylation groups identify

biological drivers and therapeutic vulnerabilities. Nature Genetics. 2022;**54**(5):649-659

[35] Nassiri F et al. A clinically applicable integrative molecular classification of meningiomas. Nature. 2021;**597**(7874):119-125

[36] White CL et al. Implementation of DNA methylation Array profiling in pediatric central nervous system tumors: The AIM BRAIN project: An Australian and New Zealand Children's Haematology/oncology group study. The Journal of Molecular Diagnostics. 2023;**25**(10):709-728

[37] Pratt D et al. High-grade glioma with pleomorphic and pseudopapillary features (HPAP): A proposed type of circumscribed glioma in adults harboring frequent TP53 mutations and recurrent monosomy 13. Acta Neuropathologica. 2022;**143**(3):403-414

[38] Jamshidi P et al. Variant allelic frequency of driver mutations predicts success of genomic DNA methylation classification in central nervous system tumors. Acta Neuropathologica. 2023;**145**(3):365-367

[39] Hoang DT et al. Prediction of DNA methylation-based tumor types from histopathology in central nervous system tumors with deep learning. Nature Medicine. 2024;**30**(7):1952-1961

[40] Koelsche C et al. Sarcoma classification by DNA methylation profiling. Nature Communications. 2021;**12**(1):498

[41] Orozco JIJ et al. Epigenetic profiling for the molecular classification of metastatic brain tumors. Nature Communications. 2018;**9**(1):4627

[42] Zuccato JA et al. Prediction of brain metastasis development with DNA methylation signatures. Nature Medicine. 2024;**30**:1-10

[43] Santana-Santos L et al. Accurate identification of primary site in tumors of unknown origin (TUO) using DNA methylation. Research Square. 2024:1-20

[44] Vos S et al. Ethical considerations for modern molecular pathology. The Journal of Pathology. 2018;**246**(4):405-414

[45] Ormond KE et al. Defining the critical components of informed consent for genetic testing. Journal of Personalized Medicine. 2021;**11**(12):1304

[46] Chauhan C, Gullapalli RR. Ethics of AI in pathology: Current paradigms and emerging issues. The American Journal of Pathology. 2021;**191**(10):1673-1683

[47] Walsh N et al. Variant reclassification and clinical implications. Journal of Medical Genetics. 2024;**61**(3):207-211

[48] Métais A et al. Clinico-pathological and epigenetic heterogeneity of diffuse gliomas with FGFR3::TACC3 fusion. Acta Neuropathologica Communications. 2023;**11**(1):14

[49] Joo JE et al. Heritable DNA methylation marks associated with susceptibility to breast cancer. Nature Communications. 2018;**9**(1):867

[50] Varshavsky M et al. Accurate age prediction from blood using a small set of DNA methylation sites and a cohort-based machine learning algorithm. Cell Reports Methods. 2023;**3**(9):100567

Chapter 3

Perspective Chapter: Computer Vision-Based Digital Pathology for Central Nervous System Tumors – State-of-the-Art and Current Advances

Daniel Hieber, Felix Holl, Vera Nickl, Friederike Liesche-Starnecker and Johannes Schobel

Abstract

Rapid advances in computer vision (CV) and artificial intelligence have opened new avenues for digital pathology, including the diagnosis and treatment of central nervous system (CNS) tumors. In addition to reviewing the state-of-the-art in CV-based digital pathology and highlighting its potential to revolutionize the field, this chapter also provides a general introduction to digital pathology and Machine Learning (ML) for neuropathologists. Although currently limited to research, the integration of CV tools into digital pathology already offers significant advantages, such as automating tissue analysis and providing quantitative assessments. The transition from research to clinical application is slowly gaining momentum. To provide neuropathologists with the necessary skills to succeed in digital pathology and ML, the chapter also discusses how physicians and researchers can create custom models and tools tailored to specific needs using tools such as nnU-Net, deepflash2, and PathML. Emphasis is placed on the importance of interdisciplinary collaboration and continued research to fully realize the potential of CV in digital pathology for CNS tumors, to address the challenges of workforce shortages and increased workloads in neuropathology.

Keywords: digital pathology, neuropathology, computer vision, central nervous system, machine learning, computational pathology

1. Introduction

Artificial intelligence (AI) and machine learning (ML) are becoming increasingly popular overall, as well as in the medical domain. With radiology as an early adapter of ML [1], especially in the form of computer vision (CV), AI already has a significant impact on medicine [2]. On the other hand, AI is only beginning its transition from research to diagnostics in pathology in general, as well as in neuropathology. Out of the 882 U.S. Food & Drug Administration (FDA) approved medical devices using ML or AI, only six are for pathological use cases, and 671 are for radiology [3].

However, this transition is now being accelerated with the release of multiple robust foundation models in 2024 [4–7]. While there is still a long road ahead in adapting AI to pathology, quite a few applications and techniques are already available to assist in the research and diagnosis of pathology. This chapter provides a broad overview of the available options and how CV can be used in digital (neuro-)pathology with a focus on central nervous system (CNS) tumors.

2. An introduction to computer vision in digital pathology

Digital pathology and the use of CV in it are no new developments. While they have been around for some time, this section will try to introduce a common definition of digital pathology for this chapter and provide an introduction to CV for medical readers. The section further highlights some of the key reasons why CV-assisted digital pathology is needed nowadays.

2.1 What is digital pathology

Digital pathology can generally be divided into two main areas: molecular data and image data. As with conventional pathology, tissue is the starting point for all further analysis. With molecular data, the tissue is analyzed regarding its genetic expression, and the resulting data is then processed using computer programs. As this work focuses on CV-based digital pathology, the image data is of main interest, with the first step being the digitization of the data.

Besides digital pathology nowadays, there is also the term computational pathology. While computational pathology is part of digital pathology, it is used to describe the usage of computer algorithms and software to analyze pathological data actively. In this chapter, the term of digital pathology is used for all matters for simplicity.

2.1.1 Digitizing pathology

With image data, the tissue slides are either stained with hematoxilyn and eosin (HE) or immunohistochemical (IHC) staining or immunofluorescence (IF) is used. However, instead of directly analyzing the resulting slides under the microscope, the data is digitized using so-called Whole-Slide Image (WSI) scanners or specialized IF scanners. To allow the same level of detail for digital analysis as with conventional microscopes, these WSIs are scanned using 20-40x magnification. This results in 100.000 x 100.000-pixel large images in general, with even larger pixel values being possible depending on the used tissue slide.

The resulting digital WSIs can be available in many different file formats depending on the scanner's manufacturer. Some of these formats are proprietary, meaning that they can only be used with software by the same vendor and its cooperation partners. However, at the foundation, most of these formats are based on the pyramidal tiled Tagged Image File (TIF) Format (TIFF). As such, the images can be transformed to the non-proprietary TIFF and, therefore, be analyzed independently of vendor-specific software.

Due to the large resolution and sheer size of the images, the resulting files can require significant storage space on hard drives. Uncompressed WSIs can take up to

40GB and more. In general, these images are already provided in a compressed format. With lossless compression algorithms like JPEG2000, the size can significantly be reduced without losing information [8].

2.1.2 Advantages of digitized pathology

At the most fundamental level, the digitization of WSIs alone already provides some major advantages over conventional pathology. The digitized WSIs can be saved in Picture Archiving and Communication Systems (PACSs), which have been used in radiology for a long time. These PACSs allow the linkage of hospital information systems and laboratory information systems, providing all relevant patient data in a single place without the need to transport paper files or search for the required information. As the data are available in these systems, independent of the actual location of the physician, pathologists can access the data remotely, allowing remote analysis to be conducted during conferences and similar events. Such remote analysis is especially useful to small clinics with only a few trained (neuro-)pathologists. Moreover, remote consultation for colleagues becomes an option without the need to send physical glass slides to other locations (and wait for them to arrive).

A further advantage is the possibility of granularly annotating the data without "damaging" it. In analog pathology, physicians often use pen markers to annotate glass slides. These are quite coarse and hide some information on the slide so that the tissue below the pen mark is no longer readable without removing the annotation first. Using specialized WSI viewers, such annotations can be created on WSIs without manipulating the original image and, therefore, losing information. Further, the annotations can be generated on a more granular level, providing more detailed information within those. **Figure 1** shows such annotations in the QuPath software on an IHC-stained WSI. The yellow annotations are created using the "wand" tool, which assists the physician with using AI to draw the annotation. These annotations can, for example, be used by junior physicians to better learn the morphological features in a histological slide or be used during diagnostics to document where the senior pathologist found relevant structures. Additionally, these digital annotations can further be used in the training of ML models on which we will focus later on.

The real advantage of digital pathology, however, comes with the exploration of ML, especially CV.

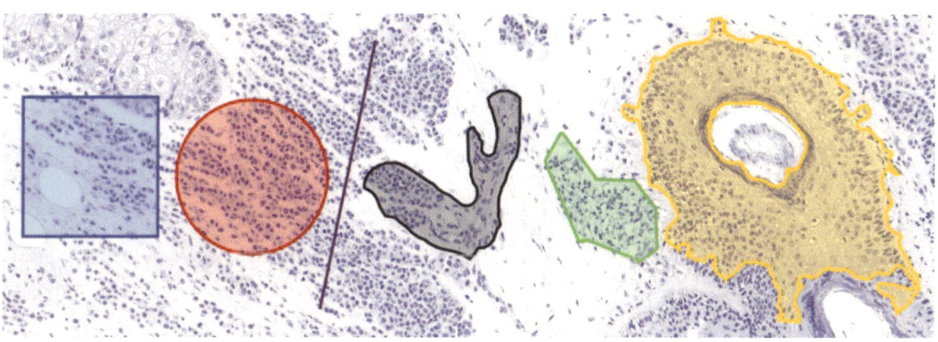

Figure 1.
Annotations using different tools in QuPath on an IHC stained image. Blue: square, Red: circle, Purple: line, Black: brush, Green: polygon, Yellow: wand. ([9], CC BY 4.0 https://creativecommons.org/licenses/by/4.0/).

2.2 What is computer vision and why do we need it in pathology

CV is a large-ranging area with many disciplines and use cases. A fitting definition comes from Müller, who defined CV as "[...] an interdisciplinary field that deals with how to automatically process, analyze, and understand images. The general aim behind computer vision is to build artificial intelligence systems which can automate visual tasks with a performance similar to or better than humans" [10]. Another definition comes from Goodfellow et al., who provided a broader definition: "Computer vision is a very broad field encompassing a wide variety of ways of processing images, and an amazing diversity of applications" [11].

2.2.1 Machine learning-based computer vision

ML-based CV is currently the most relevant in the pathological domain for tumor analysis. It can be generally separated into three groups: classification, object detection, and segmentation. The different kinds of ML-based CV are depicted in **Figure 2**.

Classification is shown in **Figure 2A**. With this CV approach an image as a whole receives one or multiple labels as per its contents. In this case, the label "Glioblastoma" was chosen, as the WSI includes the neoplastic tissue of a Glioblastoma (GBM). Other possible labels could be "HE" or "Healthy Tissue," as those also describe the content of this picture. However, such information is also easily deductible from the picture itself for a pathologist and, therefore, does not provide added value.

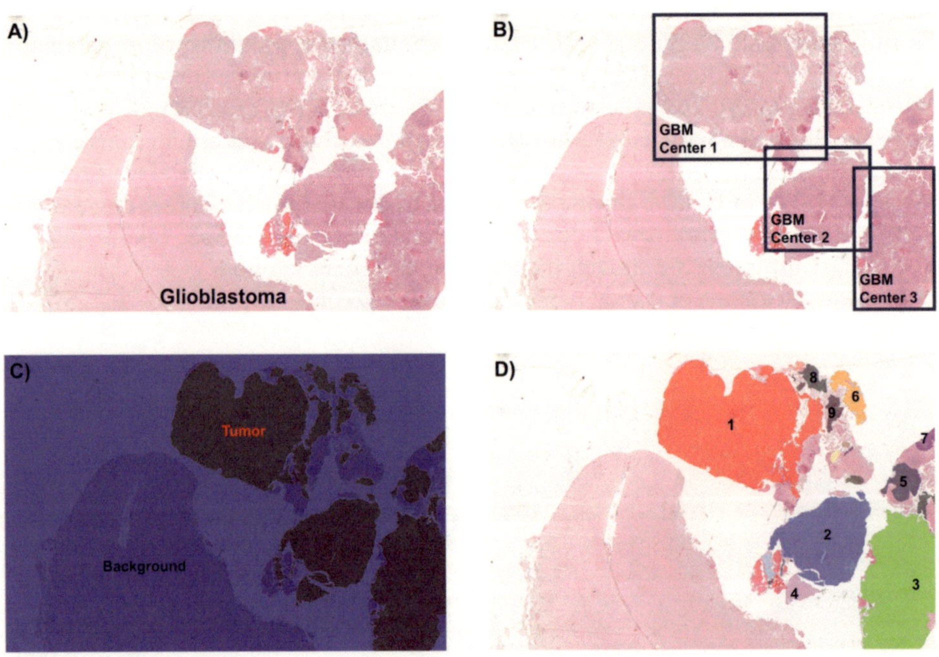

Figure 2.
Machine Learning-based Computer Vision. (A) Classification of the whole whole-slide image with one or multiple labels. (B) Object detection within an image, which detects different objects of interest and marks them with a bounding box. (C) Semantic Segmentation gives each pixel in the image a label regarding its content. (D) Instance Segmentation detecting objects of interest on a pixel level and differentiation between different objects of the same type.

Figure 2B depicts object detection. With this technique, objects of interest (in this case, the three largest tumor sections) are detected within an image and marked accordingly. Like in the figure, this is normally achieved by drawing a bounding box around the object, showing in which area of the image the object is located. This is mostly not used for tumor detection but more granular tasks like cell detection and quantification.

Semantic segmentation is the most common use case for CV in pathology (**Figure 2C**). With this technique, each pixel in the image is assigned a class. In the shown use case, only two classes are available: "Tumor" (including neoplastic tissue and necrosis) as well as "Background" (including empty areas and healthy tissue).

Figure 2D shows a version of segmentation that is less common in pathology: instance segmentation. Instead of assigning a class to each pixel in the image, we focus on a single kind of entity, in this case, the GBM. Each pixel that belongs to a GBM is then marked, and all pixels in a single group are assigned to the same instance of this entity. In the figure, these separate instances are highlighted with different colors, and the nine biggest ones are further marked with numbers.

The last type of segmentation is panoptic segmentation (not depicted in the figure). This is a combination of semantic and instance segmentation. Each pixel in the image is assigned to a class; however, all pixels are also grouped into instances.

To understand how to employ ML-based CV in the pathological domain, it is important to understand the general concept of ML first (cf. **Figure 3**). The initial step for each ML model is the concrete architecture. In this step, the internals of a new model are defined by usually taking an existing architecture and modifying it slightly to the use case. While this step only takes a couple of lines of programming code, some of the fundamental decisions are made. After the model architecture is defined, the training is conducted. In this step, large amounts of data are forwarded into the model, and it is slowly learning its task by ingesting the data repeatedly. This step requires significant computational resources for digital pathology models and can take a long time. Afterward, the trained model will be available and can be used on new data to conduct the introduced CV tasks. This step is called inference. Therefore, to apply an ML model to a use case, it is important to not only have the model's code but also the actual trained model available.

A large number of images is required to train new models sufficiently. While this sounds contradictive in (neuro-)pathology where only a few WSIs are available and labeling those takes great effort, WSIs are actually perfectly suited to be large

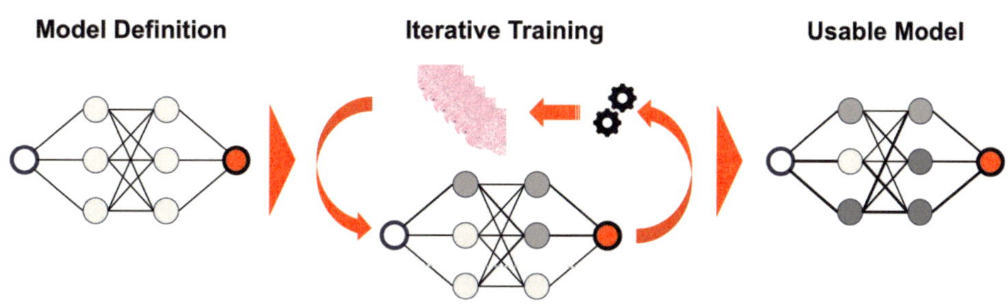

Figure 3.
Machine Learning on a meta level. Model Definition: adapting a Machine Learning architecture to the specific use case at hand. Iterative Training: training the model repeatedly on the available data while the model is slowly adapting to its task. Usable Model: the final model after the training consisting of the model architecture and the learned information.

amounts of data in themselves. WSI includes vast amounts of data in a single file, which are not practically processable by ML models as a single file. Therefore, WSIs are split into smaller sections, so-called tiles, which only show small amounts of the WSI at once. These are between 224 and 1.024 pixels in square. With this tiling technique, a WSI does not provide a single image; instead, it actually provides around 9.500 images in maximum resolution. If empty areas of the WSI are omitted, this can be approximated to 4.000 to 6.000 usable tiles per WSI. Following this, a single WSI can already provide a significant amount of data. However, the labeling of a single WSI still takes a large amount of time and a robust model still requires training on tiles of dozens to hundreds of WSIs.

2.2.2 Advantages of computer vision in pathology

The goal of CV is to "[...] build artificial intelligence systems [...] with a performance similar to or better than humans" [10]. While the advantages of a system with a performance better than a human are quite self-explanatory, systems with a performance similar to humans also already benefit pathologists.

With the worker shortage in pathology – especially in neuropathology – and the ever-increasing workload, new ways have to be found to improve existing processes in pathology [12]. While a first analysis of a slide can be done in mere seconds by a trained pathologist, the fine-grained analysis can take up much time. Moreover, sometimes, a diagnosis is not one hundred percent clear, and a second opinion is needed. While this can already be accelerated by digital pathology, as mentioned in Section 2.1.2, this second opinion can also be provided by a CV tool for every diagnosis at little time [13, 14].

In general, CV-based digital pathology can be used to automate analysis, for example, the detection of different types of tissue in WSIs [15], and speed up analysis processes, for example, by annotation regions of interest in WSIs [16]. It is even possible to annotate complete WSIs automatically using the right ML model in mere minutes compared to the hours required by manual analysis [17]. Further CV models provide objective ways to quantify expressions in WSIs, for example, Gleason scores grading [18], allowing a more robust foundation for tumor grading and treatment.

Nowadays, CV systems are already available for some use cases in pathology, for example, Paige Prostate [19], and there is a large quantity of promising research showing potential further use cases. The research in the area of CV-assisted digital pathology is steadily picking up speed, and – with the latest release of new robust foundation models for digital pathology – this trend is believed to accelerate even more [4–7].

3. Foundation models for digital pathology

The researchers at Stanford provide us with a general definition for foundation models: "A foundation model is any model that is trained on broad data [...] that can be adapted [...] to a wide range of downstream tasks [...]" [20]. To break this down, foundation models are models that were already trained on a large amount of data and can "understand" the data of this domain in a general sense. These ML models can then be specialized for new tasks in this domain with little data. This removes the need for a large amount of training data and the large computational requirements mentioned in Section 2.2.1. Instead of training a new model from the bottom up, a foundation model can be used as a solid foundation, and only a small amount of annotated data is required.

For example, training a new strong model capable of segmenting neoplastic tissue of GBMs in WSIs requires tens of thousands of annotated tiles of training data (requiring a few hundred annotated WSIs). Using a foundation model trained on HE data (not even GBM specific), sufficient results can already be achieved by a few thousand annotated tiles (which only require a few dozen WSIs). As less data is used during the training process of a new ML model, the training time is also reduced significantly.

3.1 What foundation models are available for digital pathology

In 2024, four new foundation models were released: UNI [4], CONCH [5], Virchow [6], and Prov-GigaPath [7]. Before 2024, other foundation models had already been released, including REMEDIS from Google [21], CTransPath [22], Quilt-Net [23], PLIP [24], and Phikon [25]. However, these older models were outperformed in most benchmarks by the newer foundation model generation from 2024, with only Phikon being in the top 2 in one of six benchmarks [4, 5].

Out of the four new foundation models, UNI, Virchow, and Prov-GigaPath are solely vision models. This means that the models can conduct the CV tasks introduced in Section 2. CONCH, on the other hand, is a vision-language model. As a vision-language model, CONCH can ingest image and text data and consider both in its image analysis. Besides general CV tasks such as classifying or segmenting, CONCH can also generate image captions. Using captioning, the model generates a descriptive caption for the provided image instead of only giving it predefined labels as with classification. This allows for a more detailed description of its contents compared to classification.

3.2 How to use foundation models for digital pathology

Foundation models can be used as an advanced starting point for the generation of one's own ML model. Sometimes, it is even possible to directly apply foundation models to a specific task without further training. This process, called zero-shot classification, is available for both CONCH [5] and Prov-GigaPath [7]. Furthermore, all foundation models mentioned in this chapter are available publicly as pre-trained models. This means that the model has already been trained on a large amount of data, and besides the code to recreate the model, the actual model is also available to be used.

However, even using a publicly available foundation model with a zero-shot approach still requires significant effort, decent IT knowledge, and sufficient hardware. While physicians can learn the required skills independently, using foundation models does not seem very practical. They provide a significant boost to research but do not provide direct applicability for physicians on their own.

4. Computer vision for CNS tumors in digital pathology

The options for diagnostic use by physicians are still very limited nowadays, and the focus of digital pathology overall, as well as for CNS tumors, is still mostly research-related. The aim of this section is to introduce applicable CV tools and an overview of some "ready-to-use" CV models for CNS tumors. Further, some input is provided on how to create one's own models."

4.1 CV-tools for digital pathology for CNS Tumors

While no ML-based CV tools are approved for diagnostics in neuropathology, there is a multitude of viewers and similar applications that can already be used for digital neuropathology.

In general, these solutions are combined with PACSs or allow the integration of PACSs and provide a general image viewer with the option to run some simple analysis (e.g., cell quantification). Regarding open-source/free-to-use software, these applications include tools such as QuPath [26], ORBIT [27], and OME [28]. Besides their general use as WSI viewers, these tools also allow the integration of ML algorithms to analyze the images further. The included ML algorithms, however, are only usable for research and not diagnostic. Furthermore, there is also highly specialized open-source research software like CellProfiler [29], which only has one purpose: the quantification and analysis of cells in pathological images using CV.

There is also a large number of software tools provided by larger companies such as Roche's navify [30] or Philips IntelliSite [31]. While these provide WSI viewers, which can be used for diagnostic usage and allow the integration of ML-based CV models, no FDA-approved models are available for the CNS domain. Besides the solutions of established companies, there are also applications from research institutes like the Fraunhofer ISS with the MIKAIA software [32]. As a free version, MIKAIA is a WSI viewer that allows the conversion of file formats and annotation. There is also a paid version available for research purposes, including many ML-based analysis algorithms.

Finally, some companies were founded specifically for digital pathology and specific companies just for histopathology. These include companies like KML Vision [33], 3DHISTECH [34], and Paige [35]. In general, these companies also provide some certified WSI viewers and additional unapproved algorithms, which can, therefore, only be used in research.

4.2 CV-models for digital pathology for CNS tumors

Besides using tools for digital pathology to assist in the (mostly research-centered) analysis of CNS tumors, there is also a large quantity of research on specialized CV models for CNS tumors.

Many studies have been conducted regarding the research on AI models for CV in digital pathology for CNS, as shown by the literature review by Jensen et al. [36], which highlights 68 studies for creating CV models specifically for CNS tumors. While some of the included studies are only abstracts and not all necessarily provide high-quality models, this shows a significant effort in this area. A shared characteristic of all those studies, however, is the fact that all studies were conducted preclinical and worked on retrospective data, showing the lack of application in clinical use.

Another review by Redlich et al. includes 83 studies regarding using CV for digital pathology, specifically for glioma-type tumors [37]. **Figure 4** shows the steady increase of studies from 2015 to 2023 (and the first quarter of 2024).

However, in contrast to the foundation models mentioned in Section 3.1, most of the studies do not provide the model itself, the code to recreate it, and/or did not

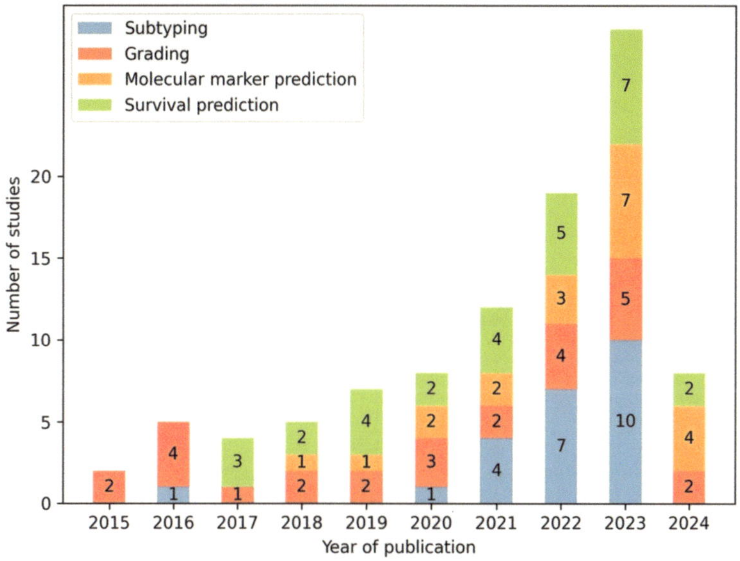

Figure 4.
Amount of studies conducted regarding the application of Computer Vision in the analysis of gliomas and the conducted task till March 18, 2024. ([37], CC BY 4.0 https://creativecommons.org/licenses/by/4.0/).

conduct reliable validation of their model's performance on other datasets. This makes those models an ill fit for any clinical use case. While studies providing their model's code or even the model itself can be a great starting point for one's own research, it is most of the time a more valid option to use foundation models as a basis for research and use the more specific studies as inspiration for the overall solution approaches.

4.3 How can we create our own models/tools

Figure 5 depicts the simplified process for the training of an ML model based on histopathological image data. The process is only symbolized using a single WSI and a few tiles. In general, many WSIs should be used to generate robust models. **Figure 5A.1**. shows the input WSI for the process, while **Figure 5A.2**. shows the corresponding label WSI marking neoplastic areas in the image. During Preprocessing areas of the WSI containing tissue are detected **Figure 5B.1** and the image is separated into tiles of smaller resolution **Figure 5B.2**. Further preprocessing steps should also be conducted on WSI and tile level, for example, color normalization [38], data augmentation [39], artifact detection [40], label cleanup [41]. However, these are omitted for simplicity in this overview. After preprocessing, tiles are selected for the training process **Figure 5C.1** and their corresponding label tiles are retrieved from the provided label WSI **Figure 5C.2**. Afterward, the training is conducted on a multitude of tiles, running the CV model over the data multiple times till the prediction (**Figure 5D** right column) fits the corresponding label (**Figure 5D** center column). When the highest possible overlap is achieved, the model training is terminated, and the resulting CV model can be used to segment complete WSIs on its own, as shown in **Figure 5E**. The process is the same for classification tasks; however, instead of an image label a "tag" or number value is supplied as the label, for example, "tumor," "gbm," 1, 2, 3.

While creating your own CV models may seem very complex at the start, there are actually some tools available to assist in their creation. The most difficult step in this

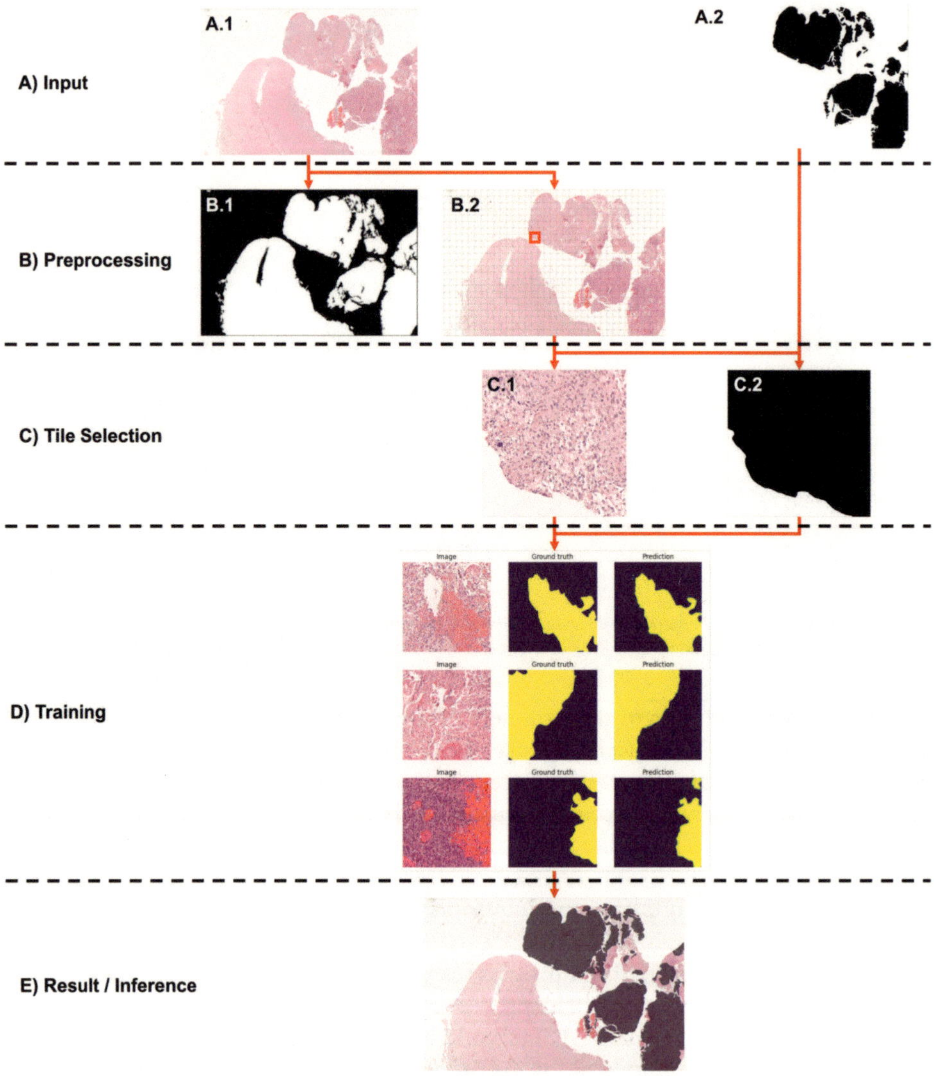

Figure 5.
Process for training a Computer Vision model based on histopathological image data. (A) Providing a Hematoxilyn and Eosin-stained whole-slide image and the corresponding label (in this case neoplastic tissue). (B) Preprocessing of the whole-slide image, detecting tissue, and tiling. (C) Select suitable tiles for the training process and return the corresponding label. (D) Training of the Computer Vision model based on many tiles and their labels (left: input tile, center: label, right: prediction). (E) Resulting segmentation for the complete whole-slide image after training.

endeavor is the data collection and preparation. While there are some tools to automate the required ML model training and creation, data preprocessing, in general, requires a large amount of manual labor.

An exception to this can be found in the Slideflow project [42]. While this program requires the installation of the Python programming language and a few different Python packages, it also provides a graphical use interface that can be used for data processing, labeling, training the ML models, and running the trained models on new data. However, compared to other solutions presented in the following part of this section, the project limits its users in their options to fully customize their approaches. Therefore, Slideflow provides a great first step for training your own CV models for digital pathology, but it should not be seen as the final solution.

4.3.1 Preparing the data

As a first step, data must be available to train a CV model. An easy way to get accustomed to ML data preparation and training can be the usage of a public dataset like the Ivy Glioblastoma Atlas (IGA) [43, 44] or The Cancer Genome Atlas (TCGA) [45]. The IGA provides labeled WSIs of GBMs from a multitude of patients, which can be used as a starting point for first models. Using software tools like PathML [46] or histolab [47] can provide valuable assistance during the required data preparation. However, both still require knowledge of the Python programming language.

4.3.2 Getting to machine learning

There are a couple of semi-automated solutions for creating and training a CV model. For classification tasks, the AUCMEDI framework [48] can be used to automatically create new CV models within a few lines of Python code. However, providing the data in the right format is a prerequisite for this. Like AUCMEDI, MONAI can be used similarly for segmentation tasks, allowing the semi-automatic creation of new segmentation CV models [49].

Providing even more automation, nnU-Net v2 [50] and deepflash2 [51] allow the creation of CV models without writing a single line of code. While both models are quite accessible to computer scientists, they still require a technical setup, and nnU-Net does not provide a graphical user interface as of yet [52]. Despite these limitations, it is possible to effectively use them as a neuropathologist effectively, and further research is ongoing to ease accessibility to medical professionals.

5. Conclusions

In conclusion, the integration of computer vision-based digital pathology represents a significant advancement in the field of CNS tumor diagnostics and treatment. This chapter has outlined state-of-the-art technologies and current advances, demonstrating how digital pathology can revolutionize pathology across various domains, including the CNS.

Despite the considerable progress, the landscape of ready-to-use solutions remains sparse, with a predominance of specialized models and applications tailored for specific research purposes. This gap underscores the importance of collaboration between physicians and the academic community. Engaging with local IT faculties and reaching out to researchers developing these models can foster fruitful partnerships, accelerating the adoption and customization of digital pathology tools in clinical settings.

As this field continues to evolve, the potential for computer vision-based applications in CNS tumor neuropathology is immense. By staying informed and actively participating in ongoing research and development, physicians can leverage these cutting-edge technologies to enhance diagnostic accuracy, improve patient outcomes, and ultimately transform the practice of neuropathology.

Conflict of interest

The authors declare no conflict of interest. The authors are in no way affiliated with the products mentioned in this chapter.

Abbreviations

AI	artificial intelligence
ML	machine learning
CV	computer vision
FDA	U.S. food & drug administration
CNS	central nervous system
HE	hematoxilyn and eosin
IHC	immunohistochemical
IF	immunofluorescence
TIF	tagged image file
TIFF	tagged image file format
PACS	picture archive and communication system
GBM	glioblastoma

Author details

Daniel Hieber[1,2,3]*, Felix Holl[1], Vera Nickl[4], Friederike Liesche-Starnecker[2] and Johannes Schobel[1]

1 DigiHealth Institute, Neu-Ulm University of Applied Sciences, Neu-Ulm, Germany

2 Department of Neuropathology, Pathology, Medical Faculty, University of Augsburg, Augsburg, Germany

3 Institute of Medical Data Science, University Hospital Würzburg, Würzburg, Germany

4 Department of Neurosurgery, Section Experimental Neurosurgery, University Hospital Würzburg, Würzburg, Germany

*Address all correspondence to: daniel.hieber@hnu.de

References

[1] Joshi G, Jain A, Araveeti SR, Adhikari S, Garg H, Bhandari M. FDA-approved artificial intelligence and machine learning (AI/ML)-enabled medical devices: An updated landscape. Electronics. 2024;**13**(3):498. Available from: https://www.mdpi.com/2079-9292/13/3/498

[2] Najjar R. Redefining radiology: A review of artificial intelligence integration in medical imaging. Diagnostics. 2023;**13**(17):2760. Available from: https://www.mdpi.com/2075-4418/13/17/2760

[3] Administration USFD. Artificial Intelligence and Machine Learning (AI/ML)-Enabled Medical Devices; 2024. Available from: https://www.fda.gov/medical-devices/software-medical-device-samd/artificial-intelligence-and-machine-learning-aiml-enabled-medical-devices

[4] Chen RJ, Ding T, Lu MY, Williamson DFK, Jaume G, Song AH, et al. Towards a general-purpose foundation model for computational pathology. Nature Medicine. 2024;**30**(3):850-862. Available from: https://www.nature.com/articles/s41591-024-02857-3

[5] Lu MY, Chen B, Williamson DFK, Chen RJ, Liang I, Ding T, et al. A visual-language foundation model for computational pathology. Nature Medicine. 2024;**30**(3):863-874. Available from: https://www.nature.com/articles/s41591-024-02856-4

[6] Vorontsov E, Bozkurt A, Casson A, Shaikovski G, Zelechowski M, Liu S, et al. Virchow: A million-slide digital pathology foundation model. arXiv. 2024 ArXiv:2309.07778 [cs, eess, q-bio]. Available from: http://arxiv.org/abs/2309.07778

[7] Xu H, Usuyama N, Bagga J, Zhang S, Rao R, Naumann T, et al. A whole-slide foundation model for digital pathology from real-world data. Nature. 2024;**630**(8015):181-188. Available from: https://www.nature.com/articles/s41586-024-07441-w

[8] Taubman DS, Marcellin MW, editors. JPEG2000: Image compression fundamentals, standards, and practice. In: Softcover Reprint of the Hardcover 1st Edition 2002, Third Printing Ed. No. 642 in the Kluwer International Series in Engineering and Computer Science. New York: Springer Science + Business Media, LLC; 2004

[9] QuPath Team. QuPath Documentation - Annotating Images. Available from: https://qupath.readthedocs.io/en/stable/docs/starting/annotating.html

[10] Müller D. Frameworks in Medical Image Analysis with Deep Neural Networks. Augsburg: University Augsburg; 2023. Available from: https://opus.bibliothek.uni-augsburg.de/opus4/104248

[11] Goodfellow I, Bengio Y, Courville A. Deep Learning. Cambridge, Massachusetts: MIT Press; 2016. 775 p. (Adaptive computation and machine learning)

[12] The Royal College of Pathologists. The Pathology Workforce. Available from: https://www.rcpath.org/discover-pathology/public-affairs/the-pathology-workforce.html

[13] Rakha EA, Toss M, Shiino S, Gamble P, Jaroensri R, Mermel CH, et al. Current and future applications

of artificial intelligence in pathology: A clinical perspective. Journal of Clinical Pathology. 2021;**74**(7):409-414. Available from: https://jcp.bmj.com/lookup/doi/10.1136/jclinpath-2020-206908

[14] McGenity C, Clarke EL, Jennings C, Matthews G, Cartlidge C, Freduah-Agyemang H, et al. Artificial intelligence in digital pathology: A systematic review and meta-analysis of diagnostic test accuracy. npj Digital Medicine. 2024;**7**(1):114. Available from: https://www.nature.com/articles/s41746-024-01106-8

[15] Niazi MKK, Parwani AV, Gurcan MN. Digital pathology and artificial intelligence. The Lancet Oncology. 2019;**20**(5):e253-e261. Available from: https://linkinghub.elsevier.com/retrieve/pii/S1470204519301548

[16] Al-Thelaya K, Gilal NU, Alzubaidi M, Majeed F, Agus M, Schneider J, et al. Applications of discriminative and deep learning feature extraction methods for whole slide image analysis: A survey. Journal of Pathology Informatics. 2023;**14**:100335. Available from: https://linkinghub.elsevier.com/retrieve/pii/S2153353923001499

[17] Chen C, Lu MY, Williamson DFK, Chen TY, Schaumberg AJ, Mahmood F. Fast and scalable search of whole-slide images via self-supervised deep learning. Nature Biomedical Engineering. 2022;**6**(12):1420-1434. Available from: https://www.nature.com/articles/s41551-022-00929-8

[18] Müller D, Meyer P, Rentschler L, Manz R, Bäcker J, Cramer S, et al. DeepGleason: A system for automated Gleason grading of prostate cancer using deep neural networks. arXiv. 2024. ArXiv:2403.16678 [cs, eess, q-bio]. Available from: http://arxiv.org/abs/2403.16678

[19] Raciti P, Sue J, Ceballos R, Godrich R, Kunz JD, Kapur S, et al. Novel artificial intelligence system increases the detection of prostate cancer in whole slide images of core needle biopsies. Modern Pathology. 2020;**33**(10):2058-2066. Available from: https://linkinghub.elsevier.com/retrieve/pii/S0893395222004756

[20] Bommasani R, Hudson DA, Adeli E, Altman R, Arora S, von Arx S, et al. On the opportunities and risks of foundation models. arXiv. 2022. ArXiv:2108.07258 [cs]. Available from: http://arxiv.org/abs/2108.07258

[21] Azizi S, Culp L, Freyberg J, Mustafa B, Baur S, Kornblith S, et al. Robust and data-efficient generalization of self-supervised machine learning for diagnostic imaging. Nature Biomedical Engineering. 2023;**7**(6):756-779. Available from: https://www.nature.com/articles/s41551-023-01049-7

[22] Wang X, Yang S, Zhang J, Wang M, Zhang J, Yang W, et al. Transformer-based unsupervised contrastive learning for histopathological image classification. Medical Image Analysis. 2022;**81**:102559. Available from: https://linkinghub.elsevier.com/retrieve/pii/S1361841522002043

[23] Ikezogwo WO, Seyfioglu MS, Ghezloo F, Geva D, Mohammed FS, Anand PK, et al. Quilt-1M: One million image-text pairs for histopathology. Advances in Neural Information Processing Systems. 2023;**36**(DB1):37995-38017

[24] Huang Z, Bianchi F, Yuksekgonul M, Montine TJ, Zou J. A visual–language foundation model for pathology image analysis using medical twitter. Nature Medicine. 2023;**29**(9):2307-2316. Available from: https://www.nature.com/articles/s41591-023-02504-3

[25] Filiot A, Ghermi R, Olivier A, Jacob P, Fidon L, Mac Kain A, et al. Scaling Self-Supervised Learning for Histopathology with Masked Image Modeling. 2023. Available from: http://medrxiv.org/lookup/doi/10.1101/2023.07.21.23292757

[26] Bankhead P, Loughrey MB, Fernández JA, Dombrowski Y, McArt DG, Dunne PD, et al. QuPath: Open source software for digital pathology image analysis. Scientific Reports. 2017;**7**(1):16878. Available from: https://www.nature.com/articles/s41598-017-17204-5

[27] Stritt M, Stalder AK, Vezzali E. Orbit image analysis: An open-source whole slide image analysis tool. PLOS Computational Biology. 2020;**16**(2):e1007313. Available from: https://dx.plos.org/10.1371/journal.pcbi.1007313

[28] Goldberg IG, Allan C, Burel JM, Creager D, Falconi A, Hochheiser H, et al. The open microscopy environment (OME) data model and XML file: Open tools for informatics and quantitative analysis in biological imaging. Genome Biology. 2005;**6**(5):R47. Available from: http://genomebiology.biomedcentral.com/articles/10.1186/gb-2005-6-5-r47

[29] Lamprecht MR, Sabatini DM, Carpenter AE. CellProfiler™: Free, versatile software for automated biological image analysis. BioTechniques. 2007;**42**(1):71-75. Available from: https://www.tandfonline.com/doi/full/10.2144/000112257

[30] Thomas M, O'Shea B, Zerbini CEH, von Meyenn M, Heinzmann S, Freund R, et al. Aiming for higher ambition: The Roche approach to cracking the code of cancer. Nature Portfolio. 2021. Available from: https://www.nature.com/articles/d42473-020-00399-z

[31] Voelker R. Digitized surgical slides. Journal of the American Medical Association. 2017;**317**(19):1942. Available from: http://jama.jamanetwork.com/article.aspx?doi=10.1001/jama.2017.5540

[32] Fraunhofer IIS. MIKAIA [Internet]. Available from: https://www.iis.fraunhofer.de/en/ff/sse/health/medical-image-analysis/mikaia.html [Accessed: August 14, 2024]

[33] KML Vision GmbH. KML Vision. Available from: https://www.kmlvision.com

[34] 3DHISTECH Ltd. 3DHISTECH. Available from: https://www.3dhistech.com

[35] Paige AI, Inc. Paige. Available from: https://paige.ai/

[36] Jensen MP, Qiang Z, Khan DZ, Stoyanov D, Baldeweg SE, Jaunmuktane Z, et al. Artificial intelligence in histopathological image analysis of central nervous system tumours: A systematic review. Neuropathology and Applied Neurobiology. 2024;**50**(3):e12981. Available from: https://onlinelibrary.wiley.com/doi/10.1111/nan.12981

[37] Redlich JP, Feuerhake F, Weis J, Schaadt NS, Teuber-Hanselmann S, Buck C, et al. Applications of artificial intelligence in the analysis of histopathology images of gliomas: A review. Npj. Imaging. 2024;**2**(1):16. Available from: https://www.nature.com/articles/s44303-024-00020-8

[38] Hoque MZ, Keskinarkaus A, Nyberg P, Seppänen T. Stain normalization methods for histopathology image analysis: A comprehensive review and experimental comparison. Information Fusion. 2024;**102**:101997. Available from: https://

linkinghub.elsevier.com/retrieve/pii/S1566253523003135

[39] Faryna K, Van Der Laak J, Litjens G. Automatic data augmentation to improve generalization of deep learning in H&E stained histopathology. Computers in Biology and Medicine. 2024;**170**:108018. Available from: https://linkinghub.elsevier.com/retrieve/pii/S0010482524001021

[40] Kanwal N, López-Pérez M, Kiraz U, Zuiverloon TCM, Molina R, Engan K. Are you sure it's an artifact? Artifact detection and uncertainty quantification in histological images. Computerized Medical Imaging and Graphics. 2024;**112**:102321. Available from: https://linkinghub.elsevier.com/retrieve/pii/S0895611123001398

[41] Bernhardt M, Castro DC, Tanno R, Schwaighofer A, Tezcan KC, Monteiro M, et al. Active label cleaning for improved dataset quality under resource constraints. Nature. Communications. 2022;**13**(1):1161. Available from: https://www.nature.com/articles/s41467-022-28818-3

[42] Dolezal JM, Kochanny S, Dyer E, Ramesh S, Srisuwananukorn A, Sacco M, et al. Slideflow: Deep learning for digital histopathology with real-time whole-slide visualization. BMC Bioinformatics. 2024;**25**(1):134. Available from: https://bmcbioinformatics.biomedcentral.com/articles/10.1186/s12859-024-05758-x

[43] Puchalski RB, Shah N, Miller J, Dalley R, Nomura SR, Yoon JG, et al. An anatomic transcriptional atlas of human glioblastoma. Science (New York, N.Y.). 2018;**360**(6389):660-663

[44] Ivy Glioblastoma Atlas. Available from: https://glioblastoma.alleninstitute.org

[45] The Cancer Genome Atlas. Available from: https://www.cancer.gov/tcga

[46] Rosenthal J, Carelli R, Omar M, Brundage D, Halbert E, Nyman J, et al. Building tools for machine learning and artificial intelligence in cancer research: Best practices and a case study with the PathML toolkit for computational pathology. Molecular Cancer Research. 2022;**20**(2):202-206. Available from: https://aacrjournals.org/mcr/article/20/2/202/678062/Building-Tools-for-Machine-Learning-and-Artificial

[47] Colling R, Pitman H, Oien K, Rajpoot N, Macklin P, CM-Path AI in histopathology working group, et al. artificial intelligence in digital pathology: A roadmap to routine use in clinical practice. The Journal of Pathology. 2019;249(2):143-150. Available from: https://pathsocjournals.onlinelibrary.wiley.com/doi/10.1002/path.5310

[48] Mayer S, Müller D, Kramer F. Standardized medical image classification across medical disciplines. arXiv. 2022. ArXiv:2210.11091 [cs, eess]. Available from: http://arxiv.org/abs/2210.11091

[49] Cardoso MJ, Li W, Brown R, Ma N, Kerfoot E, Wang Y, et al. MONAI: An open-source framework for deep learning in healthcare. arXiv. 2022. ArXiv:2211.02701 [cs]. Available from: http://arxiv.org/abs/2211.02701

[50] Isensee F, Jaeger PF, Kohl SAA, Petersen J, Maier-Hein KH. nnU-net: A self-configuring method for deep learning-based biomedical image segmentation. Nature Methods. 2021;**18**(2):203-211. Available from: https://www.nature.com/articles/s41592-020-01008-z

[51] Griebel M, Segebarth D, Stein N, Schukraft N, Tovote P, Blum R, et al.

Deep learning-enabled segmentation of ambiguous bioimages with deepflash2. Nature Communications. 2023;**14**(1):1679. Available from: https://www.nature.com/articles/s41467-023-36960-9

[52] Hieber D, Haisch N, Grambow G, Holl F, Liesche-Starnecker F, Pryss R, et al. Comparing nnU-Net and deepflash2 for histopathological tumor segmentation. In: Mantas J, Hasman A, Demiris G, Saranto K, Marschollek M, Arvanitis TN, et al., editors. Studies in Health Technology and Informatics [Internet]. IOS Press; 2024. Available from: https://ebooks.iospress.nl/doi/10.3233/SHTI240487

Section 3

Etiology and Biology

Chapter 4

Pituitary Neuroendocrine Tumors and the Role of Their Pattern of Invasion to Adjacent Structures

Diocelina Navarro-Bastida, Sergio Zavala-Vega, Noemi Gelista-Herrera, Natalia Villa-Corral, Diana Chavez-Muñoz, Ricardo Gómez-Rivera, Daniel Rembao-Bojórquez, Martha Tena-Suck, Ciltlaltepetl Salinas-Lara, Lesly Portocarrero-Ortiz, Miguel A. Ramos-Peek, Juan L. Gómez-Amador and Alma Ortiz-Plata

Abstract

Pituitary neuroendocrine tumors (PitNets) are considered benign, but can be invasive. They are classified by their size (microadenomas, macroadenomas, and giant adenomas), by their clinical manifestations (functioning, non-functioning), and by the hormonal content detected by immunocytochemistry. PitNets show slow growth, occupying the sellar region and invading adjacent structures. Their size and invasion have been analyzed using different radiological techniques, complemented by surgical observations and pathological findings. We also include the analysis of the frequency and degree of invasion of functioning and non-functioning PitNets in patients at the National Institute of Neurology and Neurosurgery in Mexico City. The analysis of the size and determination of the invasion degree of PitNets, in relation to the clinical presentation characteristics and hormonal content, allows a better understanding of the behavior of these tumors, which is crucial in planning both the surgical strategy and the follow-up, since size is related to the disease evolution.

Keywords: pituitary neuroendocrine tumor, invasive PitNets, non-functional PitNets, Hardy-Vezina classification, Knosp classification, invasion pattern

1. Introduction

Pituitary neuroendocrine tumors (PitNets; pituitary adenomas, PAs) are heterogeneous neoplasms of the central nervous system (CNS), commonly considered benign. One of the characteristics of PitNets is their slow growth, causing gradual clinical manifestations whose perception will depend on whether or not they are related to hormonal hypersecretion and the degree of invasion. In the sellar and parasellar areas, they constitute 91% of tumors and account for 10–15% of intracranial tumors [1, 2]. At the National Institute of Neurology and Neurosurgery Manuel Velasco Suárez (NINNMVS) in Mexico City, they are the second most treated tumor after meningeal tumor [3]. They come from the different cell types that constitute the anterior pituitary gland and are related to its hormonal activity [4]. There is a diverse frequency with respect to age and gender, being slightly more frequent in women

Symptoms	Frequency
Headache	128
Decreased visual acuity	117
Temporal hemianopsia	77
Hypothyroidism	48
Nausea	42
Blurry vision	39
Threw up	28
Amaurosis	28
Acromegaly	20
Dizziness	16
Amenorrhea	16
Polydipsia/polyuria	14
Ptosis	12
Galactorrhea	12
Hydrocephalus	10
Decreased libido	9
Cushing's syndrome	9
Panhypopituitarism	7
Nasal hemianopsia	5
Convulsive crisis	5
Side clinical effects	
Apoplexy	10
Death	12
Postsurgical complications	
Diabetes insipidus	47
Cerebrospinal fluid fistula	30
Hemorrhage	12
Delirium	5
Epistaxis	6

Table 1.
Clinical features and postsurgical complications of pituitary adenomas.

in some populations and in an average age range between 40 and 60 years; they are rare in children [5, 6]. In 2017, the World Health Organization (WHO) classified PitNets based mainly on their cell lineage, taking into account the transcription factors that are key to the cellular differentiation of these tumors [7]. In this way, somatotrophs (Growth hormone, GH-producing), lactotrophs (Prolactin/PRL-producing), and thyrotrophs (Thyroid-stimulating hormone/TSH-producing) come from PIT1 (pituitary-specific positive transcription factor 1) lineage; corticotrophs (Adrenocorticotropic hormone/ACTH-producing) come from TPIT lineage; and gonadotrophs (follicle-stimulating hormone/FSH-producing and leutinizing hormone/LH-producing) come from steroidogenic factor 1 (SF1) lineage. The subclassification into morphological variants is determined according to specific histological, ultrastructural, and immunohistochemical characteristics [8, 9].

In the effort to understand PitNets, they have been classified according to their size, clinical, histopathological, and molecular characteristics; however, until now, their behavior has not been completely known. Clinically, they are classified into two groups: functional (F) and non-functional (NF), depending on whether or not they are associated with endocrine syndrome. In functional PitNets, the most frequent clinical syndromes are amenorrhea-galactorrhea syndrome, acromegaly, and Cushing's disease [10]. About a third of PitNets are not associated with any clinical or biochemical evidence of hormonal excess, these are called clinically non-functional, which have an estimated prevalence of 7–41.3 cases per 100,000 population [11]. Although the majority of these tumors can secrete hormones, they are biologically inactive so that they are not clinically expressed with an endocrine syndrome [10] but they do usually present with signs and symptoms related to the local mass effect, such as headache (19–75% of cases), neurological deficits of the cranial nerves, visual field alterations as bitemporal hemianopia due to compression of optic chiasm, and hyperprolactinemia, the latter being caused due to compression of the pituitary stalk (the so-called "stalk effect"), which prevents the arrival of dopamine to the adenohypophysis and should not be misinterpreted as a prolactin-producing adenoma [6, 12, 13]. It is known that NF-PitNets are also subdivided into Null Cell (NC), which are immunohistochemically negative for hormones, and Silent (S), those in which no alteration is found in the hormonal profile, but are positive for some hormones by immunohistochemistry [14]. (**Table 1**. Clinical analysis in NINNMVS).

Two hundred twenty-one cases of PitNets (113 female and 108 male) from the National Institute of Neurology and Neurosurgery were included in the study (between the years of 2017 and 2021).

2. PitNets: Size and invasiveness

PitNets are also classified based on their size into: microadenomas if they measure <1 cm, macroadenomas > = 1 cm and up to 3 cm, and giant PitNets > = 4 cm [5]. It has been described by Hardy-Vezina and Knosp that PitNets can grow in four directions: upward (suprasellar region), downward (sphenoidal sinus: region/infrasellar), or toward one of the sides (cavernous sinus/parasellar region) [15]. Hardy et al. [16] classified adenomas according to the invasion of the sella turcica. Grade I was observed when the sella turcica was slightly enlarged, grades II and III when the sella turcica was significantly enlarged, with local destruction of the floor, and grade IV when the sella turcica was diffusely destroyed. PitNets classified from grade II to grade IV are considered invasive. Hardy also made a description of five stages (A–E) according to suprasellar extension (SSE) and invasion to adjacent structures, in which grade A describes a size of 10 mm above the sphenoid jugum, filling the chiasmatic cistern, grade B up to 20 mm, grade C up to 30 mm, grade D greater than 30 mm, and grade E with asymmetric lateral expansions. On the other hand, Knosp classifies adenomas from grade 0 to IV, according to parasellar growth. In this classification, tumor growth is evaluated, taking as reference the medial tangent of the supracavernous an intracavernous internal carotid artery, and the intercarotid line (ICL), which is the line drawn between the centers of the intra- and supracavernous ICA. In grade 0, the tumor is located within the cavernous sinus space, without invading the medial tangent of the ICA; grade I when the medial tangent of the ICA is passed without passing the ICL; grade II when the tumor extends beyond the ICL, without crossing the tangent on the lateral aspects of the ICA; grade III when the tumor extends laterally to the lateral tangent of the ICA; and grade IV when the tumor completely covers the intracavernous ICA [2]. Furthermore, it is taken into account that cranial nerves III–VI are also located in the suprasellar region, so pituitary lesions can cause disorders of the cranial nerves (III, IV, V, VI), due to involvement of the cavernous sinus and other nearby structures. Invasion into adjacent structures has been one of the factors studied to understand the biological behavior of PitNets to achieve control during disease monitoring.

Although PitNets are considered benign neoplasms, they can be aggressive and between 25 and 55% can be invasive (I) [15, 17, 18]. In the case of functional PitNets, it has not been possible to reach an agreement regarding their invasive capacity. The meaning of the word "invasion" in PitNets is controversial and there is a lot of confusion about it, since the criteria to evaluate the growth of a pituitary tumor can be according to: (1) radiological findings, (2) surgical findings, and (3) the pathological anatomy findings. The magnetic resonance imaging (MRI) of PitNets is the main technique for the evaluation since it is an important guide for the treatment and monitoring of each particular case; however, other instruments with better sensitivity are needed for microadenomas [19]. There are other imaging techniques that have been used to assess the size and extent of PitNets, such as positron emission tomography (PET), magnetic resonance spectroscopy (MRS) that detects cell proliferation, metabolic and hormonal activity, and single-photon emission computed tomography (SPET/SPECT), which have high sensitivity for neuroendocrine tumors, but there are currently few studies on the pituitary gland [20, 21].

The application of a new resource to analyze PitNets has recently been explored. This new tool, called radiomics, is a new methodology that applies computer techniques to quantify the information contained in imaging studies, applying statistical resources to propose predictive models. In this way, it is sought to make predictions about the tumor, such as consistency, histopathological characteristics, invasiveness, hormonal secretion, and response to treatment. It is proposed that radiomics can help to perform a better classification in the preoperative phase and to be able to decide the treatment and follow-up of the patient [22–24].

2.1 Classification of PitNets by degree of extension

In the NINNMVS, PitNets are classified according to their degree of extension assessed by MRI. Using Hardy-Vezina parameters, a classification of 215 cases was performed. Grade III PitNets were the most abundant with 46.04% (99/215), of which 86.8% (n = 86/99) were NF-PitNet (**Figure 1A**). The description of the extension of PitNet was observed in 177 of the 215 cases. The majority of PitNets presented

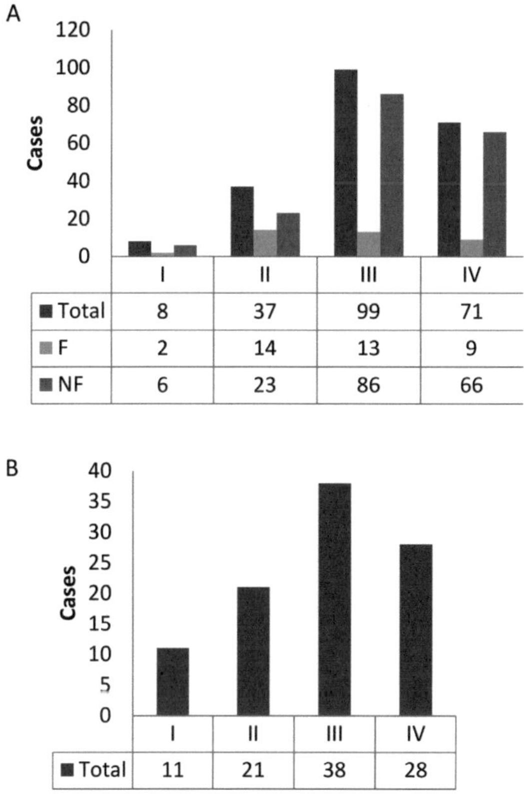

Figure 1.
Classification of PitNets according to Hardy-Vezina (A) and Knosp (B). (A) Two hundred fifteen cases were classified. Grade III were more abundant (46.04%; 99/215), of which 86.8% (n = 86/99) were NF-PitNet; (B) Ninety-eight cases were classified, of which 38 (38.7%) belonged to grade III.

suprasellar extension 66.6% (118/177), of which 63.5% belonged to grade III (75/118), with grade IIIC being the one with the greatest number of cases. Regarding parasellar extension, the majority belonged to grade IVE (**Table 2**). On the other hand, 98 cases were classified according to Knosp (**Figure 1B**). Those of grade III were the most abundant 38.7% (38/98).

The clinicopathological analysis of PitNets includes the clinical manifestations of the disease, radiological studies, surgical findings, and anatomopathological

Hardy-Vezina classification grade (n = 177)	Suprasellar extension 66.7% (n = 118)			Asymmetrical extension 33.3% (n = 59)	
	A	B	C	D	E
I	3 (2.5%)	0 (0%)	0 (0%)	0 (0%)	1 (1.7%)
II	4 (3.4%)	8 (6.8%)	10 (8.5%)	1 (1.7%)	2 (3.4%)
III	2 (1.7%)	8 (6.8%)	65 (55.1%)	6 (10.2%	6 (10.2%)
IV	0 (0%)	0 (0%)	18 (15.2%)	10 (16.9%)	33 (55.9%)

Table 2.
Grades of extension of PAs according to Hardy-Vezina classification.

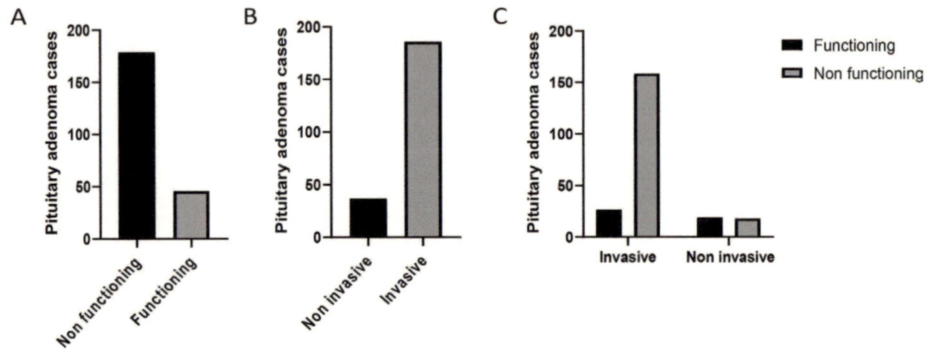

Figure 2.
Classification of pituitary adenomas by their clinical manifestations and their relationship with invasiveness (study between the years of 2017 and 2021). (A) Non-functioning pituitary adenomas are more frequent (n = 176/221; 79.6%). (B) Most of the cases are invasive (n = 184/221; 83.2%). (C) Most of the invasive pituitary adenomas are non-functioning (n = 158/221; 71.5%).

observations, which show the behavior of the PitNets. In our experience at NINNMVS, most of the PitNets studied are non-functional and invasive (**Figure 2**).

The analysis of the invasiveness and functionality of PitNets is complemented by the study of their hormonal activity using immunohistochemistry. PitNets are categorized according to their hormonal content: those that express PRL, GH, FSH/LH, TSH, ACTH, plurihormonal (PH, those that express more than one hormone), and Null Cell (NC, non-functioning tumors that did not express hormones). In our

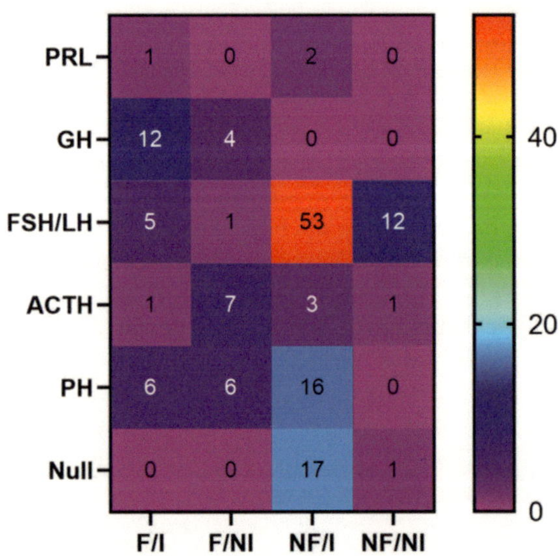

Figure 3.
Heatmap showing phenotypic analysis of PitNets with variation in hormone expression, function, and invasiveness. The x-axis indicates the secretory activity as: F = Functional; NF = Non-Functional; I = Invasive; NI = Non-Invasive. The prevalence of the six subtypes of PitNets (n = 148/221) according to their hormonal content is represented on the y-axis: PRL (prolactin); GH (growth hormone); FSH/LH (follicle-stimulating hormone, luteinizing hormone, or both); ACTH (adrenocorticotropic hormone); PH (plurihormonal) and Null (without hormone production). The change in coloration indicates the frequency of each phenotype on a rainbow color scale, where cool colors represent low values and warm colors represent high values. The number of cases of each variable is shown in each cell.

case series (n = 148), the most abundant PitNet was the gonadotrope phenotype that produces FSH and/or LH with 47.9% cases (n = 71/148), of which 74.6% (n = 53/71) belonged to the NF-I PitNet. The PH phenotype was the second with the highest proportion with 18.9% (28/148), of which 57.1% (16/28) were NF-I PitNet. And the third with 12.1% (18/148) was the Null cell phenotype, identified primarily as NF-I PitNet with 94.4% (17/18). GH, ACTH, and PRL phenotypes were the least frequent (**Figure 3**). In this study, it was observed that the highest incidence was NF-I PitNet with 61.5% (91/148), followed by F-I PitNet (PitNet invasive with hormonal detection) with 16.9% (25/148), then F-NI PitNet 12.2% (18/148) and in a lower proportion NF-NI PitNets are identified with 9.4% (14/148).

Also, differences were found regarding the age of the patients at the time of diagnosis and PitNet subtypes. The age range with the highest incidence of PitNet diagnosis for both male and female was 40 to 59 years. F-PitNet showed lower age of presentation at diagnosis (age range 19–70; average 40 years) than NF-PitNet

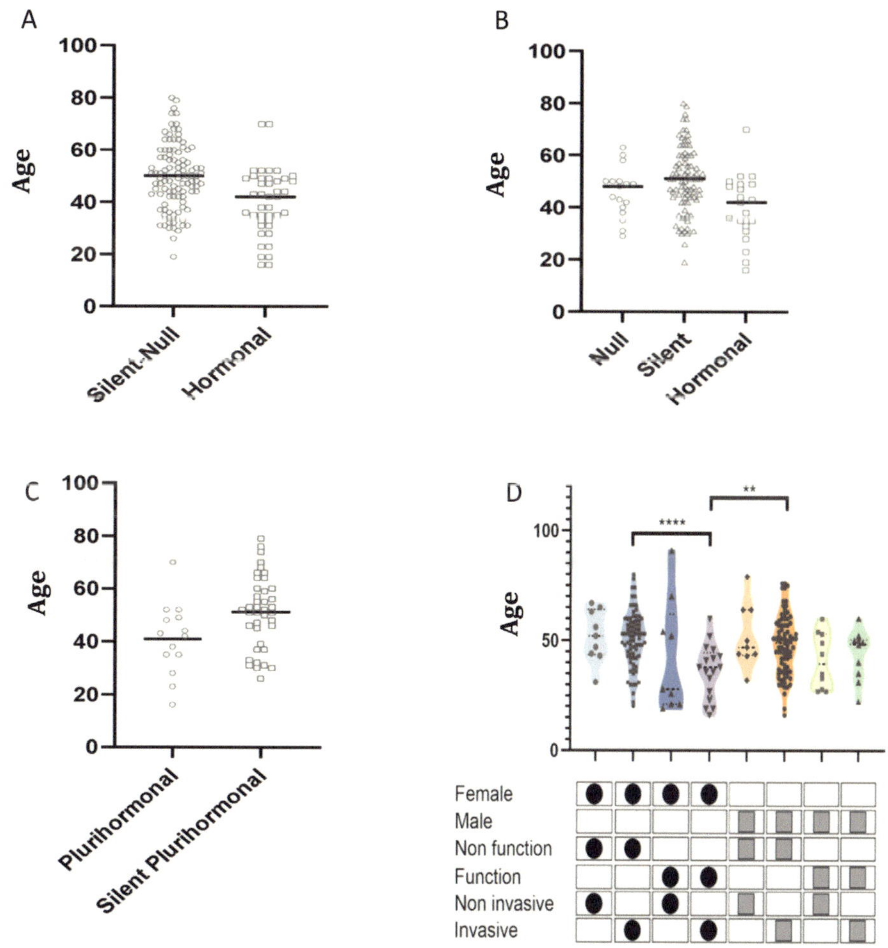

Figure 4.
Relationship between age of presentation at diagnosis and subtypes of PitNets. (A) Difference was found between the F-PitNet (hormonal) with the NF-PitNet (Silent-Null). (B) Difference was also found between the Hormonal and the Silent. (C) Plurihormonal showed a lower age of presentation than Silent-Plurihormonal. (D) Differences were found in the age of presentation between male and female, F and NF and non-invasive and invasive. Statistical difference p < 0.05.

Cell line	Invasive PAs n = 116	Suprasellar cases n = 69 (59.5%)	Ratio in % n = 69	Proportion by total in each cell line (%)	Parasellar cases n = 47 (40.5%)	Ratio in % n = 47	Proportion by total in each cell line (%)
Prl	3	2	2.8	66.6	1	2.1	33.3
GH	12	8	11.5	66.6	4	8.5	33.3
FSH and/or LH	58	29	42	50	29	61.7	50
ACTH	4	2	2.8	50	2	4.2	50
Plurihormonal	22	14	20.3	63.6	8	17	36.3
Null Cell	17	14	20.3	82.3	3	6.3	17.6

Prl = Prolactin; GH = growth hormone; FSH = follicle-stimulating hormone; LH = luteinizing hormone; ACTH = adrenocorticotropic hormone.

Table 3.
Invasion pattern of PAs by hormonal subtype.

(Silent-Null; age range 19–80; average 50 years; $p < 0.0001$, 95% CI: −14.37 - -5.33) (**Figure 4A**) and with NF-S-PitNet (age range 20–80; average 50 years; $p < 0.0009$, 95% CI -16.84 - - 4.47) (**Figure 4B**). Plurihormonal F-PitNet (age range 18–70; average 40 years) showed a statistically significant difference with plurihormonal S-PitNet (age range 30–80; mean 50 years; $p < 0.019$, 95% CI 1.71–18.79) (**Figure 4C**). Differences in the age of presentation of the condition were also observed between male and female. In female, a higher age of presentation was found in NF-I-PitNet than in FI-PitNet. Men had a higher age of presentation in NF-I-PitNet than women with FI-PitNet (**Figure 4D**).

2.2 Invasion pattern of PitNets and their hormonal activity

The invasion pattern of PitNet (PitNet-I) was oriented towards the suprasellar region with 59.4% (69/116) of the cases. For each group of PitNets according to their cell lineage assessed by immunohistochemistry, those with the highest percentage oriented to this region were the gonadotropes 42% (29/69), followed by the PH and Null Cell with the same proportion each 20.3% (14/69). Of the PitNets with parasellar orientation 40.5% (47/116), gonadrotopes showed a higher frequency 61.7% (n = 29/47). In the invasion pattern for each cell line, it was found that of the PitNets of null cells, 82.3% (14/17) were suprasellar and 50% of the gonadotropic cases (29/58) and ACTH (2/4) were parasellar (**Table 3**).

3. PitNets: The role of their invasion pattern

PitNets can grow, occupying the space adjacent to the sellar region, describing a particular pattern that may be related to the endocrinological and molecular characteristics of the tumor type. It has been reported that NF-PitNets have an incidence from 14 to 54% [11, 25] although it varies according to the population analyzed, as in the case of the Mexican population studied, in which 79.6% of the cases were NF-PitNet. This difference can be attributed to the type and size of the population in which these studies were carried out, since our work included 221 Mexican patients, treated at the National Institute of Neurology and Neurosurgery, which is a hospital concentrating on care for patients with neurological conditions. It has been found that the incidence of invasive PitNets varies from an average of 14.8%, between a range of 30–40%, and can reach up to 76% of cases [26–28]. In our study, we found that 83% of the cases were invasive PitNets, which is more consistent than what was reported by Lu et al. [28]. Therefore, it is suggested that it would be important to carry out more research that analyze factors that may be related to the development of invasiveness of PitNets depending on their population, which would be useful for preventive and therapeutic purposes [29].

Until now, it has not been found that the presentation of PitNets has a clear relationship with the gender and age of the patients. In our study, we found that the frequency of PitNets presentation in women was 51.13%, which contrasts with what was reported by Daly and Beckers [30] and Barahona et al. [30, 31] who agreed on a marked predominance of women in the incidence of PitNets (68.4 and 71.6%, respectively). However, in another study Liu et al. [26] reported that the percentage of females in its Chinese population was 57.6%. Finally, it should be noted that the population studied by Daly et al. was made up of patients of biological nationality from the United Kingdom, Switzerland, Argentina, Canada, Malta, and Iceland, and our population was exclusively natural Mexicans, which opens a question to study the possible existence of some genetic and/or environmental variants that make women more likely to develop PitNets.

In a study carried out by Slavinsky et al. [32] in which 202 NF-PitNets were included, they found that NF-I-PitNets were the most frequent (76.7; 93.1 of men and 57.8% of women), which is consistent with those found in our study because 71.5% of the PitNets in our population were NF-I-PAs, and although no differences in frequency were found between men and women in NF-PitNets, in women a significant difference was found between NF-I-PitNets and F-I-PitNets. In our study, we found that the age range with the highest incidence of PitNets diagnosis was 40–59 years, which contrasts with a work carried out by Barahona et al. [31], in which they found that the most frequent age of diagnosis was in a range of 20 to 39 years. This difference may be attributable to the fact that the majority of our population presented NF-PitNets, which generally take a long time to produce symptoms and when it does occur, it is usually very nonspecific, which lengthens and complicates the diagnostic process.

In our study, it is reported that PitNets presented at a younger age since differences were found between F-PitNets in relation to NF-PitNets and NF-S-PitNets and between plurihormonal F-PitNets compared to plurihormonal S-PitNets. These data differ with some findings reported in the literature. Torregrosa et al. [33] compared F-PitNets with S-PitNets in a population between 44.67 and 12.76 years old and found that the difference in the age ranges of their population at the time of diagnosis was not significant, reporting a mean of 44.14 and 47.3 years, respectively. This is different from what was found in our population where an important difference was observed in age, being younger in F-PitNets with a mean age of 40 years. However, they also described important inequalities in the age of diagnosis between plurihormonal F-PitNets and plurihormonal S-PAs, in a population of 48 to 16.8 years of age with a mean presentation of 39.12 years in the plurihormonal F-PitNets and 56.8 years for plurihormonal S-PitNets. This agrees with the age difference found in our study since a lower age of diagnosis (40 years) was found for PH-F-PitNets with a difference of 10 years in the mean age at the time of diagnosis, compared to the PH-S-PitNets (50 years). In another study that describes the differences between F-PitNets and NF-PitNets, a lower mean age at diagnosis for F-PitNets was reported, which is in accordance with the results of our study [34]. This is understandable, considering the symptoms that characterize F-PitNets due to hormonal action, compared to the typical presentation of NF-PitNets that manifest with more insidious symptoms attributable to mass effect. A notable aspect is the significant association that has been reported between tumor size with age, male gender, and p53 expression. In turn, tumor size and age are related to infrasellar invasion. Younger age has been observed to be a factor for early progression of residual tumor postoperatively with a tendency towards a high Mindbomb Homolog-1 (MIB-1) index, suggesting a probably high risk of recurrence in NF-PitNets [35].

It is important to highlight that invasiveness is not synonymous with aggressiveness, since the latter contemplates the sum of aspects, such as invasion, rapid tumor growth rate, resistance to standard treatment, and clinically relevant tumor growth. Unfortunately, these terms have not yet been clearly defined. Invasion has been determined through neuroimaging studies supported by the Knosp and Hardy-Vezina classifications, which are the most widely used [15] since adequate determination of PitNet invasion is crucial to plan the surgical approach and the amount of tumor resection [36]. In addition, the 2017 WHO classification for PitNets includes it as a criterion to determine whether or not a PitNet is high risk since it has been seen that up to 50% of NF macroadenomas progress within a period of 2 to 7 years [37]. It is important to take into account that several authors have emphasized that the occupation of the cavernous sinus by the tumor is not a determining factor of invasion, since it can only correspond to the expansion of the tumor, so the Knosp classification becomes important for predicting invasion of the cavernous sinus [27], which is complemented by the Hardy-Vezina classification that classifies PitNets into four grades based on their size and invasion of the sella turcica [11]. Regarding tumor growth, Raverot (2021, [28]) has defined that an unusually rapid tumor growth rate is observed when the increase in the size of the tumor in its longest diameter is ≥20%, either in the case of a single lesion or the sum of the largest diameters in a multilobulated lesion, in a time period of <6–12 months when only an annual MRI is available. Raverot gives special attention to the evaluation of tumor growth in relation to the response to treatment. As has already been demonstrated by other authors, to complete the evaluation of aggressiveness it is important to include in the histopathological analysis, the study of its hormonal activity (in order to evaluate the possible change in its secretory activity that may suggest an aggressive evolution), by immunohistochemistry for adenohypophyseal hormones, Ki67 index, and mitotic count [38, 39].

In relation to the cell subtype in our study, the most frequent PitNets were gonadotropes, with NF-PitNets being the most frequent, which is in agreement with the findings of other authors [18, 26]. However, in the study carried out by Daly et al. they found that lactotroph cell PitNets comprised approximately 50% of annual diagnoses, placing them as the most common PitNets in their population [31]. It has been reported that somatotropic PitNets cover 10–15% of cases in general, and of these the majority are functional secretory tumors [40], which is in line with what was demonstrated by our analysis, which revealed that GH-producing F-PitNets were significantly more frequent than NF-PAs. However, in another study carried out in a Chinese population, of 179 patients diagnosed with somatotropic-type PitNets, 139 were NF-PitNets [41]. Therefore, it could be suspected that factors related to the population influence the presentation of these PitNets.

On the other hand, in our analysis we found that Null Cell PitNets (NC-PitNets) are more invasive than silent PitNets (S-PitNets) in general, since invasive NC-PitNets have a frequency ratio of 17:1 with respect to non-invasive ones and S-PitNets have a frequency ratio of 5.5:1 with respect to non-invasive ones. This is supported by Haddad et al.'s [42] report since they found that NC-PitNets presented greater invasion to the cavernous sinus compared to gonadotropic S-PitNets (3.97%, 95% CI 1.04–15.14; $p = 0$). This is how a similar trend is observed in the invasion capacity of PitNets with these characteristics.

Depending on their size, PitNets are classified into microadenomas (< 10 mm) and macroadenomas (> 10 mm), where macroadenomas have a frequency of around 48% of cases [31, 37]. In our study, 96.2% of the cases were macroadenomas, classified in grades III and IV of the Hardy-Vezina and Knosp scale. This difference draws attention, making a broader investigation of the differences between populations interesting. An interesting fact was found in relation to the analysis of the expansion capacity of the PitNets. It has been reported that the expansion of the PitNets is oriented in most cases towards the suprasellar region in up to 85% of the cases. These data are distant from the growth pattern found in the PitNets that we studied since these represented the 66.7% being just over half of our population [43]. On the other hand, it was found that of the patients with suprasellar extension, 78.81% turned out to be invasive (grades III and IV of the Hardy-Vezina classification). This behavior of expansion to the suprasellar region is justified, given that classically the growth of the PitNets follows the path of least resistance. Under this premise, anatomically in the sellar region there is a central opening in the diaphragm of the sella turcica, in the direction of the suprasellar cistern [44]. However, we cannot rule out some other cause as justification for this growth pattern, because in another study it was found that more than 40% of aggressive PitNets showed invasion towards the cavernous sinus [18]. In our study, it was found that of the PitNets with parasellar extension, 93.2% were invasive. Of the PitNets classified according to Knosp, those of grade III were the most common at the time of diagnosis (38.7% of cases), unlike what was reported by Pérez et al. [45] where most of PitNets in their Spanish population were found to be in a grade II stage (31%) [45]. Additionally, it has been reported that invasion to cavernous sinus is associated with tumor size, NF-PitNet condition, high mitotic index, elevated MIB-1 immunoreaction, and p53 immunoexpression. Infrasellar invasion is related to tumor size, which in turn with MIB-1 index and mitotic figures are considered predictors of parasellar invasion. Also, p53 diffuse immunostain is considered predictor of suprasellar or subfrontal extension [35]. Invasion into adjacent structures has been observed to have surgical implications and to be a prognostic factor. It has been observed that the increase in the degree of parasellar invasion decreases the probability of gross total resection (GTR) and endocrinological remission (ER) [46]. Raverot et al. [47] classified PitNets into five grades (1a non-invasive; 1b non-invasive/proliferative; 2a invasive; 2b invasive/proliferative; and 3 metastatic) according to their size and invasion assessed by MRI, mitotic index, and immunoreaction to Ki-67 and p53. They show that 2b tumors had poor prognosis with high risk of progression and propose that this classification has prognostic value to predict PitNet behavior [47]. In a previous work carried out by our working group, the mitotic index and the expression of p53 and Ki-67 were evaluated. In this work, no relationship was found between these markers and invasive and non-invasive PitNets [48].

Additionally, in our study we found that in relation to tumor extension by secretory subtype, gonadotroph PitNets (FSH and/or LH) are the ones with the highest frequency of both suprasellar and parasellar invasion compared to the other secretory subtypes, being the majority of them non-functioning type. However, the analysis of the frequency of the extension within each subtype showed that Null Cell, Prl, GH, and plurihormonal PitNets have more suprasellar than parasellar extension. In a study of 202 cases of PitNets carried out by Le Brass et al., it was found that of the PitNets classified in grades III and IV on the Hardy scale, those that showed the highest frequency were PH-PitNets (44.4% n = 4/ 9) and GH (41.7% n = 5/12), which shows that in our population the frequency of these tumor subtypes is higher, highlighting that the number of cases per group is small, as in our study [49].

4. Conclusions

This work allowed us to investigate the behavior of PitNets in terms of their extension pattern towards surrounding structures, which could be useful in the diagnosis and follow-up of patients. Furthermore, these findings open the way to continue investigating the factors that are related to the proliferative activity and invasive capacity of pituitary adenomas, which may have particular characteristics depending on their cellular origin related to their hormonal activity.

In the cases of PitNet reviewed in patients of our institution, it was found that the age of presentation was 40 to 59 years, with a higher age of presentation in the NF-I-PAs. The most frequent PitNets were of the non-functional invasive type. It should be noted that the majority of the PitNets studied developed a suprasellar growth pattern and these in turn extend towards the anterior portion of the third ventricle. Furthermore, according to the Knosp classification, most PitNets had an invasion that was located beyond the lateral limit of the internal carotid artery (Grade III). Regarding the classification according to their cell lineage, gonadotroph-type PitNets were the most frequent in our population. They occurred in almost half of the cases and of them, the most common type was NF-I-PitNet, developing a suprasellar or parasellar tumor extension pattern in the same proportion (50%). It is striking that of the GH-PitNet, invasive functional ones are more common, which develop, in a high proportion, a pattern of suprasellar extension. Similarly, NC-PitNets, which were the third most frequent type in the population studied, showed the highest frequency of suprasellar invasion pattern. Finally, invasive ACTH adenomas were those that presented a high frequency of parasellar extension pattern, along with invasive gonadotrophs. This research work allowed us to know the behavior of PAs in terms of their extension pattern towards surrounding structures; however, it is necessary to continue investigating this type of tumor, including a greater number of cases that cover the different tumor subtypes.

Acknowledgements

This research was funded by the Consejo Nacional de Ciencia y Tecnología (grand 289912 to A. O. P.) as part of Fondo Sectorial De Investigación En Salud Y Seguridad Social SS/IMSS/ISSSTE-CONACYT and was supported by the Instituto Nacional de Neurología y Neurocirugía "Manuel Velasco Suárez."

Conflict of interest

The authors declare no conflict of interest.

Author details

Diocelina Navarro-Bastida[1,2], Sergio Zavala-Vega[3], Noemi Gelista-Herrera[3], Natalia Villa-Corral[2,4], Diana Chavez-Muñoz[2], Ricardo Gómez-Rivera[1,2], Daniel Rembao-Bojórquez[3], Martha Tena-Suck[3], Citlaltepetl Salinas-Lara[3], Lesly Portocarrero-Ortiz[5], Miguel A. Ramos-Peek[6], Juan L. Gómez-Amador[6] and Alma Ortiz-Plata[1]*

1 Laboratory of Experimental Neuropathology, National Institute of Neurology and Neurosurgery, México City, Mexico

2 Faculty of Higher Studies Iztacala, MEDICI-RED, National Autonomous University of Mexico, México City, Mexico

3 Department of Neuropathology, National Institute of Neurology and Neurosurgery, México City, Mexico

4 Autonomous University of Tlaxcala, México City, Mexico

5 Neuroendocrinology, National Institute of Neurology and Neurosurgery, México City, Mexico

6 Service of Neurosurgery, National Institute of Neurology and Neurosurgery, México City, Mexico

*Address all correspondence to: aortizplata@yahoo.com.mx

References

[1] Tsukamoto T, Miki Y. Imaging of pituitary tumors: An update with the 5th WHO classifications-part 1. Pituitary neuroendocrine tumor (PitNET)/pituitary adenoma. Japanese Journal of Radiology. 2023;**41**:789-806. DOI: 10.1007/s11604-023-01400-7

[2] Hashmi FA, Shamim MS. Pituitary adenoma: A review of existing classification systems based on anatomic extension and invasion. The Journal of the Pakistan Medical Association. 2020;**70**:368-370

[3] Aguirre-Cruz L, Rangel-López E, De la Cruz-Aguilera DL, Rodríguez-Pérez CE, Ruano L, Velásquez-Pérez L, et al. Historical distribution of central nervous system tumors in the Mexican National Institute of neurology and neurosurgery. Salud Pública de México. 2016;**58**:171-178

[4] Serioli S, Agostini L, Pietrantoni A, Valeri F, Costanza F, Chiloiro S, et al. Aggressive PitNETs and potential target therapies: A systematic review of molecular and genetic pathways. International Journal of Molecular Sciences. 2023;**24**:15719. DOI: 10.3390/ijms242115719

[5] Araujo-Castro M, Pascual-Corrales E, Ortiz-Flores AE, Escobar-Morreale HF. Pituitary-hypothalamic axis. Physiology and pathology. Medicine - Programa de Formación Médica Continuada Acreditado. 2020;**13**:846-855. DOI: 10.1016/j.med.2020.09.003

[6] Tortosa F, Webb SM. Novel aspects in histopathology of the pituitary gland. Endocrinología, Diabetes y Nutrición. 2017;**64**:152-161. DOI: 10.1016/j.endien.2017.04.001

[7] Lenders NF, Earls PE, Inder WJ, McCormack AI. The evolution in pituitary tumour classification: A clinical perspective. Endocrine Oncology. 2023;**3**:220079. DOI: 10.1530/EO-22-0079

[8] Lopes MBS. The 2017 World Health Organization classification of tumors of the pituitary gland: A summary. Acta Neuropathologica. 2017;**134**:521-535. DOI: 10.1007/s00401-017-1769-8

[9] Ortiz-Plata A, Tena-Suck ML, Pérez-Neri I, Rembao-Bojórquez D, Fernández A. Pituitary adenomas Clinico-pathological, Immunohistochemical and ultrastructural study. In: Rahimi-Movaghar V, editor. Pituitary Adenomas. Croatia: IntechOpen; 2012. pp. 49-66. DOI: 10.5772/34040

[10] Melmed S, Kaiser UB, Lopes MB, Bertherat J, Syro LV, Raverot G, et al. Clinical biology of the pituitary adenoma. Endocrine Reviews. 2022;**43**:1003-1037. DOI: 10.1210/endrev/bnac010

[11] Ntali G, Wass JA. Epidemiology, clinical presentation and diagnosis of non-functioning pituitary adenomas. Pituitary. 2018;**21**:111-118. DOI: 10.1007/s11102-018-0869-3

[12] Drummond JB, Ribeiro-Oliveira A Jr, Soares BS. Non-functioning pituitary adenomas. In: Feingold KR, Anawalt B, Blackman MR, et al., editors. Endotext [Internet]. South Dartmouth (MA): MDText.com, Inc.; 2000. Available from: https://www.ncbi.nlm.nih.gov/sites/books/NBK534880/ [Accessed: 2022 October 12]

[13] Rizzoli P, Iuliano S, Weizenbaum E, Laws E. Headache in patients with pituitary lesions: A longitudinal cohort

study. Neurosurgery. 2016;**78**:316-323. DOI: 10.1227/NEU.0000000000001067

[14] Chanson P, Raverot G, Castinetti F, Cortet-Rudelli C, Galland F, Salenave S, et al. Management of clinically non-functioning pituitary adenoma. Annales d'Endocrinologie. 2015;**76**:239-247. DOI: 10.1016/j.ando.2015.04.002

[15] Di Ieva A, Knosp E, Steiner E, Kitz K, Matula C. Pituitary adenomas with invasion of the cavernous sinus space: A magnetic resonance imaging classification compared with surgical findings. Neurosurgery. 1993;**33**:610-617. DOI: 10.1227/00006.123-19931.0000-00008

[16] Di Ieva A, Rotondo F, Syro LV, Cusimano MD, Kovacs K. Aggressive pituitary adenomas Diagnosis and emerging treatments. Nature Reviews. Endocrinology. 2014;**10**:423-435. DOI: 10.1038/nrendo.2014.64

[17] Micko A, Oberndorfer J, Weninger WJ, Vila G, Höftberger R, Wolfsberger S, et al. Challenging Knosp high-grade pituitary adenomas. Journal of Neurosurgery. 2019;**132**:1739-1746. DOI: 10.3171/2019.3.JNS19367

[18] Melmed S. Pituitary-tumor endocrinopathies. The New England Journal of Medicine. 2020;**382**:937-950. DOI: 10.1056/NEJMra1810772

[19] Yuen KCJ, Ghalib L, Buchfelder M, Hughes J, Langlois F, Molitch ME. Surveillance imaging strategies for pituitary adenomas: When, how frequent, and when to stop. Endocrine Practice. 2024;**30**:282-291. DOI: 10.1016/j.eprac.2023.12.014

[20] Yao A, Balchandani P, Shrivastava RK. Metabolic In vivo visualization of pituitary adenomas: A systematic review of imaging modalities. World Neurosurgery. 2017;**104**:489-498. DOI: 10.1016/j.wneu.2017.04.128

[21] Pînzariu O, Georgescu CE. Metabolomics in acromegaly: A systematic review. Journal of Investigative Medicine. 2023;**71**:634-645. DOI: 10.1177/10815589231169452

[22] Bioletto F, Prencipe N, Berton AM, Aversa LS, Cuboni D, Varaldo E, et al. Radiomic analysis in pituitary tumors: Current knowledge and future perspectives. Journal of Clinical Medicine. 2024;**13**:336.1-336.33615. DOI: 10.3390/jcm13020336

[23] Mendi BAR, Batur H, Çay N, Çakır BT. Radiomic analysis of preoperative magnetic resonance imaging for the prediction of pituitary adenoma consistency. Acta Radiologica. 2023;**64**:2470-2478. DOI: 10.1177/02841851231174462

[24] Koong K, Preda V, Jian A, Liquet-Weiland B, Di Ieva A. Application of artificial intelligence and radiomics in pituitary neuroendocrine and sellar tumors: A quantitative and qualitative synthesis. Neuroradiology. 2022;**64**:647-668. DOI: 10.1007/s00234-021-02845-1

[25] Bista A, Mishra D, Ghimire S, Bhandari P, Puri S. Non-functioning pituitary macroadenoma resection in twin pregnancy: A case report. Cureus. 2023;**15**:e42891. DOI: 10.7759/cureus.42891

[26] Liu J, He Y, Zhang X, Yan X, Huang Y. Clinicopathological analysis of 250 cases of pituitary adenoma under the new WHO classification. Oncology Letters. 2020;**19**:1890-1898. DOI: 10.3892/ol.2020.11263

[27] Raverot G, Ilie MD, Lasolle H, Amodru V, Trouillas J, Castinetti F, et al. Aggressive pituitary tumours and

pituitary carcinomas. Nature Reviews. Endocrinology. 2021;**17**:671-684. DOI: 10.1038/s41574-021-00550 w

[28] Lu L, Wan X, Xu Y, Chen J, Shu K, Lei T. Classifying pituitary adenoma invasiveness based on radiological, surgical and histological features: A retrospective assessment of 903 cases. Journal of Clinical Medicine. 2022;**11**:2464.13-2464.15. DOI: 10.3390/jcm11092464

[29] Ioachimescu AG. Sociodemographic factors in pituitary adenomas. Endocrinology and Metabolism Clinics of North America. 2023;**52**:705-717. DOI: 10.1016/j.ecl.2023.05.008

[30] Daly AF, Beckers A. The epidemiology of pituitary adenomas. In Endocrinology and Metabolism Clinics of North America. 2020;**49**:347-355. DOI: 10.1016/j.ecl.2020.04.002

[31] Barahona-Ulloa WF, García-Iñiguez JD, Jiménez-Encalada MG, Sacoto-Molina AM. Pituitary adenomas: Sociodemographical, clinical and therapeutic characteristics of 250 cases. Neurologia Argentina. 2021;**13**:205-211. DOI: 10.1016/j.neuarg.2021.04.002

[32] Slavinsky PT, Cervio A, Sevlever G, Arakaki J, Antico J, Katz DA. Adenomas no funcionantes: análisis etrospectivo de 202 pacientes. Revista Argentina de Endocrinología y Metabolismo. 2018;**55**:80-87. Disponible en: https://www.scielo.org.ar/scielo.php?script=sci_arttext&pid=S1851-30342018000200011&lng=es

[33] Torregrosa-Quesada ME, García-Martínez A, Sánchez-Barbie A, Silva-Ortega S, Cámara R, Fajardo C, et al. The silent variants of pituitary tumors: Demographic, radiological and molecular characteristics. Journal of Endocrinological Investigation. 2021;**44**:1637-1648. DOI: 10.1007/s40618-020-01468-2

[34] Qin J, Li K, Wang X, Bao Y. A comparative study of functioning and non-functioning pituitary adenomas. Medicine. 2021;**100**:e25306. DOI: 10.1097/MD.0000000000025306

[35] Sarkar S, Chacko AG, Chacko G. Clinicopathological correlates of extrasellar growth patterns in pituitary adenomas. Journal of Clinical Neuroscience. 2015;**22**:1173-1177. DOI: 10.1016/j.jocn.2015.01.029

[36] Ramm-Pettersen J, Berg-Johnsen J, Hol PK, Roy S, Bollerslev J, Schreiner T, et al. Intra-operative MRI facilitates tumour resection during trans-sphenoidal surgery for pituitary adenomas. Acta Neurochirurgica. 2011;**153**:1367-1373. DOI: 10.1007/s00701-011-1004-7

[37] Mavromati M, Mavrakanas T, Jornayvaz FR, Schaller K, Fitsiori A, Vargas MI, et al. The impact of transsphenoidal surgery on pituitary function in patients with non-functioning macroadenomas. Endocrine. 2023;**81**:340-348. DOI: 10.1007/s12020-023-03400-z

[38] Raverot G, Burman P, McCormack A, Heaney A, Petersenn S, Popovic V, et al. European Society of Endocrinology Clinical Practice Guidelines for the management of aggressive pituitary tumours and carcinomas. European Journal of Endocrinology. 2018;**178**:G1-G24. DOI: 10.1530/EJE-17-0796

[39] Asa SL, Mete O, Perry A, Osamura RY. Overview of the 2022 WHO classification of pituitary tumors. Endocrine Pathology. 2022;**33**:6-26. DOI: 10.1007/s12022-022-09703-7

[40] Niveiro De Jaime M, Aranda-López FI, Peiró-Cabrera G. Pathology of

pituitary adenomas. Revista Española de Patología. 2003;**36**:357-372

[41] Pangal DJ, Wishart D, Shiroishi MS, Ruzevick J, Carmichael JD, Zada G. Growth hormone secreting pituitary adenomas show distinct extrasellar extension patterns compared to nonfunctional pituitary adenomas. Pituitary. 2022;**25**:480-485. DOI: 10.1007/s11102-022-01217-z

[42] Haddad AF, Young JS, Oh T, Pereira MP, Joshi RS, Pereira KM, et al. Clinical characteristics and outcomes of null-cell versus silent gonadotroph adenomas in a series of 1166 pituitary adenomas from a single institution. JNS. 2020;**48**:E13. DOI: 10.3171/2020.3.FOCUS20114

[43] Pérez-López C, Álvarez-Escolá C, Isla GA. Therapeutic approach to non-functioning pituitary adenomas. Medicina Clínica (Barcelona). 2021;**156**:284-289. DOI: 10.1016/j.medcli.2020.08.019

[44] Chapman PR, Singhal A, Gaddamanugu S, Prattipati V. Neuroimaging of the pituitary gland: Practical anatomy and pathology. Radiologic Clinics of North America. 2020;**58**:1115-1133. DOI: 10.1016/j.rcl.2020.07.009

[45] Pérez-López C, Palpán AJ, Saez-Alegre M, Zamarrón Á, Alfonso C, Álvarez-Escola C, et al. Volumetric study of nonfunctioning pituitary adenomas: Predictors of gross Total resection. World Neurosurgery. 2021;**147**:e206-e214. DOI: 10.1016/j.wneu.2020.12.020

[46] Micko AS, Wöhrer A, Wolfsberger S, Knosp E. Invasion of the cavernous sinus space in pituitary adenomas: Endoscopic verification and its correlation with an MRI-based classification. Journal of Neurosurgery. 2015;**122**:803-811. DOI: 10.3171/2014.12.JNS141083

[47] Raverot G, Dantony E, Beauvy J, Vasiljevic A, Mikolasek S, Borson-Chazot F, et al. Risk of recurrence in pituitary neuroendocrine tumors: A prospective study using a five-tiered classification. The Journal of Clinical Endocrinology and Metabolism. 2017;**102**:3368-3374. DOI: 10.1210/jc.2017-00773

[48] Carrillo-Najar C, Rembao-Bojórquez D, Tena-Suck ML, Zavala-Vega S, Gelista-Herrera N, Ramos-Peek MA, et al. Comparative proteomic study shows the expression of Hint-1 in pituitary adenomas. Diagnostics (Basel). 2021;**11**(2):330. DOI: 10.3390/diagnostics11020330

[49] Le Bras M, Leclerc H, Rousseau O, Goudet P, Cuny T, Castinetti F, et al. Pituitary adenoma in patients with multiple endocrine neoplasia type 1: A cohort study. European Journal of Endocrinology. 2021;**185**:863-873. DOI: 10.1530/EJE-21-0630

Chapter 5

Inflammation and Its Role in the Aetiopathogenesis of Malignant Brain Tumours

Tadej Strojnik

Abstract

The role of inflammation in the aetiopathogenesis of malignant brain tumours is increasingly recognised. Chronic inflammation, characterised by a sustained immune response and tissue remodelling, contributes to the development and progression of tumours. Activated microglia and infiltrating immune cells in the brain release proinflammatory cytokines and reactive oxygen species, creating a neuroinflammatory environment that promotes tumour growth. This persistent inflammation leads to DNA damage, mutations and epigenetic changes, thus favouring malignancy. Epidemiological studies have linked chronic inflammatory diseases and infections to an increased risk of brain tumours. Underlying mechanisms include activating signalling pathways such as nuclear factor kappa B (NF-κB) and signal transducer and activator of transcription 3 (STAT3), which promote cell proliferation and survival. In contrast, inflammatory mediators promote angiogenesis and evasion of the immune system. This text discusses the role of inflammatory markers and chronic bacterial and viral infections in developing brain tumours.

Keywords: chronic inflammation, malignant brain tumours, neuroinflammation, cytokines, NF-κB, STAT3, DNA damage, epigenetics, immune evasion, prognostic markers, therapeutic strategies

1. Introduction

Inflammation is a biological response to harmful stimuli such as pathogens, damaged cells or irritants involving immune cells, blood vessels and molecular mediators. It aims to eliminate the cause of the cell injury, remove necrotic cells and initiate tissue repair. Acute inflammation is short-lived and is characterised by redness, heat, swelling and pain. It focuses on removing the damaging substances and repairing the tissue. Chronic inflammation involves immune cells such as neutrophils, macrophages and lymphocytes and is regulated by chemical mediators such as cytokines and chemokines, causing prolonged tissue destruction and healing simultaneously.

Chronic inflammation has a significant influence on the development and progression of tumours. It produces reactive oxygen and nitrogen species that cause DNA damage and mutations, thus promoting cancer. Inflammatory cytokines such as interleukin 6 (IL-6) and tumour necrosis factor-alpha (TNF-α) activate signalling pathways such as nuclear factor kappa B (NF-κB) and signal transducer and activator of transcription 3 (STAT3), which promote tumour growth and survival. Chronic inflammation promotes angiogenesis through vascular endothelial growth factor (VEGF), supports tumour invasion and metastasis by altering the extracellular matrix and creates an immunosuppressive environment that helps the tumour evade the immune system [1].

Malignant brain tumours are aggressive neoplasms that arise in or around the brain, invade the surrounding tissue and disrupt brain function, leading to significant neurological deficits and a poor prognosis. They can be primary, that is originating in the brain (e.g. gliomas, medulloblastomas), or secondary, that is metastasising from other parts of the body. Glioblastoma, a common malignant brain tumour, has a poor prognosis with an average survival time of 15 to 18 months despite aggressive treatment. Genetic, molecular, environmental and epigenetic factors play a role in developing malignant brain tumours. The most critical genetic mutations include those in tumour suppressor genes such as TP53 and oncogenes such as the epidermal growth factor (EGFR), which lead to uncontrolled cell proliferation. Epigenetic modifications such as DNA methylation and histone modification also contribute to tumour development. There are dysregulated molecular signalling pathways such as the PI3K/AKT/mTOR signalling pathway, in which several essential proteins are involved: phosphoinositide 3-kinase (PI3K), which initiates the signalling process, AKT (protein kinase B), which promotes cell survival and growth, and mTOR (mammalian target of rapamycin), which controls cell growth and protein production to promote cell survival, growth and angiogenesis [2, 3]. The tumour microenvironment (TME), consisting of immune cells, fibroblasts, endothelial cells and extracellular matrix components, promotes tumour growth, angiogenesis and evasion of the immune system. Glioblastomas, for example, exhibit extensive angiogenesis driven by VEGF and immune evasion facilitated by immunosuppressive cells such as regulatory T cells (Tregs) and myeloid-derived suppressor cells (MDSCs) [4].

Molecular profiling techniques such as RNA sequencing and DNA methylation profiling have identified different molecular subtypes of gliomas, improving the classification and understanding of tumours. The 2021 WHO classification integrates molecular features with histopathological findings and classifies tumours into specific entities such as isocitrate dehydrogenase (IDH)-mutated astrocytomas and oligodendrogliomas with 1p/19q co-deletion [5].

Understanding the role of inflammation in cancer has led to research into anti-inflammatory drugs and targeted therapies to reduce cancer risk and disease progression. Non-steroidal anti-inflammatory drugs (NSAIDs) and cyclooxygenase (COX-2) inhibitors show potential, as do targeted therapies that focus on specific inflammatory pathways, such as TNF-α and IL-6 inhibitors. Immunotherapies, including dendritic cell vaccines and mRNA vaccines, are being investigated to enhance the immune response against tumours. Significant challenges include tumour heterogeneity, the blood-brain barrier, treatment resistance and the complexity of TME. Future research will focus on personalised medicine, the combination of therapeutic modalities, the improvement of drug delivery across the blood-brain barrier and the development of biomarkers for early detection and monitoring.

2. Chronic inflammation and malignant brain tumours

2.1 Definition and characteristics of chronic inflammation

Chronic inflammation is a long-lasting and persistent inflammatory reaction lasting months to years. It often occurs when the body is unable to eliminate the cause of an acute inflammation or due to an autoimmune reaction. In contrast to acute inflammation, a rapid and short-term response to an injury or infection, chronic inflammation involves a complex interaction of immune cells and a continuous production of inflammatory mediators. A characteristic of chronic inflammation is its long duration. In contrast to acute inflammation, which usually resolves within a few days or weeks, chronic inflammation can last indefinitely. This long duration leads to ongoing tissue damage and attempts at repair, which can result in significant tissue remodelling and fibrosis. The cellular composition of chronic inflammation differs from that of acute inflammation. In chronic inflammation, the infiltrate consists mainly of macrophages, lymphocytes and plasma cells, whereas in acute inflammation, neutrophils predominate. These immune cells maintain the inflammatory response and contribute to the pathology of chronic inflammation. The production of cytokines and chemokines is a driving force in chronic inflammation. Pro-inflammatory cytokines such as tumour necrosis factor-alpha (TNF-α), interleukin-1 beta (IL-1β) and IL-6 continuously produce and maintain the inflammatory state [6]. Together with chemokines, these cytokines attract and activate other immune cells, perpetuating the inflammatory cycle. Chronic centres of inflammation often exhibit angiogenesis and fibrosis. Angiogenesis, the formation of new blood vessels, responds to the need for increased blood supply to the inflamed tissue. At the same time, the deposition of extracellular matrix components leads to fibrosis, which further alters tissue structure and function. Finally, dysregulation of the immune system is a common feature of chronic inflammation. This dysregulation can manifest as autoimmunity, in which the immune system mistakenly attacks normal tissue or cannot clear infection or other inflammatory stimuli. This persistent immune activation contributes to the chronic nature of inflammation.

2.2 Mechanisms linking chronic inflammation to tumour development

Researchers increasingly recognise chronic inflammation as a critical factor in the development of brain tumours. It is involved in various mechanisms that contribute to tumour growth and progression, making it an essential area of investigation for developing therapies. One of the most critical mechanisms linking chronic inflammation to tumour development is the persistent activation of immune cells, particularly macrophages and microglia in the brain. When chronically activated, these cells produce a range of pro-inflammatory cytokines, chemokines and reactive oxygen species (ROS). These molecules can cause DNA damage in nearby cells, leading to mutations and genomic instability, which are crucial steps in transforming normal cells into malignant cells. Studies have shown that ROS and reactive nitrogen species (RNS) generated during chronic inflammation can directly damage DNA, proteins and lipids and thus promote carcinogenesis. In addition, chronic inflammation also promotes angiogenesis in brain tumours through the production of angiogenic factors such as vascular endothelial growth factor (VEGF) [7]. This neovascularisation supplies the tumour with nutrients and oxygen, facilitating its growth and survival. Another important mechanism is the alteration of signalling pathways that regulate cell proliferation, survival and apoptosis. Chronic inflammation often leads to continuous activation of signalling pathways such as NF-κB, STAT3 and COX-2. NF-κB, an essential regulator of immune response and inflammation, can promote gene expression in cell proliferation and survival [8]. Its sustained activation in inflamed tissues promotes tumour growth and resistance to apoptosis. Similarly, activating STAT3 by inflammatory cytokines such as IL-6 contributes to oncogenesis by promoting cell proliferation and inhibiting apoptosis [9]. The dual role of the immune system in inflammation and cancer also points to a paradox in which chronic inflammation can suppress the immune system. In the tumour microenvironment, chronic inflammation recruits and activates cells such as tumour-associated macrophages (TAMs) and myeloid-derived suppressor cells (MDSCs). These cells create an immunosuppressive environment that helps the tumour evade recognition and destruction by the immune system. This immunosuppression is facilitated by the production of anti-inflammatory cytokines such as IL-10 and transforming growth factor beta TGF-β, which inhibit the activity of cytotoxic T cells and natural killer (NK) cells, thereby protecting the tumour from the immune system [10]. Persistent inflammation can induce genetic and epigenetic changes in brain cells and thus contribute to transforming normal cells into malignant cells. TME in brain tumours is profoundly affected by chronic inflammation. In this inflammatory environment, the interaction between tumour cells, immune cells and stromal cells promotes tumour growth, invasion and resistance to therapy. Epigenetic changes caused by chronic inflammation represent another link between inflammation and tumour development. Inflammatory cytokines can induce changes in DNA methylation and histone modification, leading to altered gene expression in cell cycle regulation, apoptosis and DNA repair. These epigenetic changes can stabilise the malignant phenotype of cancer cells and contribute to their aggressive behaviour. In addition to these mechanisms, chronic inflammation can alter the extracellular matrix (ECM) and promote tumour invasion and metastasis. Inflammatory cells produce matrix metalloproteinases (MMPs) and cysteine proteases such as cathepsin B, which degrade the ECM and facilitate tumour cell migration and invasion. This remodelling of the ECM is crucial for cancer metastasis as it enables tumour cells to penetrate the surrounding tissue and enter the bloodstream [11]. The complex mechanisms linking chronic inflammation to tumourigenesis include persistent activation of immune cells, DNA damage, altered signalling pathways, promotion of angiogenesis, suppression of the immune system, epigenetic changes and remodelling of the ECM. Together, these processes create an environment favouring tumours' development, progression and metastasis. Understanding these mechanisms is crucial for developing targeted therapies that can modulate the inflammatory microenvironment and potentially inhibit tumour growth and progression.

3. The role of infectious agents

3.1 Bacterial infections and common bacteria associated with brain tumours

Research has recognised that bacterial infections, including brain inflammation, are crucial in CNS disorders. Although the blood-brain barrier protects the brain, some bacteria can break through this barrier and trigger severe inflammatory reactions. Bacterial meningitis, caused by *Neisseria meningitidis*, *Streptococcus pneumoniae* and *Haemophilus influenzae*, leads to acute inflammation of the meninges with symptoms such as increased intracranial pressure and neuronal damage. Another critical infection, brain abscess, involves bacteria such as *Streptococcus* and *Staphylococcus aureus*, which form localised collections of pus. Chronic infections, although less common, also affect the CNS. Neurosyphilis caused by *Treponema pallidum* and neuroborreliosis caused by *Borrelia burgdorferi* cause significant neurological symptoms. *Helicobacter pylori*, which is often associated with gastrointestinal diseases such as peptic ulcers and stomach cancer, is particularly frequently associated with neurological disorders. Some studies suggest a possible link between infection with *H. pylori* and some other bacteria, such as *Moraxella osloensis*, and neurodegenerative diseases, such as Alzheimer's and possibly cancer, due to chronic systemic inflammation and translocation of the bacteria to the brain [12, 13]. Chronic infections with bacteria such as *Mycobacterium tuberculosis* lead to tuberculous meningitis, associated with thickened meninges and cerebral infarcts. Bacterial infections contribute to brain inflammation through direct invasion, haematogenous spread and chronic systemic inflammation. The possible link between bacterial infections and cancer emphasises the importance of further research in this area.

3.1.1 Mechanisms of bacterial-induced inflammation

Bacterial inflammation involves complex mechanisms that trigger and maintain an inflammatory reaction. The immune system recognises invading bacteria with the help of pattern recognition receptors (PRRs) such as toll like receptors (TLRs) and NOD-like receptors (NLRs), which recognise pathogen-associated molecular patterns (PAMPs) such as lipopolysaccharides (LPS), peptidoglycans and flagellin [14]. This recognition activates intracellular signalling pathways, particularly the NF-κB pathway, leading to the production of pro-inflammatory cytokines and chemokines such as TNF-α, IL-1β and IL-6, which attract immune cells to the site of infection [8]. Bacteria also trigger inflammation by activating inflammasomes that recognise intracellular PAMPs and damage-associated molecular patterns (DAMPs). Inflammasomes such as NLRP3 activate caspase-1 and convert pro-IL-1β and pro-IL-18 into active forms, further promoting the recruitment and activation of immune cells. Indirectly, bacteria cause tissue damage and release DAMPs, which are recognised by PRRs and maintain inflammation. Bacterial toxins from *Staphylococcus aureus* and *Streptococcus pneumoniae* damage host cells and release DAMPs such as high mobility group box 1 (HMGB1) and heat shock proteins (HSPs) [15]. Bacterial infections also activate the complement system, which promotes the elimination of microbes and damaged cells. Complement fragments C3a and C5a increase the permeability of blood vessels and attract immune cells, which promotes inflammation. Activated immune cells produce reactive oxygen species (ROS) and reactive nitrogen species (RNS) during bacterial-induced inflammation. While these molecules are antimicrobial, their excessive production can damage cellular components, release more DAMPs and perpetuate inflammation [16]. Persistent bacterial infections can lead to chronic inflammation that contributes to diseases such as cancer. Persistent inflammation and resulting DNA damage in the epithelial cells of the stomach have been linked to gastric cancer due to chronic *Helicobacter pylori* infection. Bacterial-induced inflammation involves PRR recognition of bacterial components, activation of inflammatory pathways and inflammasomes, complement system involvement, and ROS and RNS production. These mechanisms initiate and maintain inflammation, which, if unresolved, can lead to chronic inflammation and associated diseases.

3.1.2 Case studies on the link between bacterial infections and brain tumours: exploring the role of the bacterial microbiome and the brain-gut connection

Epidemiological and clinical studies indicate a possible link between bacterial infections and brain tumours. *Propionibacterium acnes* has occasionally been found in certain gliomas and is associated with chronic inflammation and other cancers. *Borrelia burgdorferi*, the causative agent of Lyme disease, has been associated with CNS lymphomas, possibly due to chronic inflammation [17]. *Moraxella osloensis*, although less common, has been detected in brain infections and associated with gliomatosis cerebri, suggesting that chronic bacterial infections may contribute to brain tumours. These findings underscore the possible link between chronic bacterial infections and brain tumours and highlight the role of persistent inflammation in tumorigenesis. The brain-gut axis, a complex communication network between the gastrointestinal tract and the CNS, involves neuronal, hormonal and immunological pathways, with the gut microbiome playing a crucial role. The gut microbiome, made up of trillions of microorganisms, influences brain health *via* the vagus nerve and modulates the immune system, affecting systemic inflammation and brain health. Dysbiosis, an imbalance in the gut microbiome, can lead to systemic inflammation and promote the development of tumours. Certain gut bacteria influence response to chemotherapy and immunotherapy, with a diverse gut microbiome associated with better treatment outcomes. The gut microbiome also influences the blood-brain barrier (BBB). Some bacteria strengthen it, while dysbiosis weakens it, allowing harmful substances to enter the brain. Interventions that target the gut microbiome, such as probiotics, prebiotics and dietary changes, can complement the treatment of brain tumours by reducing inflammation, boosting immune function and improving the effectiveness of treatment [18, 19].

3.2 Viral infections and common viruses associated with brain tumours

3.2.1 Overview of oncogenic viruses and viral mechanisms of inducing inflammation and carcinogenesis

Several oncogenic viruses are associated with cancer by transforming normal cells into malignant ones through genetic integration, chronic inflammation and immune escape. The human papillomavirus (HPV), particularly high-risk types such as HPV-16 and HPV-18, is associated with cervical cancer, anogenital cancer and oropharyngeal cancer. HPV integrates its genome into the host's DNA and produces the oncoproteins E6 and E7 that disrupt tumour suppressor proteins p53 and pRb, leading to uncontrolled cell division and malignancy [20]. Epstein-Barr virus (EBV) is associated with cancers such as Burkitt's lymphoma, Hodgkin's lymphoma and nasopharyngeal carcinoma. EBV infects B cells and epithelial cells and causes lifelong latent infections. EBV proteins such as latent membrane protein 1 (LMP1) and EBV nuclear antigen 1 (EBNA1) drive oncogenesis by manipulating gene expression and immune response to promote cell proliferation and survival [21]. Hepatitis B (HBV) and hepatitis C viruses (HCV) contribute significantly to the development of liver cancer. HBV integrates its DNA into the host genome, disrupts cell function and promotes oncogenesis through the HBx protein. HCV causes chronic inflammation and oxidative stress, leading to liver damage and fibrosis, with its core protein modulating cellular signalling pathways involved in cancer [22, 23]. Human T-cell lymphotropic virus type 1 (HTLV-1) is associated with adult T-cell leukaemia/lymphoma (ATL). HTLV-1 integrates into host DNA and activates signalling pathways involving the Tax protein that promote cell proliferation and inhibit apoptosis, contributing to genetic instability [24]. Persistent viral infections cause genetic and epigenetic changes in host cells, contributing to carcinogenesis. For example, chronic EBV or HPV infection can lead to methylation of tumour suppressor gene promoters, resulting in gene silencing and uncontrolled cell growth. Oncogenic viruses cause cancer through direct genetic integration, chronic inflammation, modulation of host cell signalling, immune escape and genetic and epigenetic alterations.

3.2.2 Epidemiological studies on viruses in brain tumour patients

Epidemiological studies have increasingly investigated the possible links between viral infections and the development of brain tumours. These studies have provided valuable insights into how certain viruses may contribute to the development of brain tumours *via* mechanisms such as chronic inflammation, immunosuppression and direct genetic alterations of host cells. EBV is strongly associated with primary central nervous system lymphomas (PCNSL), especially in immunocompromised patients. Several studies have shown that EBV DNA is present in the tumour cells of PCNSL patients. EBV genomes are present in a significant proportion of PCNSL cases, particularly in patients with AIDS, suggesting that EBV may play a role in the development of these tumours by contributing to the oncogenic transformation of B cells in the brain [25]. HPV DNA has been found in glioma tissues in several epidemiological studies, suggesting a possible link. In addition, HPV DNA has been detected in a subset of glioblastoma samples, indicating that the virus may play a role in the development or progression of these aggressive brain tumours. Polyomaviruses have been associated with brain tumours, including the JC virus (JCV) and the BK virus (BKV). JCV, in particular, is associated with progressive multifocal leukoencephalopathy (PML) and has been detected in brain tumour tissue. In one study, the presence of JCV DNA was detected in a significant number of medulloblastomas and glioblastomas, suggesting that JCV may contribute to the development of these tumours through its ability to induce chromosomal instability and disrupt standard cell cycle control [26]. Cytomegalovirus (CMV) has been found in glioblastoma tissue, raising the question of its involvement in developing brain tumours and suggesting a possible link between CMV infection and the development of glioblastomas. Further research has confirmed these initial findings and indicated that CMV may contribute to the development of tumours by promoting inflammatory responses and influencing the tumour environment [27]. In another study, researchers demonstrated the presence of three herpes viruses: HSV-2, Epstein-Barr virus (EBV) and HHV-6 and a human enterovirus in glioma tissues. Interestingly, although the study detected the viruses in the tumour tissues, the patient's plasma showed no signs of viral infection. Five patients had small amounts of HSV-1 and HSV-2 immunoreactivity in their sera, even though these viruses could not be detected in their tumour tissue. The study concluded that common viruses such as HSV-1, HSV-2 and EBV are chronically present in the sera of patients with glioblastoma but not necessarily in the tumour tissue, suggesting a possible link between the chronic presence of viruses in the blood and the progression of glioma. The results were specific to glioblastoma multiforme and not to lower-grade gliomas [28]. Epidemiological evidence supports the possible involvement of various viruses in developing brain tumours.

4. Molecular and cellular signalling pathways

4.1 Inflammatory signalling pathways

4.1.1 NF-κB pathway in brain tumours

The NF-κB signalling pathway is crucial for regulating immune responses, inflammation, cell proliferation and survival. Its dysregulation is associated with various types of cancer, including brain tumours. In brain tumours, particularly gliomas, the NF-κB pathway promotes tumour growth, progression and resistance to therapy. The NF-κB family comprises five transcription factors: RelA (p65), RelB, c-Rel, NF-κB1 (p50/p105) and NF-κB2 (p52/p100). These factors form different dimers that regulate inflammation, immunity, cell proliferation and survival genes. Usually, the NF-κB dimers are kept inactive in the cytoplasm by inhibitor of nuclear factor kappa B (IκB) proteins [29]. When stimuli such as cytokines or stress signals activate it, the IκB proteins degrade, allowing NF-κB to enter the cell nucleus and regulate gene transcription. In gliomas, NF-κB is often constitutively active due to genetic alterations, cytokine production and ROS. Genetic mutations in the NF-κB signalling pathway's components or upstream signalling molecules such as EGFR lead to persistent activation [8]. Tumour and immune cells produce cytokines such as TNF-α and IL-1β, activating NF-κB. ROS from tumour and inflammatory cells also activate NF-κB by degrading IκB. NF-κB promotes the growth of brain tumours through several mechanisms. It regulates genes that drive cell cycle progression and inhibit apoptosis, promoting cell proliferation and survival. NF-κB also induces the expression of VEGF and thus promotes angiogenesis to supply the tumour with nutrients and oxygen. NF-κB modulates the immune response by inducing immunosuppressive cytokines and molecules such as PD-L1, contributing to immune defence. In addition, NF-κB activation increases the expression of matrix metalloproteinases (MMPs) and thus facilitates invasion and metastasis. Influencing the NF-κB signalling pathway offers therapeutic potential for brain tumours. Inhibitors of the IkappaB kinase (IKK) complex can prevent NF-κB activation, while antioxidants can reduce ROS levels and thus indirectly inhibit NF-κB. Cytokine inhibitors targeting TNF-α and IL-1β are also being researched. These strategies aim to reduce tumour growth and improve the effectiveness of treatments such as chemotherapy and radiotherapy [30].

4.1.2 JAK/STAT pathway in brain tumours

The Janus kinase/signal transducer and activator of the transcription (JAK/STAT) signalling pathway is essential for transmitting extracellular signals to the nucleus, leading to DNA transcription and cellular responses. This signalling pathway significantly influences cellular processes such as proliferation, differentiation and immune response. In brain tumours, particularly gliomas, dysregulation of the JAK/STAT signalling pathway contributes to tumour development and progression. The JAK/STAT signalling pathway is activated when cytokines and growth factors bind to their receptors and activate the JAKs. These JAKs phosphorylate STAT proteins, which then dimerize and translocate to the nucleus to regulate gene expression. IL-6 is an important cytokine in this process, binding to its receptor and triggering JAK activation and STAT3 phosphorylation. In gliomas, dysregulated JAK/STAT signalling, particularly involving STAT3, promotes cell proliferation and survival by upregulating genes such as c-Myc, cyclin D1, Bcl-2 and Bcl-xL [31]. This persistent activation leads to uncontrolled tumour growth and resistance to apoptosis. The pathway also mediates inflammation in the tumour microenvironment, with IL-6-induced STAT3 activation leading to cytokine production and chemokines that recruit immune cells to the tumour site [32]. This inflammatory environment can paradoxically promote tumour growth and suppress effective antitumour immunity. In addition, STAT3 activation promotes angiogenesis by upregulating VEGF, ensuring adequate blood supply for tumour growth. Furthermore, the JAK/STAT signalling pathway is crucial for maintaining glioma stem cells' stemness and self-renewal capacity (GSCs), which contribute to tumour development, maintenance and recurrence. Inhibition of STAT3 has been shown to reduce the stem cell properties of glioma stem cells, highlighting their role in tumour proliferation [33]. The potential of interfering with the JAK/STAT signalling pathway as a treatment for gliomas is promising. Several inhibitors targeting JAKs or STAT3 are currently under investigation in preclinical and clinical trials.

4.1.3 Role of cytokines and chemokines in brain tumours

Cytokines and chemokines are essential messengers of the immune system that influence immune reactions, inflammation and the progression of tumours. In brain tumours, particularly gliomas and glioblastomas, these molecules significantly influence the tumour microenvironment and contribute to growth, invasion, angiogenesis and immune evasion. Pro-inflammatory cytokines such as interleukin-6 (IL-6), tumour necrosis factor-alpha (TNF-α) and interleukin-1 beta (IL-1β) play a crucial role in brain tumours. IL-6 promotes tumour growth and survival by activating the JAK/STAT3 signalling pathway and maintaining glioma stem cells [9]. TNF-α activates the NF-κB signalling pathway and promotes cell proliferation, survival and invasion by upregulating matrix metalloproteinases (MMPs) [34]. IL-1β promotes angiogenesis, invasion and metastasis by inducing pro-angiogenic factors such as VEGF and MMPs, thus contributing to tumour aggressiveness. Anti-inflammatory cytokines such as interleukin-10 (IL-10) and transforming growth factor-beta (TGF-β) also impact brain tumours. IL-10 suppresses immune responses and promotes immune tolerance, contributing to immune evasion and a poor prognosis. TGF-β acts as an immunosuppressant in gliomas, inhibiting antitumour immune activity and promoting tumour invasion and angiogenesis [35]. Chemokines such as the CXCL12/CXCR4 axis, CCL2 (MCP-1) and CCL5 (RANTES) are crucial for the biology of brain tumours. The CXCL12/CXCR4 axis promotes angiogenesis and metastasis by recruiting endothelial progenitor cells and facilitating tumour cell colonisation [36]. CCL2 recruits tumour-associated macrophages (TAMs), which support tumour growth and suppress antitumour immunity. CCL5 attracts regulatory T cells (Tregs) and myeloid-derived suppressor cells (MDSCs), contributing to an immunosuppressive tumour environment and promoting tumour progression and resistance to therapy [37]. Cathepsins, particularly cathepsin B and cathepsin D, are lysosomal proteases involved in tumour progression, invasion and metastasis. Cathepsin B is overexpressed in gliomas, degrades the extracellular matrix and activates other proteases and signalling pathways that promote invasion and metastasis [38]. Cathepsin D promotes cell proliferation and resistance to apoptosis and correlates with aggressive tumour behaviour and resistance to therapy. Esterases, including acetylcholinesterase (AChE) and butyrylcholinesterase (BChE), modulate the tumour microenvironment and influence tumour growth, proliferation, migration and invasion. Due to the observed altered cholinesterase activity in gliomas, researchers are investigating the potential antitumour effects of cholinesterase inhibitors. Understanding the role of cytokines, chemokines, cathepsins and esterases in brain tumours provides valuable insights into potential therapeutic targets for treating these malignancies [39].

4.2 Cellular mechanisms

4.2.1 The role of microglia and macrophages in brain inflammation and tumour development

Microglia and macrophages are crucial in the brain's immune response, particularly in inflammation and tumour development. As integral components of the brain tumour microenvironment, they contribute significantly to tumour growth, progression and modulation of the immune response.

Microglia, the resident macrophages of the central nervous system (CNS), arise from yolk sac precursors during embryonic development and serve as the brain's primary immune cells. Microglia are activated in response to brain injury or infection and adopt a proinflammatory or anti-inflammatory phenotype. In their proinflammatory role, they produce cytokines such as TNF-α, IL-1β and IL-6 that contribute to the inflammatory environment in brain tumours and promote tumour cell proliferation and survival [40]. Alternatively, activated microglia (M2 phenotype) produce anti-inflammatory cytokines such as IL-10 and TGF-β that support tissue repair but can also promote tumour growth by suppressing antitumour immune responses and promoting angiogenesis. Microglia also promote tumour cell invasion and metastasis by producing matrix metalloproteinases (MMPs) that degrade the extracellular matrix (ECM), facilitating tumour cell migration. They also secrete growth factors such as VEGF that promote angiogenesis and ensure blood supply to the growing tumour. Tumour-associated microglia suppress the activation and function of T cells and other immune cells, helping brain tumours evade the immune system.

Macrophages in brain tumours include resident microglia and peripheral macrophages recruited from the bloodstream and often referred to as tumour-associated macrophages (TAMs) [41]. Chemokines such as monocyte chemoattractant protein-1 (CCL2 (MCP-1)) and stromal cell-derived factor 1 (CXCL12 (SDF-1)) recruit peripheral macrophages to the tumour [42]. Tumour and stromal cells produce these chemokines. Once in the tumour microenvironment, macrophages can transition to the M1 (proinflammatory) or M2 (anti-inflammatory) phenotype, with the M2 phenotype more commonly associated with tumour promotion. M1 macrophages have antitumor properties because they produce high proinflammatory cytokines and ROS that can kill tumour cells. However, immunosuppressive conditions often limit their presence in the tumour microenvironment. M2 macrophages support tumour growth by producing anti-inflammatory cytokines, promoting tissue remodelling and enhancing angiogenesis. They also secrete factors that inhibit the antitumour immune response, thus helping to evade the tumour's immune system. Macrophages interact with tumour and stromal cells to create a supportive microenvironment for growth and progression by secreting growth factors, cytokines and proteases that remodel the ECM and promote tumour cell invasion.

Microglia and macrophages play critical roles in brain inflammation and tumour development. Their dual function of promoting inflammation and suppressing immune responses makes them key components of the tumour microenvironment.

4.2.2 The importance of astrocytes and other glial cells in brain tumours

Astrocytes and other glial cells, such as oligodendrocytes and ependymal cells, play an essential role in maintaining the homeostasis of the brain. Reactive astrocytes promote tumour growth by secreting growth factors such as hepatocyte growth factor (HGF) and transforming growth factor-beta (TGF-β), thereby promoting the proliferation and survival of glioma cells in response to brain injury or disease [43]. They also alter the tumour microenvironment by releasing extracellular matrix components and cytokines that facilitate tumour invasion and angiogenesis, such as matrix metalloproteinases (MMPs), which degrade the extracellular matrix. In addition, astrocytes create an immunosuppressive environment by secreting anti-inflammatory cytokines such as IL-10 and TGF-β, which inhibit the activation and function of immune cells and help tumour cells evade immune recognition [44]. Astrocytes regulate extracellular glutamate levels *via* glutamate transporters. Dysregulation can lead to excitotoxicity, which damages both tumour and normal brain cells. Some studies suggest that astrocytes have a direct antitumour effect by producing molecules that induce apoptosis of tumour cells or inhibit their proliferation. For example, astrocytes produce Fas ligand (FasL), which can trigger apoptosis in Fas-expressing tumour cells [45]. Oligodendrocytes form and maintain myelin in the central nervous system. They can influence tumour progression and promote the invasion of tumour cells. Ependymal cells facilitate the spread of tumours through the cerebrospinal fluid and contribute to the spread of tumour cells to distant brain and spinal cord areas. Astrocytes and other glial cells play a multifaceted role in the biology of brain tumours. Astrocytes and other glial cells play a multifaceted role in the biology of brain tumours and influence tumour growth, invasion and immune system evasion through various mechanisms.

4.2.3 Tumour microenvironment and inflammation in brain tumours

The tumour microenvironment (TME) plays a crucial role in the development, progression and resistance to brain tumour therapy, especially in gliomas and glioblastomas. It consists of tumour cells, stromal and immune cells, components of the extracellular matrix (ECM) and signalling molecules such as cytokines and chemokines. Tumour cells interact with stromal cells (fibroblasts, endothelial cells, pericytes) and immune cells (macrophages, microglia, T cells, MDSCs) to modulate the TME and promote survival and proliferation. The ECM provides structural support and biochemical signals and facilitates tumour invasion and metastasis when remodelled. Inflammation, a hallmark of cancer, significantly affects the TME. Chronic inflammation within the TME promotes tumour development and progression through multiple mechanisms. Pro-inflammatory cytokines such as IL-6, TNF-α and IL-1β activate key signalling pathways (NF-κB and JAK/STAT) that promote tumour cell proliferation, survival and invasion. Chemokines such as CCL2 and CXCL12 recruit immune cells, including macrophages and lymphocytes, into the TME. Tumour-associated macrophages (TAMs) and microglia can adopt a tumour-promoting phenotype (M2) and secrete factors that promote tumour growth, angiogenesis and immune evasion [42]. Tumours also create an immunosuppressive microenvironment by recruiting regulatory T cells (Tregs) and MDSCs, supported by cytokines such as IL-10 and TGF-β [1]. Chronic inflammation produces angiogenic factors such as VEGF, which promote the formation of new blood vessels and supply the tumour with oxygen and nutrients. Inflammatory cells in the TME produce matrix metalloproteinases (MMPs) that degrade the ECM, promoting tumour invasion and metastasis while releasing growth factors that promote tumour progression [46]. Cathepsins, particularly cathepsin B and D, contribute significantly to TME by promoting tumour progression, invasion and metastasis. Cathepsin B is overexpressed in gliomas and promotes tumour invasion by degrading ECM components. Cathepsin D promotes cell proliferation and resistance to apoptosis, and its overexpression is associated with aggressive tumour behaviour and resistance to therapy. Influencing inflammation and proteolytic activity within the TME offers potential therapeutic strategies for treating brain tumours [47].

5. Blood markers for inflammation in brain tumours

5.1 Common inflammatory markers

Inflammatory markers in the blood reflect systemic inflammation and provide valuable information about tumours' presence, progression and disease course. One important marker is C-reactive protein (CRP), produced by the liver in response to cytokines such as IL-6. Elevated CRP levels are expected in patients with brain tumours and are associated with poor prognosis and aggressive disease [48, 49]. Interleukin-6 (IL-6) is another critical marker that tumour cells, microglia and astrocytes produce. Elevated IL-6 levels in glioma patients correlate with tumour progression and poor clinical outcomes, as IL-6 promotes cell proliferation and survival *via* the JAK/STAT3 signalling pathway [50]. Tumour necrosis factor-alpha (TNF-α) is a proinflammatory cytokine that regulates immune cells, inflammation and apoptosis. In brain tumours, TNF-α contributes to the inflammatory microenvironment and is associated with increased tumour aggressiveness and poor prognosis. It promotes tumour cell proliferation and invasion and their resistance to apoptosis *via* the NF-κB signalling pathway [51]. Interleukin-1 beta (IL-1β) is a proinflammatory cytokine that promotes angiogenesis, invasion and metastasis by inducing the expression of proangiogenic factors such as VEGF and MMPs. Glioma patients frequently exhibit elevated levels of IL-1β [52]. Fibrinogen is another marker, an acute-phase protein involved in coagulation and inflammation. High fibrinogen levels in glioma patients are associated with increased tumour burden, poor prognosis and shorter survival time. Fibrinogen promotes tumour growth by facilitating angiogenesis and metastasis [53]. Soluble intercellular adhesion molecule 1 (sICAM-1) plays a role in leukocyte adhesion and migration. Elevated sICAM-1 levels in glioma patients are associated with tumour growth and poor prognosis. sICAM-1 increases the invasive potential of tumour cells and facilitates metastasis by promoting cell-cell and cell-matrix interactions [54]. Erythrocyte sedimentation rate (ESR) is a nonspecific marker that measures the rate at which red blood cells sediment within 1 hour. Elevated ESR values indicate inflammation and correlate with increased tumour burden and poor prognosis in glioma patients [49]. Procalcitonin levels typically increase in response to bacterial infections, sepsis and various cancers, including brain tumours. This marker reflects systemic inflammatory reactions and possible paraneoplastic syndromes [48]. The neutrophil-lymphocyte ratio (NLR) indicates systemic inflammation and immune responses by calculating the blood's ratio of neutrophils to lymphocytes. Elevated NLR values are associated with poor prognosis in glioma patients and demonstrate an aggressive tumour phenotype and an immunosuppressive environment [55]. Overall, inflammatory markers such as CRP, IL-6, TNF-α, IL-1β, fibrinogen, sICAM-1, ESR, procalcitonin and NLR are critical for diagnosing, prognosis and monitoring brain tumours. Elevated levels of these markers reflect the systemic inflammatory response associated with tumour growth and provide insight into disease aggressiveness and patient outcomes.

6. Interaction between inflammation and genetic factors

6.1 Genetic predispositions affecting inflammation and tumour risk

Genetic predispositions significantly influence inflammation and the risk of developing brain tumours. Inherited genetic mutations and polymorphisms are associated with increased susceptibility to chronic inflammation and tumour development, particularly in gliomas and glioblastomas. These genetic factors affect tumour development and have prognostic significance, impacting patient outcomes and determining therapeutic strategies. Important genetic predispositions are as follows:

TP53 gene mutations: The TP53 gene encodes the tumour suppressor protein p53, which regulates the cell cycle and apoptosis. Mutations in TP53, which frequently occur in gliomas, impair the function of p53, which leads to uncontrolled cell proliferation and increased tumour susceptibility. These mutations are also associated with chronic inflammation, which promotes tumour development [56]. Prognostically, TP53 mutations are often associated with poorer outcomes as they can contribute to resistance to conventional therapies and more aggressive tumour behaviour.

PTEN gene mutations: The PTEN gene, a tumour suppressor, negatively regulates the phosphatidylinositol 3-kinase and Akt/protein kinase B (PI3K/AKT) signalling pathway, which is critical for cell growth and survival. PTEN mutations or deletions, frequently observed in glioblastomas, lead to hyperactivation of the PI3K/AKT signalling pathway and promote cell survival and proliferation. These mutations also increase inflammatory reactions in the tumour microenvironment [57]. Prognostically, loss of PTEN function is associated with a poorer prognosis as it promotes tumour growth and survival, leading to increased tumour aggressiveness and lower patient survival.

NF1 gene mutations: Neurofibromatosis type 1 (NF1), caused by mutations in the NF1 gene, encodes the tumour suppressor neurofibromin, which inhibits the rat sarcoma signalling (RAS) pathway. NF1 mutations lead to uncontrolled cell growth and an increased risk of glioma, particularly in individuals with neurofibromatosis type 1. These mutations are associated with increased inflammatory responses in the tumour microenvironment [58]. Prognostically, patients with NF1 mutations often have a higher risk of developing multiple tumours and may experience more rapid tumour progression.

IDH1/IDH2 mutations: Mutations in the isocitrate dehydrogenase genes IDH1 and IDH2 are common in low-grade gliomas and secondary glioblastomas. These mutations produce the oncometabolite 2-hydroxyglutarate (2-HG), which disrupts cellular metabolism and epigenetic regulation. IDH mutations are associated with a distinct metabolic and inflammatory tumour microenvironment that influences tumour behaviour and prognosis [59, 60]. Prognostically, IDH mutations are generally associated with a better outcome than wild-type IDH, as tumours with these mutations tend to be less aggressive and more responsive to treatment.

Genetic predispositions that modulate inflammation play an essential role in the prognosis of brain tumour patients. Mutations in tumour suppressor genes such as TP53, PTEN and NF1, not only influence the inflammatory milieu but also impact patients' clinical outcomes. TP53 and PTEN mutations, for example, are generally associated with more aggressive tumour behaviour and a poorer prognosis. IDH mutations often lead to better outcomes because they make these tumours less aggressive.

Understanding these genetic factors provides valuable insights into the mechanisms of tumour development and offers potential biomarkers for prognostic assessment.

6.2 Epigenetic changes due to chronic inflammation in brain tumours

Inflammation-related epigenetic changes can influence gene expression and thus contribute to tumour development, progression and resistance to therapy.

DNA methylation: Chronic inflammation often leads to hypermethylation of CpG islands in the promoter regions of tumour suppressor genes, silencing them. Hypermethylation of the O-6-methylguanine-DNA methyltransferase (MGMT) promoter in gliomas, particularly glioblastomas, is a critical epigenetic alteration that affects tumour sensitivity to alkylating chemotherapeutic agents such as temozolomide (TMZ). MGMT is a DNA repair enzyme that removes alkyl groups from guanine, protecting cells from the damaging effects of alkylating agents. The hypermethylation of the MGMT promoter silences the gene, leading to reduced production of the MGMT protein. As a result, the tumour cells can no longer effectively repair the DNA damage caused by chemotherapy, making them more susceptible to the cytotoxic effects of chemotherapy. Studies have shown that hypermethylation of the MGMT promoter is a favourable prognostic marker in glioma patients. Patients with hypermethylated MGMT promoters tend to have better clinical outcomes due to the higher efficacy of alkylating agents in these tumours [61]. More recent studies continue to investigate the role of MGMT methylation in optimising treatment strategies and understanding resistance mechanisms. Given the critical role of MGMT methylation in glioma prognosis and treatment response, various therapeutic approaches are being explored, such as combination therapies combining TMZ with DNA repair inhibitors (e.g. polyadenosine diphosphate ribose polymerase (PARP) inhibitors), which could enhance the cytotoxic effect of TMZ in MGMT-methylated tumours. Researchers are investigating drugs that can induce or stabilise MGMT promoter methylation to increase the proportion of tumour cells with silenced MGMT and sensitise them to alkylating agents. Hypermethylation of the MGMT promoter is an important prognostic marker and predictor of response to alkylating chemotherapy in gliomas. Conversely, chronic inflammation can lead to global DNA hypomethylation that activates transposable elements and oncogenes, further promoting tumour progression [62]. This process is associated with genomic instability and poorer clinical outcomes.

Mutations in isocitrate dehydrogenase (IDH) genes: Mutations in IDH genes are common in gliomas and result in 2-hydroxyglutarate (2-HG) production. This oncometabolite inhibits DNA demethylation enzymes and leads to widespread hypermethylation, impairing gene expression in cell differentiation and proliferation, and contributes to the glioma CpG island methylator phenotype (G-CIMP). IDH mutations are generally associated with a better prognosis than IDH wild-type, as they tend to be less aggressive and more responsive to treatment.

Histone modifications: Chronic inflammation affects histone acetylation and deacetylation, affecting chromatin structure and gene expression. Histone acetyltransferases (HATs) and histone deacetylases (HDACs) play a central role in this process. Inflammatory cytokines can modulate these enzymes, leading to either gene activation or suppression. Increased HDAC activity, often triggered by inflammatory signals, can suppress tumour suppressor genes and promote tumourigenesis [63, 64]. High HDAC activity is associated with a poorer prognosis due to increased tumour growth and resistance to apoptosis. Histone methylation, particularly at lysine residues, is another critical epigenetic change affected by chronic inflammation. Methylation of histone H3 at lysine 9 (H3K9me) and lysine 27 (H3K27me) is associated with transcriptional repression and is frequently observed in brain tumours. It contributes to silencing genes that control the cell cycle and apoptosis [65]. These changes are often associated with more aggressive tumours and poorer outcomes.

Non-coding RNAs: Chronic inflammation can alter the expression of microRNAs (miRNAs) and long non-coding RNAs (lncRNAs), which regulate gene expression post-transcriptionally. In gliomas, inflammation-induced dysregulation of miRNAs such as miR-21, miR-155 and miR-221/222 has been associated with tumour growth, invasion and resistance to therapy. These miRNAs can target tumour suppressor genes and pathways involved in apoptosis and cell cycle regulation, thereby promoting tumourigenesis [66]. Dysregulated miRNAs are often associated with poor prognosis as they promote malignancy and therapy resistance of tumours. LncRNAs such as HOTAIR and MALAT1 are upregulated in response to inflammatory signals in gliomas and contribute to tumour growth and metastasis by modulating chromatin structure and gene expression [67]. These lncRNAs are associated with a more aggressive tumour phenotype and poorer patient outcomes.

Chronic inflammation induces various epigenetic changes in brain tumours, including DNA methylation, histone modifications and dysregulation of non-coding RNAs. These changes are crucial in tumour development, progression and resistance to therapy.

7. Therapeutic implications

7.1 Anti-inflammatory treatments and their potential in brain tumours

Chronic inflammation significantly impacts the tumour microenvironment in brain tumours, especially gliomas and glioblastomas. Interfering with inflammatory processes is a promising strategy to inhibit tumour growth, reduce disease progression, and improve treatment outcomes.

Non-steroidal anti-inflammatory drugs (NSAIDs): NSAIDs inhibit cyclooxygenase (COX) enzymes, reducing the production of prostaglandins that mediate inflammation and pain. Overexpression of COX-2 is common in gliomas and is associated with a poor prognosis. Studies show that NSAIDs such as aspirin inhibit tumour cell proliferation and induce apoptosis in glioma cells, with long-term use of NSAIDs associated with a lower risk of glioblastoma [68].

Corticosteroids: Corticosteroids such as dexamethasone have a strong anti-inflammatory effect by suppressing cytokine production and inhibiting leukocyte infiltration into the tumour microenvironment. They often treat peritumoral oedema and alleviate symptoms in brain tumour patients. However, long-term use can lead to significant side effects such as immunosuppression and metabolic complications [1, 69].

Targeted anti-inflammatory therapies: IL-6 inhibitors such as tocilizumab target pro-inflammatory cytokines involved in glioma progression. On the other hand, TNF-α inhibitors have been shown to possibly induce GBM. NF-κB pathway inhibitors reduce inflammation and induce apoptosis in tumour cells, improving the treatment outcome in glioblastoma patients [70].

Immunomodulatory therapies: Immune checkpoint inhibitors such as pembrolizumab and nivolumab improve the immune system's ability to recognise and attack tumour cells. Researchers are investigating their effectiveness in combination with anti-inflammatory treatments. Toll-like receptor (TLR) agonists can modulate inflammation and activate immune responses against tumour cells, possibly complementing conventional therapies [71, 72].

Auranofin: A gold-containing compound traditionally used in the treatment of rheumatoid arthritis. Auranofin inhibits thioredoxin reductase, which leads to increased oxidative stress and apoptosis in cancer cells. It also exhibits anti-inflammatory properties by inhibiting NF-κB signalling. Studies show that auranofin increases the sensitivity of glioblastoma cells to radiotherapy and chemotherapy [73].

8. Current clinical trials and new therapies

In clinical trials, researchers investigate immunotherapy approaches such as chimeric antigen receptor T-cell (CAR-T) therapy and targeted therapies such as IDH and BRAF inhibitors such as vemurafenib and dabrafenib. Pembrolizumab, when used together with bevacizumab, has not been proven to improve survival rates in patients with glioblastoma.

Recent studies have investigated dual *CAR T-cell therapy* targeting EGFR and IL13Rα2 and showed a promising reduction in tumour size in glioblastoma with controllable neurotoxicity [74]. In another study, researchers combined CAR T cells with bispecific T cell engagers for glioblastoma and observed significant tumour shrinkage and controllable side effects [75].

Dendritic cell vaccines stimulate the immune system to recognise and attack tumour cells by presenting tumour-specific antigens. Clinical studies such as those on DCVax®-L and ICT-107 have extended progression-free and overall survival. Challenges include tumour heterogeneity and immune evasion, but personalised vaccines based on a patient's tumour profile are very promising [76].

Viral vectors: Viral vectors introduce therapeutic genes into tumour cells, induce cell death, enhance the immune response, or inhibit tumour growth. Oncolytic viruses such as DNX-2401 and gene therapies with vectors such as TOCA 511 and G47Δ have shown their potential in clinical trials. Future research aims to improve the specificity of vectors, overcome immune responses, and integrate these therapies into multimodal treatment strategies [77].

mRNA vaccines: mRNA vaccines, known for their success in preventing diseases such as COVID-19, are now being researched for treating cancer, including gliomas. These vaccines use mRNA to encode tumour-specific antigens and stimulate an immune response against the tumour cells. mRNA vaccines introduce synthetic mRNA encoding tumour-specific antigens into the body's cells. These cells produce the encoded proteins and present them on their surface with the help of molecules of the major histocompatibility complex (MHC). This presentation triggers an immune response that activates dendritic cells and cytotoxic T lymphocytes (CTLs) to attack and kill tumour cells expressing these antigens. In addition, mRNA vaccines promote the formation of memory T cells that provide long-term protection against tumour recurrence. They are naturally degraded in the body and can be produced quickly and flexibly, enabling the development of personalised vaccines based on the individual tumour profile. In addition, mRNA vaccines can trigger strong immune responses, which is crucial for targeting immunosuppressive tumours such as gliomas. Preclinical studies have shown the potential of mRNA vaccines for glioma treatment [78].

Anti-inflammatory treatments and new therapies, such as NSAIDs, targeted therapies, immunomodulatory treatments, and novel agents, can be combined with immunotherapies and personalised approaches to increase their effectiveness. The heterogeneity of brain tumours, the blood-brain barrier, resistance to therapy, and the complex tumour microenvironment pose a significant challenge. Future research will focus on personalised medicine, combination therapies, novel drug delivery systems, immunotherapy, epigenetic therapies, and the development of biomarkers. Understanding and targeting the tumour microenvironment will be crucial for developing effective treatments.

9. Conclusion

Inflammation plays a decisive role in the development and progression of brain tumours such as gliomas and glioblastomas. Chronic inflammation creates a tumour-friendly environment and offers therapeutic intervention opportunities. Anti-inflammatory treatments and targeted therapies have the potential to reduce tumour growth. Challenges include tumour heterogeneity and evasion of the immune system, but personalised vaccines based on a patient's tumour profile are promising. Biomarkers for inflammation in brain tumours can improve early diagnosis and treatment monitoring. Overcoming resistance mechanisms and influencing multiple signalling pathways involved in tumour growth should improve overall treatment outcomes. Novel delivery systems are crucial for improving the delivery of therapeutics across the blood-brain barrier. In addition, understanding the interactions within the tumour microenvironment is critical to disrupting the supportive niche that tumours rely on for growth and survival. Integrating personalised medicine, advanced immunotherapies such as dendritic cells and mRNA vaccines, and novel drug delivery systems promises to improve treatment efficacy and patient outcomes significantly.

Acknowledgements

I want to express my sincere gratitude to Prof. Tamara T. Lah from the National Institute of Biology in Ljubljana for our productive collaboration in brain tumour research over the years. I am also extremely thankful to my patients for their trust and inspiration and my family for their unwavering support and understanding.

Conflict of interest

The authors declare no conflict of interest.

Author details

Tadej Strojnik
Faculty of Medicine University of Maribor, Neurosurgical Institute Fram Slovenia, Alma Mater Europaea University Maribor Slovenia, Maribor, Slovenia

*Address all correspondence to: tadej.strojnik@almamater.si

References

[1] Zhao H, Wu L, Yan G, Chen Y, Zhou M, Wu Y, et al. Inflammation and tumor progression: Signaling pathways and targeted intervention. Signal Transduction and Targeted Therapy [Internet]. 2021;**6**(1):1-15. Available from: /pmc/articles/PMC8273155/

[2] Shin D, Cho KH. Critical transition and reversion of tumorigenesis. Experimental & Molecular Medicine [Internet]. 2023;**55**(4):692-705. Available from: https://www.nature.com/articles/s12276-023-00969-3

[3] Glaviano A, Foo ASC, Lam HY, Yap KCH, Jacot W, Jones RH, et al. PI3K/AKT/mTOR signaling transduction pathway and targeted therapies in cancer. Molecular Cancer [Internet]. 2023;**22**(1):1-37. DOI: 10.1186/s12943-023-01827-6

[4] Lin H, Liu C, Hu A, Zhang D, Yang H, Mao Y. Understanding the immunosuppressive microenvironment of glioma: Mechanistic insights and clinical perspectives. Journal of Hematology & Oncology [Internet]. 2024;**17**(1):31. Available from: /pmc/articles/PMC11077829/

[5] Antonelli M, Poliani PL. Adult type diffuse gliomas in the new 2021 WHO classification. Pathologica [Internet]. 2022;**114**(6):397. Available from: /pmc/articles/PMC9763975/

[6] Megha KB, Joseph X, Akhil V, Mohanan PV. Cascade of immune mechanism and consequences of inflammatory disorders. Phytomedicine [Internet]. 2021;**91**:153712. Available from: /pmc/articles/PMC8373857/

[7] Ohnishi S, Ma N, Thanan R, Pinlaor S, Hammam O, Murata M, et al. DNA damage in inflammation-related carcinogenesis and cancer stem cells. Oxidative Medicine and Cellular Longevity [Internet]. 2013;**2013**:3-6. Available from: /pmc/articles/PMC3870134/

[8] Liu T, Zhang L, Joo D, Sun SC. NF-κB signaling in inflammation. Signal Transduction and Targeted Therapy [Internet]. 2017;**2**(1):1-9. Available from: https://www.nature.com/articles/sigtrans201723

[9] Huang B, Lang X, Li X. The role of IL-6/JAK2/STAT3 signaling pathway in cancers. Frontiers in Oncology [Internet]. 2022;**12**:2-3. Available from: /pmc/articles/PMC9800921/

[10] Otegbeye F, Ojo E, Moreton S, Mackowski N, Lee DA, De Lima M, et al. Inhibiting TGF-beta signaling preserves the function of highly activated, in vitro expanded natural killer cells in AML and colon cancer models. PLoS One [Internet]. 2018;**13**(1):2-10. Available from: /pmc/articles/PMC5771627/

[11] Raskov H, Gaggar S, Tajik A, Orhan A, Gögenur I. The matrix reloaded—The role of the extracellular matrix in cancer. Cancers (Basel) [Internet]. 2023;**15**(7):2-16. Available from: /pmc/articles/PMC10093330/

[12] Gorlé N, Bauwens E, Haesebrouck F, Smet A, Vandenbroucke RE. *Helicobacter* and the potential role in neurological disorders: There is more than *Helicobacter pylori*. Frontiers in Immunology [Internet]. 2020;**11**:2-4. Available from: /pmc/articles/PMC7901999/

[13] Strojnik T, Kavalar R, Gornik-Kramberger K, Rupnik M, Robnik SL, Popovic M, et al. Latent brain infection

with Moraxella osloensis as a possible cause of cerebral gliomatosis type 2: A case report. World Journal of Clinical Oncology [Internet]. 2020;**11**(12):1064. Available from: /pmc/articles/PMC7769709/

[14] Li D, Wu M. Pattern recognition receptors in health and diseases. Signal Transduction and Targeted Therapy [Internet]. 2021;**6**(1):1-24. Available from: https://www.nature.com/articles/s41392-021-00687-0

[15] Cicchinelli S, Pignataro G, Gemma S, Piccioni A, Picozzi D, Ojetti V, et al. PAMPs and DAMPs in sepsis: A review of their molecular features and potential clinical implications. International Journal of Molecular Sciences [Internet]. 2024;**25**(2):19-30. Available from: /pmc/articles/PMC10815927/

[16] Lugrin J, Rosenblatt-Velin N, Parapanov R, Liaudet L. The role of oxidative stress during inflammatory processes. Biological Chemistry [Internet]. 2014;**395**(2):203-230. DOI: 10.1515/hsz-2013-0241/html

[17] Uldry PA, Regli F, Ferrazzini M. Primary lymphoma of the nervous system following radiculoneuritis caused by Borrelia burgdorferi: Study of a case. Schweizer Archiv für Neurologie und Psychiatrie (1985). 1988;**139**(1):31-38

[18] Lin B, Ye Z, Ye Z, Wang M, Cao Z, Gao R, et al. Gut microbiota in brain tumors: An emerging crucial player. CNS Neuroscience & Therapeutics [Internet]. 2023;**29**(Suppl. 1):84. Available from: /pmc/articles/PMC10314108/

[19] Parker A, Fonseca S, Carding SR. Gut microbes and metabolites as modulators of blood-brain barrier integrity and brain health. Gut Microbes [Internet]. 2020;**11**(2):135. Available from: /pmc/articles/PMC7053956/

[20] Yim EK, Park JS. The role of HPV E6 and E7 Oncoproteins in HPV-associated cervical carcinogenesis. Cancer Research and Treatment: Official Journal of Korean Cancer Association [Internet]. 2005;**37**(6):319. Available from: /pmc/articles/PMC2785934/

[21] Cao Y, Xie L, Shi F, Tang M, Li Y, Hu J, et al. Targeting the signaling in Epstein-Barr virus-associated diseases: Mechanism, regulation, and clinical study. Signal Transduction and Targeted Therapy [Internet]. 2021;**6**(1):1-33. Available from: https://www.nature.com/articles/s41392-020-00376-4

[22] Xu Q, Gu S, Liang J, Lin Z, Zheng S, Yan J. The biological function of hepatitis B virus X protein in hepatocellular carcinoma. Oncology Research [Internet]. 2019;**27**(4):509. Available from: /pmc/articles/PMC7848407/

[23] Mahmoudvand S, Shokri S, Taherkhani R, Farshadpour F. Hepatitis C virus core protein modulates several signaling pathways involved in hepatocellular carcinoma. World Journal of Gastroenterology [Internet]. 2019;**25**(1):42. Available from: /pmc/articles/PMC6328967/

[24] Mohanty S, Harhaj EW. Mechanisms of oncogenesis by HTLV-1 tax. Pathogens [Internet]. 2020;**9**(7):1-28. Available from: /pmc/articles/PMC7399876/

[25] Gandhi MK, Hoang T, Law SC, Brosda S, O'Rourke K, Tobin JWD, et al. EBV-associated primary CNS lymphoma occurring after immunosuppression is a distinct immunobiological entity. Blood [Internet]. 2021;**137**(11):1468. Available from: /pmc/articles/PMC7976507/

[26] Gunasegaran B, Ashley CL, Marsh-Wakefield F, Guillemin GJ, Heng B. Viruses in glioblastoma: An update on

evidence and clinical trials. BJC Reports [Internet]. 2024;**2**(1):1-21. Available from: https://www.nature.com/articles/s44276-024-00051-z

[27] Yang T, Liu D, Fang S, Ma W, Wang Y. Cytomegalovirus and glioblastoma: A review of the biological associations and therapeutic strategies. Journal of Clinical Medicine [Internet]. 2022;**11**(17):5221. Available from: /pmc/articles/PMC9457369/

[28] Strojnik T, Duh D, Lah TT. Prevalence of neurotropic viruses in malignant glioma and their Onco-modulatory potential. In Vivo (Brooklyn) [Internet]. 2017;**31**(2):221. Available from: /pmc/articles/PMC5411749/

[29] Oeckinghaus A, Ghosh S. The NF-κB family of transcription factors and its regulation. Cold Spring Harbor Perspectives in Biology [Internet]. 2009;**1**(4):2-5. Available from: /pmc/articles/PMC2773619/

[30] Guo Q, Jin Y, Chen X, Ye X, Shen X, Lin M, et al. NF-κB in biology and targeted therapy: New insights and translational implications. Signal Transduction and Targeted Therapy [Internet]. 2024;**9**(1):1-37. Available from: https://www.nature.com/articles/s41392-024-01757-9

[31] Ou A, Ott M, Fang D, Heimberger AB. The role and therapeutic targeting of JAK/STAT signaling in glioblastoma. Cancers [Internet]. 2021;**13**(3):437. Available from: https://www.mdpi.com/2072-6694/13/3/437/htm

[32] Johnson DE, O'Keefe RA, Grandis JR. Targeting the IL-6/JAK/STAT3 signalling axis in cancer. Nature Reviews Clinical Oncology [Internet]. 2018;**15**(4):234. Available from: /pmc/articles/PMC5858971/

[33] Jin J, Grigore F, Chen CC, Li M. Self-renewal signaling pathways and differentiation therapies of glioblastoma stem cells (review). International Journal of Oncology [Internet]. 2021;**59**(1):1-11. Available from: http://www.spandidos-publications.com/10.3892/ijo.2021.5225/abstract

[34] Tang D, Tao D, Fang Y, Deng C, Xu Q, Zhou J. TNF-alpha promotes invasion and metastasis via NF-kappa B pathway in oral squamous cell carcinoma. Medical Science Monitor Basic Research [Internet]. 2017;**23**:141. Available from: /pmc/articles/PMC5391804/

[35] Komai T, Inoue M, Okamura T, Morita K, Iwasaki Y, Sumitomo S, et al. Transforming growth factor-β and interleukin-10 synergistically regulate humoral immunity via modulating metabolic signals. Frontiers in Immunology [Internet]. 2018;**9**(JUN):14. Available from: /pmc/articles/PMC6010538/

[36] Strazza M, Mor A. Consider the chemokines: A review of the interplay between chemokines and T cell subset function. Discovery Medicine [Internet]. 2017;**24**(130):31. Available from: /pmc/articles/PMC8266128/

[37] Kumar V, Patel S, Tcyganov E, Gabrilovich DI. The nature of myeloid-derived suppressor cells in the tumor microenvironment. Trends in Immunology [Internet]. 2016;**37**(3):208. Available from: /pmc/articles/PMC4775398/

[38] Strojnik T, Zajc I, Bervar A, Židanik B, Golouh R, Kos J, et al. Cathepsin B and its inhibitor stefin a in brain tumors. Pflügers Archiv. 2000;**439**(7):122-123

[39] Naro GR, Noverati N, Craig T. The role of C1-esterase inhibitors in the

management of vasogenic edema in glioblastoma. Case Reports in Medicine [Internet]. 2020;**2020**:1-4. Available from: https://pubmed.ncbi.nlm.nih.gov/32082381/

[40] Cole AP, Hoffmeyer E, Chetty SL, Cruz-Cruz J, Hamrick F, Youssef O, et al. Microglia in the brain tumor microenvironment. Advances in Experimental Medicine and Biology [Internet]. 2020;**1273**:197-208. Available from: https://pubmed.ncbi.nlm.nih.gov/33119883/

[41] Guadagno E, Presta I, Maisano D, Donato A, Pirrone CK, Cardillo G, et al. Role of macrophages in brain tumor growth and progression. International Journal of Molecular Sciences [Internet]. 2018;**19**(4):4-9. Available from: /pmc/articles/PMC5979398/

[42] Deshmane SL, Kremlev S, Amini S, Sawaya BE. Monocyte chemoattractant protein-1 (MCP-1): An overview. Journal of Interferon & Cytokine Research [Internet]. 2009;**29**(6):313. Available from: /pmc/articles/PMC2755091/

[43] Luo J. TGF-β as a key modulator of astrocyte reactivity: Disease relevance and therapeutic implications. Biomedicine [Internet]. 2022;**10**(5):1-9. Available from: /pmc/articles/PMC9138510/

[44] Norden DM, Fenn AM, Dugan A, Godbout JP. TGFβ produced by IL-10 redirected astrocytes attenuates microglial activation. Glia. 2014;**62**(6):881-895

[45] Gratas C, Tohma Y, Van Meir EG, Klein M, Tenan M, Ishii N, et al. Fas ligand expression in glioblastoma cell lines and primary astrocytic brain tumors. Brain Pathology [Internet]. 1997;**7**(3):863. Available from: /pmc/articles/PMC8098208/

[46] Niland S, Riscanevo AX, Eble JA. Matrix metalloproteinases shape the tumor microenvironment in cancer progression. International Journal of Molecular Sciences [Internet]. 2022;**23**(1):1-8. Available from: /pmc/articles/PMC8745566/

[47] Rudzińska M, Parodi A, Soond SM, Vinarov AZ, Korolev DO, Morozov AO, et al. The role of cysteine cathepsins in cancer progression and drug resistance. International Journal of Molecular Sciences. 2019;**20**(14):3602 [Internet]. Available from: https://www.mdpi.com/1422-0067/20/14/3602/htm

[48] Dharmajaya R, Sari DK. Role and value of inflammatory markers in brain tumors: A case controlled study. Annals of Medicine and Surgery [Internet]. 2021;**63**:102107. Available from: /pmc/articles/PMC7890138/

[49] Strojnik T, Smigoc T, Lah TT. Prognostic value of erythrocyte sedimentation rate and C-reactive protein in the blood of patients with glioma. Anticancer Research. 2014;**34**(1):339-347

[50] Singh M, Raghav A, Gautam KA. Role of the circulatory interleukin-6 in the pathogenesis of gliomas: A systematic review. World Journal of Methodology [Internet]. 2022;**12**(5):428. Available from: /pmc/articles/PMC9516551/

[51] Wang QW, Lin WW, Zhu YJ. Comprehensive analysis of a TNF family based-signature in diffuse gliomas with regard to prognosis and immune significance. Cell Communication and Signaling: CCS [Internet]. 2022;**20**(1):10-13. Available from: /pmc/articles/PMC8744324/

[52] Fathima Hurmath K, Ramaswamy P, Nandakumar DN.

IL-1β microenvironment promotes proliferation, migration, and invasion of human glioma cells. Cell Biology International [Internet]. 2014;**38**(12):1415-1422. DOI: 10.1002/cbin.10353

[53] Wang PF, Meng Z, Song HW, Yao K, Duan ZJ, Li SW, et al. Higher plasma fibrinogen levels are associated with malignant phenotype and worse survival in patients with glioblastomas. Journal of Cancer [Internet]. 2018;**9**(11):2024 Available from: /pmc/articles/PMC5995933/

[54] Yoo KC, Kang JH, Choi MY, Suh Y, Zhao Y, Kim MJ, et al. Soluble ICAM-1 a pivotal communicator between tumors and macrophages, promotes mesenchymal shift of glioblastoma. Advanced Science [Internet]. 2022;**9**(2):2102768. DOI: 10.1002/advs.202102768

[55] Ma L, Li G, Wei M. Neutrophil-to-lymphocyte ratio and its changes are related to grade II–IV glioma recurrence. Cancer Management and Research [Internet]. 2020;**12**:9429. Available from: /pmc/articles/PMC7533248/

[56] Kandoth C, McLellan MD, Vandin F, Ye K, Niu B, Lu C, et al. Mutational landscape and significance across 12 major cancer types. Nature. 2013;**502**(7471):333-339 [Internet]. Available from: https://www.nature.com/articles/nature12634

[57] Sansal I, Sellers WR. The biology and clinical relevance of the PTEN tumor suppressor pathway. Journal of Clinical Oncology [Internet]. 2004;**22**(14):2954-2963. Available from: https://pubmed.ncbi.nlm.nih.gov/15254063/

[58] Gutmann DH, Ferner RE, Listernick RH, Korf BR, Wolters PL, Johnson KJ. Neurofibromatosis type 1. Nature Reviews. Disease Primers [Internet]. 2017;**3**:17004. Available from: https://pubmed.ncbi.nlm.nih.gov/28230061/

[59] Turcan S, Rohle D, Goenka A, Walsh LA, Fang F, Yilmaz E, et al. IDH1 mutation is sufficient to establish the glioma hypermethylator phenotype. Nature [Internet]. 2012;**483**(7390):479-483. Available from: https://pubmed.ncbi.nlm.nih.gov/22343889/

[60] Yan H, Parsons DW, Jin G, McLendon R, Rasheed BA, Yuan W, et al. IDH1 and IDH2 mutations in gliomas. New England Journal of Medicine [Internet]. 2009;**360**(8):765-773. DOI: 10.1056/NEJMoa0808710

[61] Hegi ME, Diserens AC, Gorlia T, Hamou MF, de Tribolet N, Weller M, et al. MGMT gene silencing and benefit from temozolomide in glioblastoma. The New England Journal of Medicine [Internet]. 2005;**352**(10):997-1003. Available from: https://pubmed.ncbi.nlm.nih.gov/15758010/

[62] Ehrlich M. DNA hypomethylation in cancer cells. Epigenomics [Internet]. 2009;**1**(2):239. Available from: /pmc/articles/PMC2873040/

[63] Lu C, Ward PS, Kapoor GS, Rohle D, Turcan S, Abdel-Wahab O, et al. IDH mutation impairs histone demethylation and results in a block to cell differentiation. Nature [Internet]. 2012;**483**(7390):474-478. Available from: https://www.nature.com/articles/nature10860

[64] Barneda-Zahonero B, Parra M. Histone deacetylases and cancer. Molecular Oncology [Internet]. 2012;**6**(6):579-589. Available from: https://pubmed.ncbi.nlm.nih.gov/22963873/

[65] Cheng Y, He C, Wang M, Ma X, Mo F, Yang S, et al. Targeting epigenetic regulators for cancer therapy: Mechanisms and advances in clinical trials. Signal Transduction and Targeted Therapy [Internet]. 2019;**4**(1):1-39. Available from: https://www.nature.com/articles/s41392-019-0095-0

[66] Banelli B, Forlani A, Allemanni G, Morabito A, Pistillo MP, Romani M. MicroRNA in glioblastoma: An overview. International Journal of Genomics [Internet]. 2017;**2017**(1):7639084. DOI: 10.1155/2017/7639084

[67] Arun G, Aggarwal D, Spector DL. MALAT1 long non-coding RNA: Functional implications. Noncoding RNA [Internet]. 2020;**6**(2):1-7. Available from: /pmc/articles/PMC7344863/

[68] Chang CY, Pan PH, Li JR, Ou YC, Der WJ, Liao SL, et al. Aspirin induced glioma apoptosis through Noxa upregulation. International Journal of Molecular Sciences [Internet]. 2020;**21**(12):1-15. Available from: /pmc/articles/PMC7352791/

[69] Afshari AR, Sanati M, Aminyavari S, Shakeri F, Bibak B, Keshavarzi Z, et al. Advantages and drawbacks of dexamethasone in glioblastoma multiforme. Critical Reviews in Oncology/Hematology. 2022;**172**: 103625

[70] Kraemer LS, Humes RJ, Syed AS, Tritsch AM. A rare but morbid occurrence: Development of glioblastoma multiforme during tumor necrosis factor inhibitor therapy. Cureus [Internet]. 2022;**14**(5):1-3. Available from: /pmc/articles/PMC9199570/

[71] Ser MH, Webb MJ, Sener U, Campian JL. Immune checkpoint inhibitors and glioblastoma: A review on current state and future directions. Journal of Immunotherapy and Precision Oncology [Internet]. 2024;**7**(2):97-110. DOI: 10.36401/JIPO-23-34

[72] Nayak L, Molinaro AM, Peters K, Clarke JL, Jordan JT, de Groot J, et al. Randomized phase II and biomarker study of Pembrolizumab plus bevacizumab versus Pembrolizumab alone for patients with recurrent glioblastoma. Clinical Cancer Research [Internet]. 2021;**27**(4):1048-1057. Available from: https://pubmed.ncbi.nlm.nih.gov/33199490/

[73] Haas B, Schütte L, Wos-Maganga M, Weickhardt S, Timmer M, Eckstein N. Thioredoxin confers intrinsic resistance to cytostatic drugs in human glioma cells. International Journal of Molecular Sciences [Internet]. 2018;**19**(10):6-8. Available from: /pmc/articles/PMC6212897/

[74] Bagley SJ, Logun M, Fraietta JA, Wang X, Desai AS, Bagley LJ, et al. Intrathecal bivalent CAR T cells targeting EGFR and IL13Rα2 in recurrent glioblastoma: Phase 1 trial interim results. Nature Medicine [Internet]. 2024;**30**(5):1320-1329. Available from: https://pubmed.ncbi.nlm.nih.gov/38480922/

[75] Choi BD, Gerstner ER, Frigault MJ, Leick MB, Mount CW, Balaj L, et al. Intraventricular CARv3-TEAM-E T cells in recurrent glioblastoma. The New England Journal of Medicine [Internet]. 2024;**390**(14):1290-1298. Available from: https://pubmed.ncbi.nlm.nih.gov/38477966/

[76] Gatto L, Di Nunno V, Tosoni A, Bartolini S, Ranieri L, Franceschi E. DCVax-L vaccination in patients with glioblastoma: Real promise or negative trial? The debate is open. Cancers (Basel) [Internet]. 2023;**15**(12):4-6. Available from: /pmc/articles/PMC10296384/

[77] Asija S, Chatterjee A, Goda JS, Yadav S, Chekuri G, Purwar R. Oncolytic immunovirotherapy for high-grade gliomas: A novel and an evolving therapeutic option. Frontiers in Immunology [Internet]. 2023;**14**:5-7. Available from: /pmc/articles/PMC10050572/

[78] Mendez-Gomez HR, DeVries A, Castillo P, von Roemeling C, Qdaisat S, Stover BD, et al. RNA aggregates harness the danger response for potent cancer immunotherapy. Cell [Internet]. 2024;**187**(10):2521-2535.e21. Available from: https://pubmed.ncbi.nlm.nih.gov/38697107/

Chapter 6

Mid-Intensity 30.5 GHz Continuous Wave Exposure of Glioblastoma Organoids

Cristiano Palego, Christopher Hancock, Elena Rampazzo, Luca Persano, Arianna Casciati, Mirella Tanori, Mariateresa Mancuso and Caterina Merla

Abstract

In this chapter, we delve into the therapeutic potential of 30.5 GHz millimeter waves on 3D glioblastoma organoids. We specifically investigated mild thermal radiation effects in the context of new emerging focused energy delivery and bio-electromagnetic approaches. Our in-house developed exposure system, coupled with a rigorous dosimetry protocol and extensive multi-physics modeling, supported biological endpoint evaluation in terms of transcriptional profiling, cell morphological changes, and cell phenotypic characterization. Crucially, the induced thermal effect was minimal, aligning closely with our simulation models and indicating the precise control of energy delivery. Notably, a 0.1 W power level enhanced the efficacy of Temozolomide, significantly increasing cell apoptosis while not affecting the differentiation status of glioblastoma organoid cells. This combination suggests a new avenue for glioblastoma treatment, leveraging millimeter wave-induced mechanisms that warrant further investigation. Our findings underscore the promise of this minimally invasive technique, offering a glimpse into future glioblastoma therapies.

Keywords: continuous waves, dosimetry, energy delivery, glioblastoma organoids, millimeter waves, thermal effect, transcriptomics

1. Introduction

Glioblastoma multiforme (GBM) remains one of the most aggressive and treatment-resistant forms of brain cancer, with a median survival time of 15 months [1]. Significant breakthroughs in GBM treatment have remained elusive since establishment of the current standard line of treatment – which includes surgery, radiation therapy, and chemotherapy – two decades ago [2].

To overcome these challenges, innovative, energy-based treatment modalities are being explored as alternatives or complements to traditional interventions.

IntechOpen

These emerging approaches, including focused ultrasound (FUS), tumor-treating fields (TTFs), high-frequency irreversible electroporation (H-FIRE), and microwave or millimeter wave-induced hyperthermia, leverage electromagnetic and electromechanical mechanisms to target tumor cells with precision and minimal invasiveness.

Focused ultrasound (FUS) energy delivery can be guided through intraoperative MRI and is being explored as a non-invasive method to manage blood-brain barrier opening (BBBO) and enhance the delivery and effectiveness of chemotherapeutic agents [3]. FUS BBBO also disrupts the immunosuppressive glioblastoma microenvironment, potentially aiding in tumor cell detection and initiating an antitumor immune response [4]. Sonodynamic therapy [5] is undergoing a phase 1 clinical trial [6] and uses FUS to make 5-aminolevulinic acid (5-ALA) – a drug designed for visualizing tumors during surgery which is safe for normal brain tissue – cytotoxic to GBM cells in multiple areas of the brain. Histotripsy, a form of cavitation that allows fast mechanical ablation with high-energy ultra-short ultrasound pulses, has shown potential in preclinical models [7].

Tumor-treating fields (TTFs) employ low-intensity, intermediate-frequency alternating electric fields to obstruct mitosis selectively in cancer cells [8]. These fields disrupt spindle formation and chromosome segregation for rapidly dividing tumor cells while largely sparing normal tissues. This non-invasive technique has shown promise in clinical trials [9] for newly diagnosed and recurrent glioblastoma, offering a unique mechanism of action that complements traditional therapies.

Other EM approaches aim at cell microenvironment modulation while avoiding direct thermal loading [10–15]. Recent advancements in the use of Pulsed Electric Fields (PEF) for treating brain cancer have focused on their impact on brain cells, including both healthy and cancerous cells. High-Frequency Irreversible Electroporation (H-FIRE), a novel approach employing bipolar electric pulses, has emerged as a promising method for inducing tissue necrosis and cell death while minimizing side effects typically associated with monopolar pulses, such as neuronal stimulation and muscle contraction [10]. The goal is to optimize treatment parameters, particularly for brain tumors like GBM, by achieving effective cell ablation without damaging surrounding healthy tissues.

Research has demonstrated that GBM cells respond to irreversible electroporation or to H-FIRE when exposed to electric fields that exceed a tissue-specific lethal threshold, leading to cell death. This method offers several benefits, including the absence of cytotoxic effects, precise targeting of tumor tissues, a non-thermal ablation mechanism, and preservation of nerves and major blood vessels [11]. Preclinical studies have confirmed the safety and efficacy of these techniques for treating GBM [12]. Interestingly, primary brain tumors containing glioma stem-like cells (GSC) show higher sensitivity to H-FIRE than normal astrocytes, highlighting a potential therapeutic opportunity. However, neuronal stem cells (NSC) exhibit similar sensitivity to these electric pulses, emphasizing the need for personalized cell-specific characterization in clinical applications [13].

H-FIRE has also shown promise as both a monotherapy and in combination with other treatments for malignant glioma. Studies in orthotopic rat models have demonstrated statistically significant improvements in overall survival and increased immune response markers in treated groups compared to controls. Moreover, H-FIRE at appropriate doses can cause a transient disruption of the BBB, lasting up to 72 hours post-treatment, which may enhance the efficacy of chemotherapy by allowing better drug penetration into the brain [14].

The ability of H-FIRE to selectively ablate cancer stem cells and potentially transform the tumor microenvironment from immunosuppressive to antitumor through Damage Associated Molecular Pattern (DAMP) signaling is particularly exciting. This capability suggests that H-FIRE could be fine-tuned to improve patient outcomes, particularly for those with primary brain tumors, by prolonging overall survival through the targeted destruction of cancer stem cells [15].

While non-thermal EM approaches such as TTFs and H-FIRE offer promising avenues for glioblastoma treatment, other methods intentionally seek to induce thermal stress to achieve therapeutic effects. Among these, microwave ablation has been less researched for brain tumors compared to FUS. This is due to its poorer resolution and the risk of generating heat that can harm surrounding healthy brain tissue, potentially leading to neurological deficits. However, achieving efficient ablation without causing skull heating for off-centre targets remains a challenge even for minimally invasive FUS energy delivery. This issue persists even with hyperthermia [3], where the targeted temperature rise (T_{MAX} = 40–45°C) is lower than for ablation (T_{MAX} > 56°C). Despite these challenges, hyperthermia is a compelling approach due to its role as a potent radio-sensitizer, showing potential to improve treatment outcomes and reduce radiation toxicity. Studies have demonstrated that hyperthermia prior to radiotherapy impairs DNA repair, inhibits survival pathway activation, and reduces glioma stem cell proliferation both *in vitro* and *in vivo* [16, 17].

In this context, exploring mild hyperthermia ($\Delta T \sim 10°C$, $T_{MAX} < 35°C$) through millimeter wave (MMW) stimulation is promising. MMW energy delivery is becoming more technologically appealing due to the proliferation of 5G/6G communications and the increasing availability of components. It considerably increases lateral spatial resolution in available electrosurgery tools (e.g. 14.5 GHz [18]) while enabling signal depth of penetration over several cell layers. Additionally, MMW stimulation can potentially elicit or couple with non-thermal dynamics, including absorption dynamics, protein vibration, resonance, unfolding, and hydration [19]. Like other methods that disrupt the tumor microenvironment and generate reactive oxygen species from sono- or radio-sensitizers, MMW may offer a unique interaction mechanism and complement other therapeutical approaches. MMW can be delivered to brain tumor by endoscopy yielding limited invasiveness and a focused treatment as required in this terrible pathology [20].

Our study specifically investigates the potential of combining mild temperature increases with chemotherapy, using mid-intensity (P < 5 W) MMW radiation at 30.5 GHz on glioblastoma organoids. These 3D structures, derived from primary patient GBM cells, mimic real tumors' complexity and cellular heterogeneity, reflecting individual tumor variability. We aim to (1) identify the threshold input power density causing stress or modifications in organoids; (2) assess the effects of MMW signals within the mid-thermal regime; and (3) explore non-thermal effects in this frequency range. This comprehensive approach successfully highlights cell and molecular responses in a relevant 3D glioblastoma model, advancing the potential of 30.5 GHz MMW as a novel coadjutant treatment option.

2. Materials and methods

2.1 30.5 GHz source development

Creo-Medical, UK developed the 30.5 GHz generator in **Figure 1** for the present organoid work and potentially supporting future *in vivo* MMW stimulation

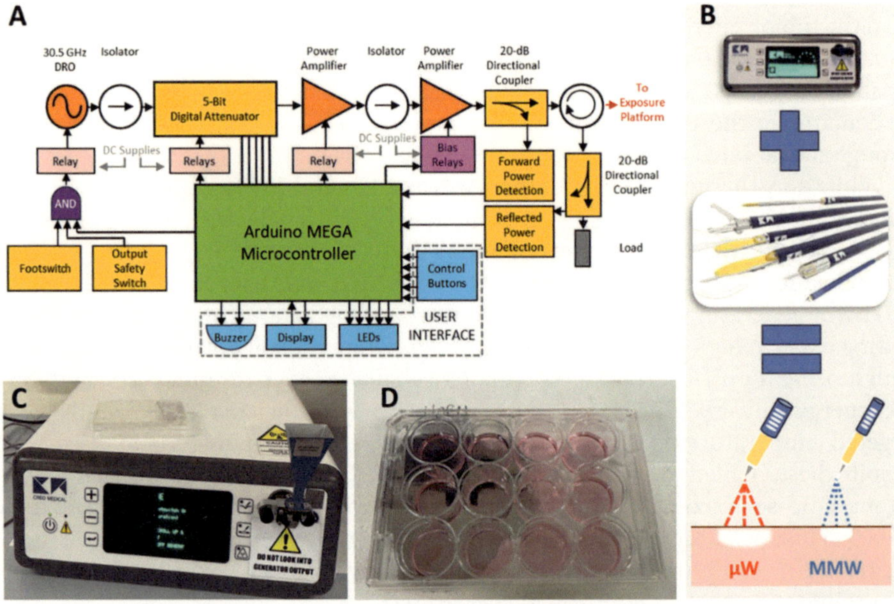

Figure 1.
(A): The 30.5 GHz CW source and control unit developed by Creo Medical to support organoid irradiation in this work and (B): Future minimally invasive MMW procedures with enhanced lateral resolution than in current microwave range settings. (C): Closeup view of experimental setup with Ka-band horn antenna and (D) the single-well container that hosts organoids at its centre and in placed in direct contact of the antenna.

applications. This advanced continuous wave (CW) source comprises a complete millimeter wave line-up including a mechanically tunable dielectric resonator oscillator (DRO-3404, 30–31 GHz, POUT~11.5 dBm), a pre-amplifier (ERZ-HPA-2000-400-24, Gain = 20 dB), and a Power Amplifier (Qorvo's TGA2595-CP). The signal is amplified from the initial 11.5 dBm to an expected 22 dBm after the pre-amplifier, and finally to 36.5 dBm (4.5 W) at the Power Amplifier output.

To ensure system integrity and performance, isolators were added to prevent reflected power from damaging sensitive components such as the oscillator and pre-amplifier. Thermal management is achieved by assembling the pre-amplification line-up onto an aluminum plate, which secures each component and acts as a heatsink.

Onboard power supplies and regulation enable the system to operate with only an external mains AC connection (85–250 V), while handling power delivery to each component. The onboard controller automatically sets power supplies and bias conditions for active components. Integrated power detectors support monitoring of forward and reflected power levels, allowing output control via a digital attenuator. Therefore, MMW power attenuation and waveform duration can be entirely managed by the user through an intuitive microcontroller-digital display interface based on an Arduino MEGA, ensuring precise experiment execution and reproducibility.

Housed in its own enclosure, the generator connects to the exposure platform – a Ka-band (26.5–40 GHz) Pasternack PE9850/2F-20 horn antenna – via a quick-release waveguide (WG22). The 30.5 GHz source's power capacity ensures the delivery of sufficient energy at the exposure platform, with its flexible timing control allowing for varied delivery formats in a range of bioelectric experiments.

Two formats were selected for organoid exposure: CW1 (0.1 W Root Mean Square for 20 minutes) and CW2 (0.2 W RMS for 10 minutes). This aimed at comparing different MMW exposure conditions while maintaining the same E = 120 J delivered energy. Sham groups were included in the experiments and were exposed in the same setup with no MMW power being delivered.

2.2 Optimization of MMW setup for organoid irradiation

2.2.1 Numerical modeling/optimization approach and optimized setup

The optimal exposure setup for millimeter wave (MMW) radiation stimulation of glioblastoma organoids was determined through a judicious combination of numerical dosimetry and experimental thermal probing [20]. The key criteria guiding the optimization process were: (1) Impedance matching: quantified by the reflection coefficient (S_{11} scattering parameter), with values at or below −10 dB indicating suitable power transfer; (2) Specific Absorption Rate (SAR) homogeneity: measured by the coefficient of variation (CV), which is the ratio of the standard deviation of the SAR to its mean value over a chosen volume.

Parametric full-wave simulations were conducted using CST Microwave Studio to model the electromagnetic (EM) and thermal behavior of the setup. Organoids were modeled as dielectric cylinders with a diameter of 2 mm, a height of 0.7 mm, and centres spacing of 5 mm, reflecting experimental conditions. We used complex permittivity values similar to gray matter (ε' = 20, tgδ = 0.3, [21]) with a slightly different (lower) conductivity. This is justified by the fact that organoid tissue is evidently different from the brain due to the lack of additional heterogeneous cell types and their growth within a culture media that is quite different from the Cerebrospinal Fluid in its composition. The optimized configuration [20] is shown in **Figure 2**. Using a single 22 mm diameter well in a 12 multi-well plate provided the best balance between transferring MMW power to the samples and minimizing variations in energy absorption across the sample for the well placed in direct contact with the horn antenna. The optimal height of the culture medium in the well was determined to be 3 mm.

2.2.2 Organoid number, impedance matching and SAR inhomogeneity

Millimeter wave (MMW) power transfer is governed by impedance matching between the antenna's output and the sample setup. This involves matching the fundamental Transverse Electric (TE10) mode, launched by the WG22 rectangular waveguide through the horn antenna's flare, with the dielectric properties of the holder/culture/organoid stack. The culture medium, forming the bulk of the sample volume, largely determines the S_{11} response with organoid presence and number exerting a secondary influence.

The number of irradiated organoids n was two, with a spacing of by 5 mm when placed in the holder centre, thus balancing the need for multiple samples with the challenges of culturing a larger number. Critically, the analysis summarized in **Figure 2**, shows that adding up to n = 10 organoids increases their fractional volume (F) to no more than 2%. Therefore, a dielectric mixture model was used to predict the corresponding reflection coefficient degradation would be bound to 0.1 dB, confirming their negligible mismatching impact.

However, **Figure 2** also suggests that even this modest effect can cause large variations in energy absorption by different parts of the sample, resulting in SAR

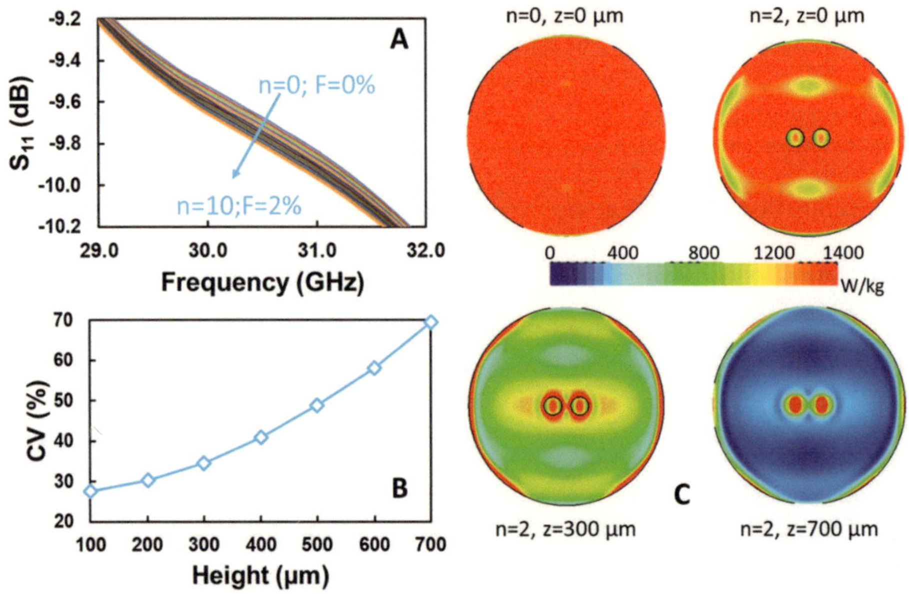

Figure 2.
(A): Ka-bad impedance matching response considering dependence from organoid number and fractional volume (B): SAR coefficient of variation for organoid slices at different heights along vertical z-axis. (C): Comparison of SAR distribution for the unloaded medium, and for the medium with two GBM organoids, again at different sampled z heights as from the parametric analysis in Ref. [20].

inhomogeneity. Indeed, the presence of organoids significantly affects the SAR distribution, with substantial variations in homogeneity observed along the height (z-axis) of the organoid due to abrupt changes in electrical properties at the boundaries between the organoids, the culture medium, and the container. The "meniscus effect" [20] also impacts SAR homogeneity and impedance matching. The curved liquid surface at the well edges increases interface curvature and reduces central medium height, leading to greater organoid fractional volume, thus exacerbating both SAR CV and reflection coefficient degradation.

2.2.3 Thermal modeling and experimental validation

Coupled EM/thermal simulations predicted the temporal evolution of temperature distribution within the sample holder and the organoids. SAR levels in the organoids were evaluated slice by slice at 100 μm intervals. SAR values were averaged over 1 mm^3 cubes to match the sensing volume of thermal probes employed for experiments. These were conducted using a fiber optic probe (Lumasense, US) with two sensors 5 mm apart, complemented by thermo-camera imaging for broader area coverage and hotspot characterization.

The SAR(T) dependence was derived by fitting measured temperature curves to the standard bio-heat transfer model for three different power levels and a short (2 s) CW power on-time, which minimizes convective and radiative transfer. This relationship was then extrapolated to longer exposure times and lower power levels, supporting SAR extraction in CW1 and CW2 measurement conditions, both in unloaded media and media containing organoids. To validate our simulation approach, measured and simulated temperature and SAR values without organoids were compared. Measurements and simulations were scaled to a common reference power of 0.5 W, revealing only a 10% deviation between predicted and observed values, which fell within the range of measurement standard deviation.

Measured temperature increases (4.5°C for CW1, 7.2°C for CW2) closely matched simulated values (4.4°C and 8.8°C respectively), with thermo-camera results (3.8°C and 9.5°C) providing further confirmation [20]. The higher temperature increase despite shorter exposure time in CW2 suggests that the achieved temperature increase depends more on maximum power (or energy rate) than on exposure time or total delivered energy.

This validated method allowed for fine-tuning of the experimental setup, optimizing parameters such as holder type, holder-antenna distance, and medium height. The final optimized single-well setup, as described in Section 2.1.1 (**Figure 2**), features a 3 mm medium height in direct contact with the antenna. Furthermore, this approach enabled parametric studies of coefficient of variation (CV) in organoid slices, including centre versus edge effects. The overall procedure was ultimately validated by comparing measured temperature increases (using two independent measurement approaches) with simulated values.

2.2.4 Further optimization results

The validated modeling procedure yielded the results in **Figure 2** along with a detailed parametric analysis of the exposure setup [20]. We observed the highest absorbance at organoid centres, gradually decreasing towards the edges. Nevertheless, the SAR coefficient of variation (CV) increased with z peaking at the surface due to dielectric discontinuity at the organoid/medium interface. Interestingly, the SAR pattern with organoids at one height may more closely resemble the distribution without organoids at a different height. This highlights how organoids alter the overall SAR distribution in the well. Along with the previous observation on CV's height dependence, this outlines the complexity of propagation and absorption homogeneity in the investigated multiple medium setting.

This setup provides a foundation for consistent and well-controlled exposure of organoids, supporting future MMW radiation studies. While the impedance matching and SAR CV were fully characterized for the tested two-organoid scenario, this approach can be readily extended to any number of organoids.

2.3 Biological methods

2.3.1 GBM organoid generation and treatment

The primary GBM culture employed within this study was obtained after written informed consent for the donation of tumor tissues under the auspices of the protocol for the acquisition of human brain tissues obtained from the Ethical Committee of the Padova University-Hospital. Cells were isolated from tumor biopsies taken at surgery according to previously reported protocols [22, 23] and cultured in DMEM-F12 supplemented with 10% BIT9500 (StemCell Technologies Inc., Vancouver, Canada), 20 ng/ml basic Fibroblast Growth Factor (bFGF) and 20 ng/ml Epidermal Growth Factor (EGF; both from Cell Guidance Systems Ltd., Cambridge, UK) in an atmosphere of 2% oxygen, 5% carbon dioxide and balanced nitrogen in a H35 hypoxic cabinet (Don Whitley Scientific Ltd., Shipley, UK) [24].

Organoids were established by embedding 100.000 primary cells (or 1 mm^3-sized tumor fragments) in 10 µl Matrigel® (Corning®, Corning, NY) droplets to be polymerized in a standard 37°C incubator. Then freshly generated organoids were cultured in the above-described media in normoxic conditions (21% oxygen) until 21 days before being exposed to specific CW protocols. GBM organoids were routinely monitored for their growth and half-medium changed at least twice a week to ensure their proper growth. After CW exposure, GBM organoids were cultured for additional 24 hours for obtaining transcriptional data, for 72 hours for histological purposes, or treated with 500 µM Temozolomide (Selleck Chemicals, Houston, TX) for 5 days before being analyzed for any induction of cell death.

2.3.2 Transcriptional and histological analyses

Transcriptional data of control and CW-exposed organoids were obtained from at least two different organoids/experimental replicate after 24 hours from treatment. In particular, after proper extraction (miRNeasy Kit, Qiagen, Hilden, Germany), total RNAs were hybridized to Gene Chip™ WT Clariom™ S arrays (Affymetrix, Santa Clara, CA) according to manufacturer's instructions and analyzed as described by using default Affymetrix microarray analysis parameters and normalized by Repeated Measure Analysis (RMA) [20]. Differentially expressed genes between CW-exposed and control organoids were identified using Limma (FDR < 0.05 and fold change ≥2).

For histology, control and treated organoids were fixed for 30 minutes in 4% formaldehyde in PBS, washed, and impregnated in 30% sucrose for at least 20 hours before being embedded in Tissue-Tek® OCT Compound (Sakura Finetek USA, Inc., Torrance, CA) and cryosectioned to obtain 10 µm thick slides. Hematoxylin and eosin staining was performed according to standard procedures. For immunofluorescence, organoid slides were blocked in 5% BSA (Sigma-Aldrich, St. Louis, MO), 1% goat serum (Vector Laboratories, Newark, CA) PBS solution, and then stained with primary antibodies: Hif-1α (Sigma-Aldrich, Saint Louis, MO) Nestin (Merck, Darmstadt, Germany), βIII-tubulin (Covance Laboratories Inc. Princeton, NJ), S100, Ki67 and GFAP (all from Agilent Dako from Agilent Technologies, Santa Clara, CA); Cleaved Caspase 3 (Cell Signaling Technology, Danvers, MA).

After incubation with the most appropriate Alexa-dye conjugated secondary antibodies (Thermo Fisher Scientific, Waltham, MA), slides were counterstained with DAPI (Sigma-Aldrich, Saint Louis, MO). For both histology and immunofluorescence, images were collected with a Zeiss Axio Imager M1 epifluorescence microscope (Zeiss, Oberkochen, Germany). Images were analyzed and cellular nuclei were counted by the Analyze plugin of ImageJ (https://imagej.nih.gov). Graphs were generated by GraphPad Prism 8.0.1 software (GraphPad, La Jolla, CA) and data analyzed with the included statistical tools. Bar graphs display data arranged as mean ± standard error of the mean (SEM).

3. Results

3.1 Present organoids model of GBM with respect to clinical approaches

Glioblastoma multiforme (GBM) is one of the most aggressive and lethal forms of brain cancer, with limited treatment options and a very poor prognosis, as stated in the Introduction. The development of organoid models for GBM has been a significant advancement in the field of cancer research, particularly in studying the disease's biology, drug response, and potential treatment strategies. Here's where current GBM organoid models stand with respect to clinical approaches for: (1) modeling tumor heterogeneity, (2) acting as drug screening tool or support to therapy development, (3) studying tumor microenvironment interactions.

3.1.1 Modeling tumor heterogeneity

For the first point, GBM organoids are excellent at recapitulating the heterogeneity of GBM tumors, including the presence of different cell types, genetic mutations, and microenvironmental features that are critical to the disease. This heterogeneity is often missed in traditional 2D cell cultures but is essential for understanding the complexity of GBM.

This aspect is crucial for the development of personalized medicine, where treatments can be tailored to the specific characteristics of a patient's tumor. The ability to model the patient's tumor may more accurately help in predicting responses to therapies and in the identification of new therapeutic targets.

3.1.2 Acting as drug screening tool

For the second aspect, GBM organoids offer a platform for high-throughput drug screening, allowing researchers to test a wide range of compounds in a setting that closely mimics the tumor environment. This can lead to the identification of novel drugs or drug combinations that may be effective against GBM. Although still mostly in preclinical stages, this approach has the potential to streamline the drug development process, bringing new therapies to clinical trials faster. Organoids could also help in the development of individualized treatment regimens, potentially improving outcomes by selecting the most effective drugs for each patient.

3.1.3 Studying tumor microenvironment interactions

Finally, for the third point, GBM organoids can be co-cultured with other cell types, such as immune cells or cells of the blood-brain barrier, allowing for a more comprehensive study of the tumor microenvironment. This is particularly important in GBM, where interactions between the tumor and its surrounding environment play a crucial role in disease progression and treatment resistance. Insights gained from these studies can inform the development of therapies that target not just the tumor cells but also the supportive microenvironment, potentially overcoming resistance mechanisms and leading to more effective treatments.

3.1.4 Current clinical integration

Glioblastoma multiforme (GBM) organoids are a significant improvement over traditional models, and they are still complex and labour-intensive to produce and maintain. Additionally, there can be variability in organoid formation, which might affect the reproducibility of results. Despite their potential, the translation of findings from GBM organoid models to clinical practice is still in its early stages. While organoids provide a more realistic model for studying GBM, clinical trials are needed to validate findings and determine the actual therapeutic benefit in patients. However, there is growing interest in integrating organoid models into clinical workflows, especially for personalized medicine approaches. For example, organoids derived from a patient's tumor could be used to test drug responses *ex vivo* before administering treatments *in vivo*, as proposed in our study.

3.2 Proximity of organoid to *in vivo* model

3.2.1 GBM organoids well resemble human tumor structure and phenotype

In order to obtain more reliable *in vitro* models of GBM, able to better resemble the morphological and phenotypic characteristics GBM tumors *in vivo*, we exploited the availability of fresh GBM specimens and further processed them, eventually generating GBM organoids to be subjected to the above selected therapeutic frequencies. To this end, we adapted to our purposes the already available protocols for the generation of cerebral and brain tumor organoids [25, 26], allowing the reproducible generation of the GBM organoid models described within this section. In particular, after surgical removal of the tumor, GBM biopsies were mechanically and enzymatically dissociated as previously described [22] to obtain either small sized tumor fragments ($\leq 1\ mm^3$) or single cell suspensions (**Figure 3A**, panel (i)).

Then, 100.000 GBM cells (or one fragment) were dissolved into 10 μl of Matrigel and plated onto sterile parafilm molds to allow their polymerization as small droplets/domes (**Figure 3A**, panel (ii)). After polymerization, these "organoid precursors" were transferred in the culturing media and allowed to grow until being processed for histology and immunofluorescence analyses (**Figure 3A**, panel (iii)). GBM organoids progressively acquired an increasingly compact morphology, thus achieving their "mature" structure after 20–30 days in culture, eventually resembling the histology of the patient tumor biopsy they were derived from (**Figure 3B** and **C**). Accordingly, tumor fragments-generated GBM organoids displayed a similar behavior, with cancer cells progressively invading the polymerized structure and finally acquiring the same rounded organoid shape and histology, although in a greater timeframe (**Figure 3D**).

We previously demonstrated that within the GBM mass, phenotypically defined cancer cells are spatially distributed along at least three different layers including a tumor core characterized by necrosis and prominent hypoxia, which hosts the most immature and stem-like cell subpopulations, a peripheral layer composed of more differentiated cells (even characterized by a mixed glial-neuronal lineage) and a transition layer between them, characterized by highly proliferating cancer cells [24, 27, 28]. Nevertheless, we should not forget the possible presence of an additional more peripheral layer in which cancer cells invade the normal brain parenchyma, easily recognizable through 5-ALA administration [29]. Interestingly, after 30 days of growth, GBM organoids display a regular rounded shape with a low cellularized core surrounded by a thick and denser organoid margin (**Figure 3B**), well resembling human GBM tumors at MRI.

Phenotypically, GBM organoids are characterized by a heterogenic distribution of different cell phenotypes including: a widespread high expression of the neural stem cell marker Nestin, a higher stabilization of the Hif-1α protein in the inner portions of the organoid [24], a prominent presence of GFAP expressing cells in which are homogeneously distributed cancer cells displaying a mixed neuronal phenotype (e.g. also

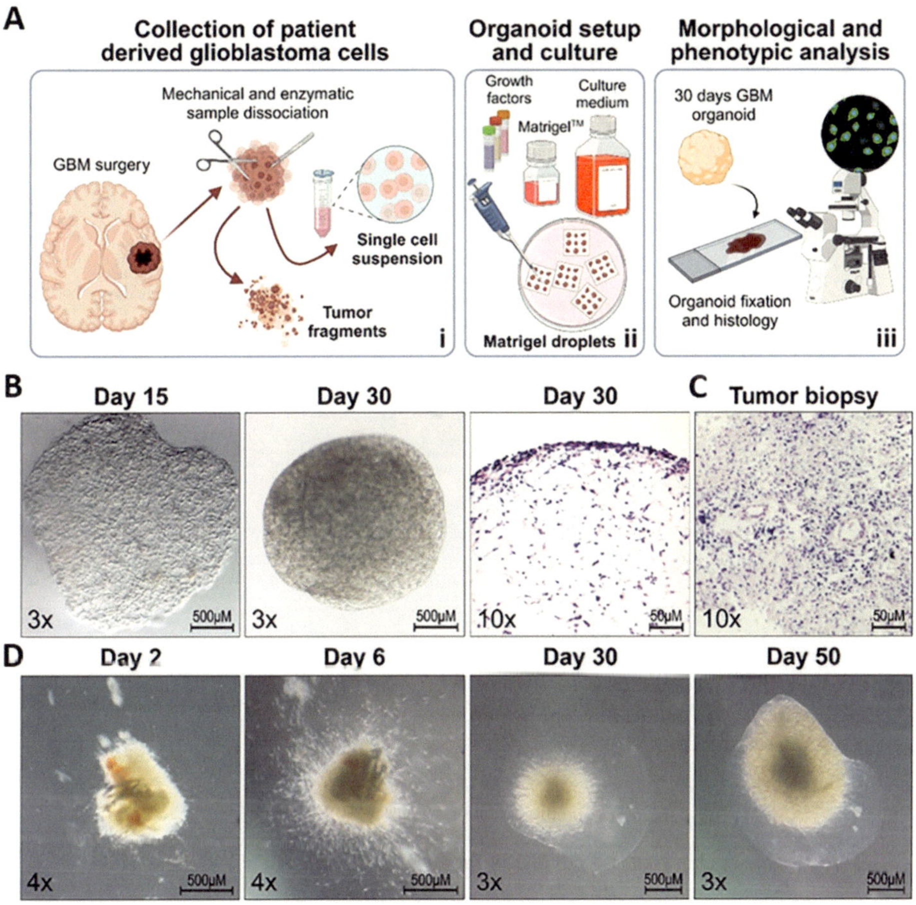

Figure 3.
GBM organoid generation and growth. (A): Cartoon summarizing the process of GBM organoid generation and phenotypic characterization, including (i) the collection of human GBM samples from patients and their initial gross processing as minced tissue fragments (diameter ≤ 1 mm) and single-cell suspensions; (ii) GBM organoid preparation and culture by inclusion of cells (10–200 × 10^3) or fragments into Matrigel® droplets and their subsequent long-term culture in the appropriate supplemented media; (iii) GBM organoid fixation, cryosectioning, and histological and immunophenotypic evaluation. Panel (A) was created with Biorender.com. (B, C): Representative stereotactic images of GBM organoids during time (day 15–30, (B) left panels) and their histological (hematoxylin and eosin staining) characterization (day 30, (B) right panel) and comparison with the original tumor tissue GBM cells were derived from (C). (D): Representative stereotactic images of tumor fragments-derived GBM organoid growth during time (day 2–50).

expressing βIII-tubulin), and a relatively low proliferation index (Ki67$^+$ cells), more compatible with the proliferation rate of GBM cells within human tumors (**Figure 4**).

3.2.2 30.5 GHz CW treatment affects GBM cell survival and sensitize organoids to TMZ chemotherapy

To test *in vitro* the therapeutic efficacy of the simulated CW exposures, a series of 21 days grown organoids were exposed to either CW1 and CW2 treatment protocols or maintained in control conditions before being analyzed in terms of transcriptional modulations, histology, and cell death. In particular, after 72 h from treatment,

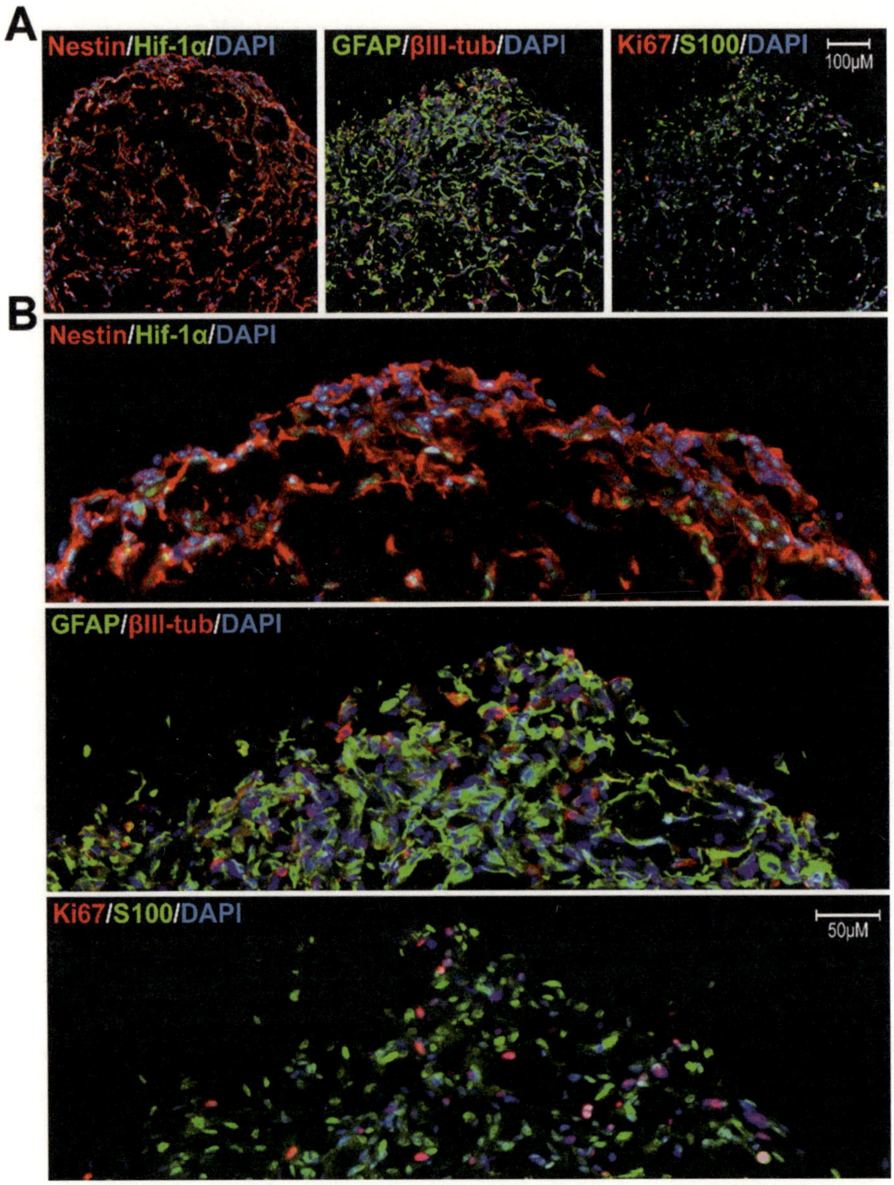

Figure 4.
Phenotypic characterization of GBM organoids. Representative immunofluorescence images (A, original magnification 10x) and their relative magnification (B) showing the spatial expression of a series of GBM phenotypic and proliferation markers, including Nestin (red) and Hif-1α (green), GFAP (green) and β-III-tubulin (red), and Ki67 (red) and S100 (green). Cell nuclei have been counterstained with DAPI (blue).

CW-exposed organoids did not show any evident variation in size, structure, and histology (**Figure 5A**). However, immunofluorescence analysis revealed that CW stimulation was sufficient to trigger a pro-apoptotic response of GBM cells residing within the organoids, with CW2 displaying the most severe effects (**Figure 5A** and **C**).

In this context, the gene expression profiling of GBM organoids collected after 24 was able to identify 257 differentially expressed genes (DEGs) between sham and CW1 exposed organoids, and 183 DEGs between sham and CW2 exposed organoids.

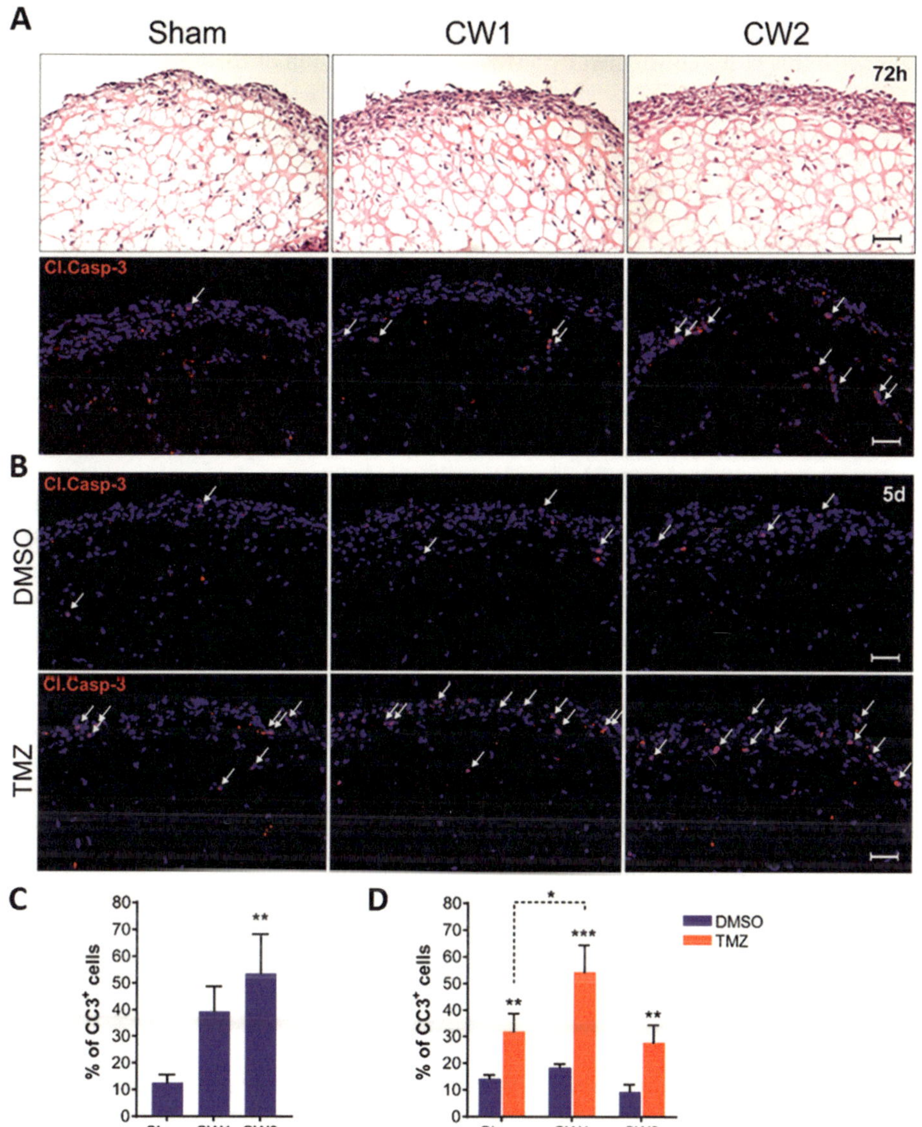

Figure 5.
*GBM organoid treatment and evaluation of CW effects. (A): Representative hematoxylin and eosin (top) or Cleaved Caspase 3 (Cl.Casp-3, red nuclei indicated by arrows) immunofluorescence (bottom) staining of GBM organoids after 72 h from being treated with the sham, CW1, or CW2 exposing protocols. (B): Cleaved Caspase 3 immunofluorescence analysis displaying GBM organoids treated for 5 days with DMSO (top) or TMZ (bottom), both added to the culturing medium 24 h from sham or CW1/CW2 exposures. Original magnification: 10x; bar: 50 μm. (C, D): Relative quantifications of Cl. Casp-3⁺ cells in samples as in A (C) and B (D). In (C), *p < 0.05, by one-way ANOVA with Tukey's multiple comparisons test relative to the sham group. In (D), asterisks over a column (**p < 0.01 and ***p < 0.001) indicate a significant difference relative to matched DMSO-treated groups by unpaired t-test. Asterisks over brackets (*p < 0.05) by one-way ANOVA with Tukey's multiple comparisons test.*

Since the delivered energy was equal in the two different treatments, we aimed to identify the common perturbed genes; by intersecting the two different gene lists we retrieved 143 upregulated - and 22 downregulated genes commonly affected by 30.5 GHz CW exposure. Pathway enrichment analysis through GSEA identified

CW-exposed organoids as characterized by an increased expression of genes related to the response to DNA damage, the activation of DNA repair mechanisms, and cell cycle, with this latter confirmed by a significant expansion of the Ki67^{+} GBM cell populations within the CW treated organoids [20]. More specifically, the majority of the upregulated DEGs were related to the regulation of chromatin conformation and replication machinery. While the few downregulated genes did not significantly enrich for any cellular process. Based on these results, we evaluated the possibility of exploiting the effects displayed by the stimulation with CWs through the combination of a temporally defined chemotherapeutic intervention with TMZ. In particular, we exposed GBM organoids to CWs as described and, after 24 hours, treated them for an additional 5 days with TMZ, with the aim of specifically targeting the CW-induced cell proliferation boost. Remarkably, CW pre-treatment dramatically sensitized GBM organoids to TMZ (**Figure 5B** and **D**), independently of any transient induction of cell death observed at earlier timepoints (**Figure 5C**).

3.3 Benefits of mid-intensity thermal sensitization

The MMW irradiation increases the temperature by a few degrees, but this rise remains within the normal temperature range for cells. In fact, their temperature does not exceed 37°C, which is the physiological temperature for cells and tissues. Therefore, the effects observed, as well as their combination with chemotherapeutic agents, cannot simply be attributed to a thermal mechanism similar to that used in hyperthermia applications [20]. In our study, we also noted a stronger effect of TMZ after CW1 exposure, which resulted in a lower temperature increase compared to CW2 exposure, thus supporting our hypothesis. However, the mechanisms underlying the observed effects could be highly complex, and at this point, it is not possible to completely rule out the role of temperature. Clearly, further experiments are necessary to clarify this issue. Nonetheless, the slight temperature increase is beneficial for therapeutic purposes, as it is less invasive and painful for potential future applications in humans.

4. Discussion

The primary objective of this study was to demonstrate the potential of mid-intensity, CW stimulation while determining energy delivery formats that yield significant endpoints in a glioblastoma organoid model. Our findings not only achieved this goal but also outlined the need for further investigation in this field.

The extinguishing effect of CW stimulation when cells are not re-exposed could not be within the scope of the present study. This limitation was not solely due to time constraints but also stemmed from the uncertainty surrounding the number of repeated stimulations organoids can undergo while still providing meaningful results. Future research should rely on additional cell biology experiments aimed at elucidating this aspect by implementing a rigorous evaluation of several close-range experimental timepoints within the proposed actionable timeframe as it could significantly impact the design of therapeutic protocols. Nevertheless, this will require dedicated effort and time.

Our results showed that CW2 induced more pronounced apoptosis and less proliferation in the mid-term range (72 hours after exposure), likely due to the milder temperature increase compared to CW1, which delivers higher power. Consequently, the CW/TMZ combination more effectively induced apoptosis for the CW1 protocol, as CW1 favors proliferation, which is then targeted by TMZ. These observations underscore the complex interplay between CW parameters, cellular responses, and chemotherapeutic efficacy. Identifying the optimal window for TMZ administration post-exposure, along with fine-tuning signal intensity and exposure duration, could lead to an enhanced chemotherapeutic response for TMZ or other alkylating agents.

While our focus on TMZ provided valuable insights, future studies should expand the scope to include different chemotherapeutic drugs with diverse mechanisms of action. Moving beyond agents that directly affect proliferating cells could offer a more comprehensive understanding of how CW stimulation interacts with various treatment modalities targeting cancer cell migration and infiltration, rather than proliferation. Future studies could explore the effects of CW stimulation combined with matrix metalloproteinase inhibitors, which impede tumor invasion, or anti-angiogenic agents that restrict tumor vascularization. Additionally, examining the interaction between CW exposure and immunomodulatory therapies could unveil potential synergies in activating antitumor immune responses. These diverse approaches may uncover unexpected therapeutic opportunities and provide a more holistic strategy for combating the complex nature of GBM.

5. Conclusions

In summary, we comprehensively characterized an exposure setup for 30.5 GHz CW suitable for experiments on 3D GBM organoids, in terms of numerical/experimental dosimetry and thermal regimen. From our characterization, we demonstrated the possibility to use this exposure modality (especially CW1 protocol) as a therapeutic adjuvant in a future possible treatment for GBM. Our approach impacts the functioning and behavior of GBM cells by inducing a statistically significant increase of proliferation, as confirmed by both transcriptional and functional analyses. This result leads to the enhancement of a subsequent TMZ administration and to future and innovative combination therapies for GBM.

While the present study did not demonstrate direct MMW radiation-induced cell differentiation pathways, the growing body of literature on EM-based microenvironment manipulation suggests promising avenues for future research. These emerging approaches may lead to the development of therapeutic modalities that selectively target GBM cancer stem cells, potentially increasing their susceptibility to conventional treatments and addressing one of the major challenges in GBM therapy.

Acknowledgements

The authors gratefully acknowledge the support from Bangor University's School of Computer Science and Engineering for the open-access publication of this contribution. The work in this chapter was supported by Project ECS 0000024 Rome Technopole, -CUP B83C22002820006, NRP Mission 4 Component 2 Investment 1.5, Funded by the European Union -NextGenerationEU. This work was also supported by CARIPARO Foundation project number 20/16.

Conflict of interest

CH was employed by Creo Medical Limited. The remaining authors declare no conflict of interest.

Author details

Cristiano Palego[1*], Christopher Hancock[2], Elena Rampazzo[3], Luca Persano[3], Arianna Casciati[4], Mirella Tanori[4], Mariateresa Mancuso[4] and Caterina Merla[4]

1 Bangor University, Bangor, United Kingdom

2 Creo Medical Ltd., Bath, United Kingdom

3 University of Padova, Padova, Italy

4 ENEA, Rome, Italy

*Address all correspondence to: c.palego@bangor.ac.uk

References

[1] Rong L, Li N, Zhang Z. Emerging therapies for glioblastoma: Current state and future directions. Journal of Experimental & Clinical Cancer Research. 2022;**41**(1):142. DOI: 10.1186/s13046-022-02349-7

[2] Stupp R, Mason WP, van den Bent MJ, Weller M, Fisher B, Taphoorn MJ, et al. Radiotherapy plus concomitant and adjuvant temozolomide for glioblastoma. *New England Journal of Medicine*. 2005;**352**:987-996. DOI: 10.1056/NEJMoa043330

[3] Meng Y, Hynynen K, Lipsman N. Applications of focused ultrasound in the brain: From thermoablation to drug delivery. *Nature Reviews Neurology*. 2021;**17**:7-22. DOI: 10.1038/s41582-020-00418-z

[4] Aldape K, Brindle KM, Chesler L, Chopra R, Gajjar A, Gilbert MR, et al. Challenges to curing primary brain tumours. Nature Reviews Clinical Oncology. 2019;**16**(8):509-520. DOI: 10.1038/s41571-019-0177-5

[5] Bonosi L, Marino S, Benigno UE, Musso S, Buscemi F, Giardina K, et al. Sonodynamic therapy and magnetic resonance-guided focused ultrasound: New therapeutic strategy in glioblastoma. *Journal of Neuro-Oncology*. 2023;**163**:219-238. DOI: 10.1007/s11060-023-04333-3

[6] National Library of Medicine, ClinicalTrials.gov, Sonodynamic Therapy in Patients With Recurrent GBM (GBM 001) [Internet]. 2023. Available from: https://clinicaltrials.gov/study/NCT06039709?term=shayan% 20moosa& rank=1 [Accessed: 2024-06-24]

[7] Roberts JW, Powlovich L, Sheybani N, LeBlang S. Focused ultrasound for the treatment of glioblastoma. Journal of Neuro-Oncology. 2022;**157**:237-247. DOI: 10.1007/s11060-022-03974-01

[8] Carrieri FA, Smack C, Siddiqui I, Kleinberg LR, Tran PT. Tumor treating fields: At the crossroads between physics and biology for cancer treatment. Frontiers in Oncology. 2020;**10**:575992. DOI: 10.3389/fonc.2020.575992

[9] Shah PP, White T, Khalafallah AM, Romo CG, Price C, Mukherjee D. A systematic review of tumor treating fields therapy for high-grade gliomas. Journal of Neuro-Oncology. 2020;**148**:433-443. DOI: 10.1007/s11060-020-03563-z

[10] Campelo SN, Popelka S, Anderson RS. Structure of protein-surface interaction layers in polymer brushes. APL Bioengineering. 2023;8:026117. DOI: 10.1063/j.0198382

[11] Lorenzo MF, Arena CB, Davalos RF. Maximizing local access to therapeutic delivery in glioblastoma. Part III: Irreversible electroporation and high-frequency irreversible electroporation for the eradication of glioblastoma. In: Codon Publications, editors. Glioblastoma. 1st ed. Brisbane: Codon Publications; 2017. p. 19. DOI: 10.15586/codon.glioblastoma.2017

[12] Murphy KR, Rogers A, Pavlovic D. Bioelectrochemistry and biophysical analysis of cell interaction. Bioelectrochemistry. 2022;**144**:108001. DOI: 10.1016/j.bioelechem.2021.108001

[13] Ivey JW, Wasson EM, Alinezhadbalalami N, Kanitkar A, Debinski W, Sheng Z, et al.

Characterization of ablation thresholds for 3D-cultured patient-derived glioma stem cells in response to high-frequency irreversible electroporation. Research (Washington, D.C.). 2019;**2019**:8081315. DOI: 10.34133/2019/8081315

[14] Campelo SN, Popelka S, Kim BS. Advances in cancer immunotherapy. Frontiers in Oncology. 2023;**13**:1171278. DOI: 103389/fonc.2023.1171278

[15] Partridge B, Long CJ, Hainline B. Neuromodulation techniques in behavioral neuroscience. Journal of Neuroscience Methods. 2020;**330**:108630. DOI: 10.1016/j.jneumeth.2020.108630

[16] Frey B, Weiss E-M, Rubner Y, Wunderlich R, Ott OJ, Sauer R, et al. Old and new facts about hyperthermia-induced modulations of the immune system. International Journal of Hyperthermia. 2012;**28**(6):528-542. DOI: 10.3109/02656736.2012.677933

[17] Zhu L, Altman MB, Laszlo A, Straube W, Zoberi I, Hallahan DE, et al. Ultrasound hyperthermia technology for radiosensitization. Ultrasound in Medicine & Biology. 2019;**45**(5):1025-1043. DOI: 10.1016/j.ultrasmedbio.2018.12.007

[18] Hancock CP, Chaudhry S, Wall P, Goodman AM. Proof of concept percutaneous treatment system to enable fast and finely controlled ablation of biological tissue. Medical & Biological Engineering & Computing. 2007;**45**(6):531-540. DOI: 10.1007/s11517-007-0184-z

[19] Sugiyama J-I, Tokunaga Y, Hishida M, Tanaka M, Takeuchi K, Satho D, et al. Nonthermal acceleration of protein hydration by sub-terahertz irradiation. Nature Communications. 2023;**14**:2825. DOI: 10.1038/s41467-023-38462-0

[20] Rampazzo E, Persano L, Karim N, Hodgking G, Pinto R, Casciati A, et al. On the effects of 30.5 GHz sinusoidal wave exposure on glioblastoma organoids. Frontiers in Oncology. 2024;**14**:1307516. DOI: 10.3389/fonc.2024.1307516

[21] ITTS Foundation Tissue Properties [Internet]. 2011. Available from: https://itis.swiss/virtual-population/tissue-properties/database/ [Accessed: 2024-08-04]

[22] Pistollato F, Persano L, Della Puppa A, Rampazzo E, Basso G. Isolation and expansion of regionally defined human glioblastoma cells in vitro. Current Protocols in Stem Cell Biology. 2011;**17**:3.4.1-3.4.10. DOI: 10.1002/9780470151808.sc0304s172

[23] Porcù E, Maule F, Manfreda L, Mariotto E, Bresolin S, Cani A, et al. Identification of homoharringtonine as a potent inhibitor of glioblastoma cell proliferation and migration. Translational Research. 2023;**251**:41-53. DOI: 10.1016/j.trsl.2022.06.0173

[24] Pistollato F, Abbadi S, Rampazzo E, Persano L, Della Puppa A, Frasson C, et al. Intratumoral hypoxic gradient drives stem cells distribution and MGMT expression in glioblastoma. Stem Cells. 2010;**28**(5):851-862. DOI: 10.1002/stem.4152

[25] Lancaster MA, Knoblich JA. Generation of cerebral organoids from human pluripotent stem cells. Nature Protocols. 2014;**9**(10):2329-2340. DOI: 10.1038/nprot.2014.158

[26] Hubert CG, Rivera M, Spangler LC, Wu Q, Mack SC, Prager BC, et al. A three-dimensional organoid culture system derived from human glioblastomas recapitulates the hypoxic gradients and cancer stem cell

heterogeneity of tumors found in vivo. Cancer Research. 2016;**76**(8):2465-2477. DOI: 10.1158/0008-5472.CAN-15-2402

[27] Persano L, Rampazzo E, Della Puppa A, Pistollato F, Basso G. The three-layer concentric model of glioblastoma: Cancer stem cells, microenvironmental regulation, and therapeutic implications. ScientificWorldJournal. 2011;**11**:1829-1841. DOI: 10.1100/2011/736480

[28] Della Puppa A, Persano L, Masi G, Rampazzo E, Sinigaglia A, Pistollato F, et al. MGMT expression and promoter methylation status may depend on the site of surgical sample collection within glioblastoma: A possible pitfall in stratification of patients? Journal of Neuro-Oncology. 2012;**106**(1):33-41. DOI: 10.1007/s11060-011-0639-9

[29] Rampazzo E, Della Puppa A, Frasson C, Battilana G, Bianco S, Scienza R, et al. Phenotypic and functional characterization of glioblastoma cancer stem cells identified through 5-aminolevulinic acid-assisted surgery [corrected]. Journal of Neuro-Oncology. 2014;**116**(3):505-513. DOI: 10.1007/s11060-013-1348-3

Chapter 7

Heterogeneity of Glioblastoma

Samuel Guzman

Abstract

Glioblastomas are IDH-wildtype, WHO grade 4 tumors with a poor prognosis. The tumor biology is heterogeneous with distinct subpopulations that can likely contribute to overall tumor diversity in this group. Molecular techniques are allowing for sub classification of this tumor type, which can hopefully allow for identification of therapeutic targets. DNA methylation has subclassified GBMs into 5 groups, while techniques like spatial transcriptomics/RNA seq have found intratumoral heterogeneity in single neoplasms. Future data has to correlate these findings to clinical data and tumor location in the brain to allow the underlying biology to be better assessed and targeted. Multileveled analysis is beginning to be performed and showing great progress.

Keywords: glioblastoma, high grade glioma, neoplasm, oncology, molecular, transcriptomics

1. Introduction

Glioblastoma, IDH-wildtype, is the most frequent intracranial tumor in adults that accounts for 15% of total cases [1]. This tumor is aggressive with a 5 year survival of 16% [1], with minimal response to chemotherapy and radiation. Glioblastomas are currently diagnosed as one large heterogeneous group of tumors, with few targetable molecular mutations identified although molecular changes can impact the prognosis of the patient. Notably, some mutations such as a glioblastoma with an FGFR3-TACC3 mutation correlating with a longer survival. Glioblastomas demonstrate inter-tumor heterogeneity (differences between different tumors being compared) as well as intra-tumor heterogeneity (regional population differences of the same tumor), which is thought to play a big role in the tumor's response to therapy and overall aggressiveness [1, 2].

This chapter details the features of glioblastoma in adult patients from the pathological and mechanistic perspectives.

The topics are discussed in the following order:

- Diagnostic Neuropathology of Glioblastoma
- Glioblastoma Subclassification by Transcriptomics
- Glioblastoma Subclassification by DNA Methylation
- Advancements in Glioblastoma Understanding with Spatial Biology

IntechOpen

2. Neuropathology diagnosis

The way astrocytomas are diagnosed has been updated in the 5th edition of the WHO classification for Central Nervous System Tumors [1]. To diagnose a glioblastoma, the tumor must be IDH-wildtype and occur in an adult. When a tumor is IDH mutant, the most common IDH mutation observed is a point mutation at IDH1 R132H, although mutations at IDH2 can occur albeit infrequently. The occurrence of these mutations is more common in individuals under 55 years old, and despite having a similar histology as a glioblastoma, IDH-wildtype, they have a much better prognosis. In an adult, a high grade glioma with an IDH mutation is diagnosed as an Astrocytoma, IDH-mutant, WHO grade 4. A glioblastoma also must lack characteristic histone modifications that can be diagnostic for other tumor entities such as H3K27M (Diffuse midline glioma, H3 K27M-altered) and H3 G34R (Diffuse hemispheric glioma, H3 G34-mutant), depending on their location.

Glioblastoma is an aggressively infiltrative tumor that occurs in the subcortical white matter, where it follows the white matter tracts of structures such as the corpus callosum, and can even involve deep gray matter structures. Based on its morphology, the tumor is expected to exhibit necrotic areas, such as palisading necrosis, along with microvascular proliferation. Additionally, Glioblastoma, IDH-wildtype neoplasms display a variety of architectural patterns that are associated with molecular findings, as explained below.

Gemistocytic astrocytic neoplasms consist of abundant glassy, non-fibrillary cytoplasm that shows GFAP positivity. Most cases are associated with an IDH and TP53

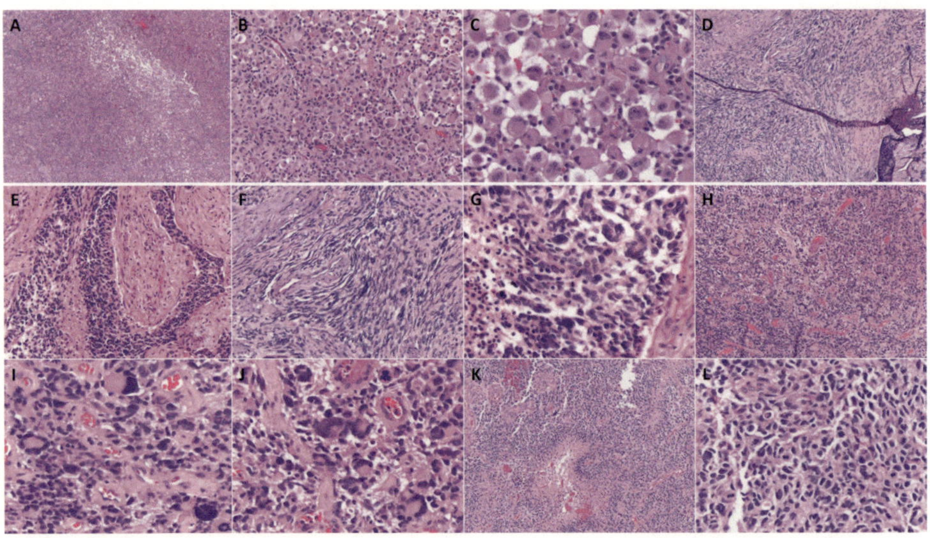

Figure 1.
Case 1 (A–C). A. (H&E, x 40), B. (H&E, x 200), C. (H&E, x 400). This is a glioblastoma, IDH-wildtype, WHO grade 4 with a prominent epithelioid component that exemplifies the discohesive nature of the tumor cells with abundant glassy cytoplasm. Case 2(D-G). D. (H&E, x 100), E. (H&E, x 200), F. (H&E, x 400), G. (H&E, x 400). This is a glioblastoma, IDH-wildtype, WHO grade 4 that is consistent with a gliosarcoma subtype as can be seen with biphasic pattern with sarcomatous features. Case 3 (H-J). H. (H&E, x 100), I. (H&E, x 400), J. (H&E, x 400). This is a glioblastoma, IDH-wildtype with giant cell features and history of Li-Fraumeni Syndrome with histology that illustrates the frequent giant cells which are surrounded by bizarre shaped tumor cells. Case 4 (K-L). K. (H&E, x 100) L. (H&E, x 400). This is a glioblastoma, IDH-wildtype, WHO grade 4 with prominent neuronal features, that shows irregular carrot shaped cells that appear neuronal.

mutation [3, 4]. The diagnosis requires that over 20% of the tumor is made up of this specific cell type. Giant cell glioblastomas have large multinucleated tumor cells, with bizarre cells and severe nuclear atypia, which can be seen on **Figure 1(H-J)**, and have microsatellite instability mutations, as seen with IHC staining for PMS2, MSH2, MSH6, MLH1. Intraoperatively, these tumors can appear similar to a metastasis because of their well-defined borders and reticulin deposits [5, 6]. Granular cell glioblastomas are composed of large histiocytic appearing tumor with eosinophilic granules in the cytoplasm that weakly stain for CD68 but are negative for CD163 [7]. These tumors are nearly always IDH-wildtype. Gliosarcomas are biphasic tumors with mesenchymal and glial components as can be seen in **Figure 1(D-G)**. Most commonly, they take on sarcomatous features with heavy reticulin and collagen [6, 8]. These tumors are also thought to have a worse prognosis than other glioblastoma, as they can have extracranial metastasis as well as invade the dura. Small cell glioblastoma is another IDH-wildtype tumor that is composed of a high density, monotonous tumor that is highly proliferative and is EGFR amplified [9]. Epithelioid GBM is IDH-wildtype with a BRAF V600E mutation in ~50% of the cases, that is composed of polygonal to rounded, loosely cohesive tumor cells with prominent nucleoli and is illustrated in **Figure 1(A–C)** [10]. These tumors can also resemble pleomorphic xanthoastrocytomas, WHO grade 3. Finally, there are glioblastomas with a primitive neuronal component, which are composed of hyperchromatic, irregularly shaped cells, that occasionally form nodules within the tumor, as well as possibly forming Homer Wright rosettes [11]. Some of these features can be seen in **Figure 1(K-L)**. These tumors are usually IDH-wildtype and can express NMYC gene amplifications. This tumor can also seed in the CSF.

The immunohistochemistry panel used to diagnose a glioma typically includes stains for GFAP, OLIG2, IDH1, ATRX, P53, and Ki-67 (MIB-1) [1]. A GFAP (glial fibrillary acidic protein) stain highlights the intermediate filaments that are present in glial cells. Olig2 (oligodendrocyte transcription factor) is a precursor glial marker. An IDH1 stain highlights the IDH1 R132H point mutation most commonly seen with gliomas. ATRX (Alpha-Thalassemia/intellectual Disability syndrome X-linked) is usually lost in glioblastomas and P53 can be overexpressed, although these stains can be variable. The Ki-67 (MIB-1) stain is a proliferative index marker that can be variable in a GBM with areas showing a higher rate compared to areas with a lower rate. Additionally, these stains emphasize the heterogeneity present in this tumor group.

If any of the following molecular results are present, a diagnosis of glioblastoma can be made even without morphologic criteria: EGFR amplification, gain of chromosome 7 with loss of chromosome 10 alterations, and/or TERT promoter mutation [1]. A prognostic marker that is assessed is the promoter methylation status of MGMT (O6-methylguanine DNA methyl transferase), which encodes a DNA repair protein and can blunt alkylating drug effects from drugs such as temozolomide. Cases exhibiting MGMT promoter methylation tend to have a more favorable prognosis [1]. About 40–50% of Glioblastomas, IDH-wildtype, have an MGMT promoter methylation [1].

3. Transcriptomic subclassification

In order to learn more about this heterogeneous group of tumors, many groups have turned to gene expression-based methods to further sub-classify the tumors. Verhaak et al. [12] developed a gene expression-based molecular classification system for GBM that was composed of Proneural, Neuronal, Classical, and Mesenchymal subtypes, which were assessed by transcriptomic microarray analysis of cases from

The Cancer Genome Atlas (TCGA). Each subtype correlates to a unique set of somatic mutations that can further support the categorization. The aggressiveness of the tumor as well as responses to treatment also correlate with the molecular subtype. Notably, this research was done before IDH1 mutant tumors were separated out from the Glioblastoma designation. Wang et al. [13] revised this molecular classification system and only focused on the IDH-wildtype glioblastomas. This most significantly altered the proneural subtype as 30% of the cases in this group were IDH1 mutant, compared to the other subtypes being IDH1-wildtype.

3.1 Classical subtype

According to Verhaak's study [12], the classical subtype of glioblastoma has chromosome 7 amplification that is paired with a loss of chromosome 10 in 100% of cases. A high level of EGFR amplification is found in 97% of cases. This subtype is usually negative for TP53 mutations, as compared to other GBM subtypes. There is also a frequent CDKN2A homozygous deletion in this group. Other precursor factors as well as neural stem cell markers commonly identified in this group are: Notch (NOTCH3, JAG1, and LFNG) and Sonic hedgehog (SMO, GAS1, and GLI2) as well as FGFR3, PDGFA, AKT2, NES. Wang et al. [13] later added the following genes to the list: PTPRA, ELOVL2, SOX9, PAX6, CDK4, SEPT11, MEOX2.

3.2 Mesenchymal subtype

The mesenchymal subtype has the poorest prognosis and is most enriched with macrophages/microglial cells, necrosis and have reactive astrocytes nearby. This subtype has focal hemizygous deletion at 17q11.2, containing the NF1 gene and mutations of CASP1/4/5/8, ILR4, CHI3L1, TRADD, TLR2/4, RELB, MET. These cases also have higher activity of CD44 and MERTK. In addition, Wang et al. [13] also revealed the following significant gene alterations: BCL3, TGFBI, ITGB1, LOX, COL1A2, VDR, IL6, MMP7. The tumor-associated macrophages are reprogrammed by tumor cells through cytokines and soluble factors, which promote invasion, angiogenesis and, in some cases, immunosuppression.

3.3 Proneural subtype

The proneural subtype was noted to have a population IDH1 point mutation in the Verhaak system [12]. There was also a focal amplification of 4q12, which harbors the PDGRA gene. This PDGRA amplification is much higher than the other subtypes. This subtype also has frequent TP53 mutations. There were also fewer +7/−10 chromosomal alterations in this subtype as well as high OLIG2 expression. This subtype also has increased expression of developmental genes such as: SOX, DCX, DLL3, ASCL1 and TCF4. Later research by Wang et al. [13] revealed the following genes as significant once the IDH-mutant cases were taken out of the study: GARBR3, HOXD3, ERBB3, SOX10, CDKN1C, PDGFRA, HDAC2, and EPHB1. **Figure 2** illustrates the heatmap from the Wang et al. study [13].

3.4 Neural subtype

The neural subtype was the fourth group that the Verhaak system outlined but was later removed in the Wang system. This group was thought to include an adjacent

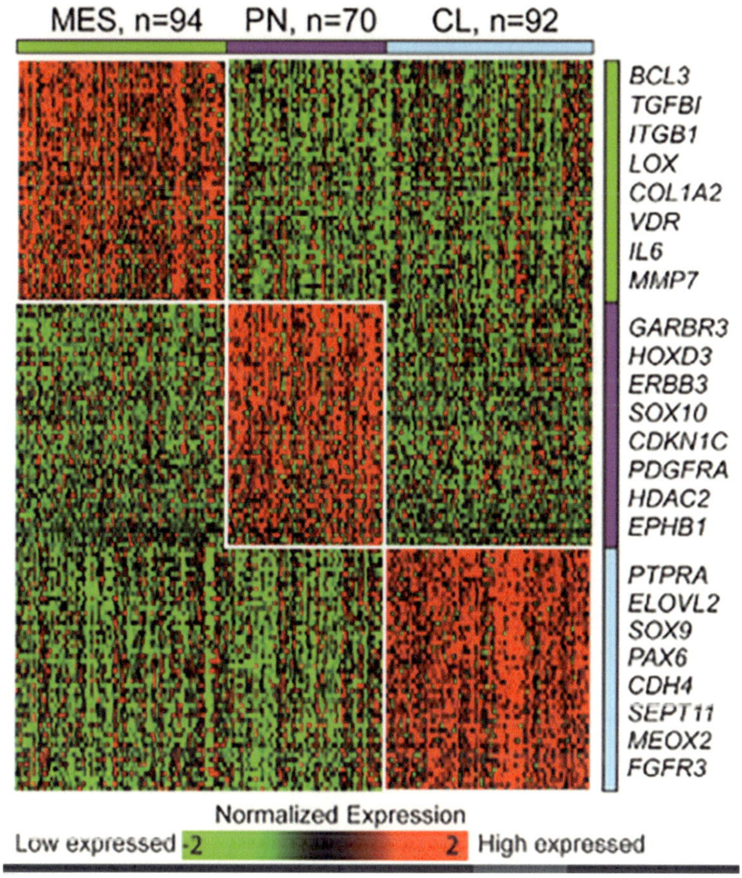

Figure 2.
Heatmap of 50-gene signature by gene expression subtype. Representative genes are shown for each subtype. Image reprint from Wang et al. "Tumor Evolution of Glioma-Intrinsic Gene Expression Subtypes Associates with Immunological Changes in the Microenvironment."

tumor edge and was not truly representative of a subtype of glioblastoma. This is a non-tumor specific category that is likely related to the margin of tumor and contamination.

The gene-based approach to categorizing glioblastoma was helpful in analyzing large numbers of tumors for the most clinically relevant genes that exist within each group. This helps explain the inter-tumoral heterogeneity that exists between tumors of this category and gain an idea of the underlying mechanism taking place. These bulk RNA methods (RNAseq and microarray) were helpful in identifying the proneural subgroup as having a good prognosis as well as a consistent IDH mutation finding. The glioblastoma group no longer includes that IDH mutant gliomas for these reasons.

4. DNA methylation classification

DNA methylation patterns are used to identify different cell types in the brain based on developmental origin and subtyping brain tumors [14, 15]. This diagnostic platform was incorporated in the WHO 2021, and is the sole method to be used to classify some tumor types such as high-grade glioma with pleomorphic and pseudopapillary features (HPAP) [1]. DNA methylation is a chemical modification that involves adding methyl groups to DNA, which occurs at cytosine residues within a CpG dinucleotide. DNA methylation is also important in regulating gene expression and in maintaining genome stability.

4.1 Novel glioblastoma subgroups

More recently, DNA methylation profiles have helped to subgroup the glioblastoma category. A recent study by Reuss et al. [16] analyzed 10,782 tumors that were diagnosed as glioblastoma, according to the WHO 2021 definition, with DNA methylation by v12.8 version of the brain tumor classifier [16]. They identified 9 methylation classes of glioblastoma, IDH-wildtype that appeared distinct and correlated with various mutations, as well as copy number variations. A T-SNE from the paper is shown in **Figure 3**. The 9 groups are: adult-type high grade glioma, IDH-wildtype, subtype B (HGG_B), adult-type high grade glioma, IDH-wildtype, subtype E (HGG_E), adult-type high grade glioma, IDH-wildtype, subtype F (HGG_F), glioblastoma, IDH-wildtype, RTK1 subtype (GBM RTK1), glioblastoma, IDH-wildtype, RTK2 subtype (GBM RTK2), glioblastoma, IDH-wildtype, typical mesenchymal type (GBM MES, TYP), glioblastoma, IDH-wildtype, atypical mesenchymal type (GBM MES, ATYP), glioblastoma, IDH-wildtype, with primitive neuronal component (GBM PNC), high-grade diffuse glioma of the midline/posterior fossa, H3/IDH-wildtype (GBM-CBM). The most frequently identified subtypes are GBM MES TYP, GBM RTK1 and GBM RTK2 [16, 17].

4.2 Correlation with existing molecular features

Interestingly, methylation subgroups correlate with molecular findings. EGFR amplification was identified most frequently in the following subgroups: GBM RTK2

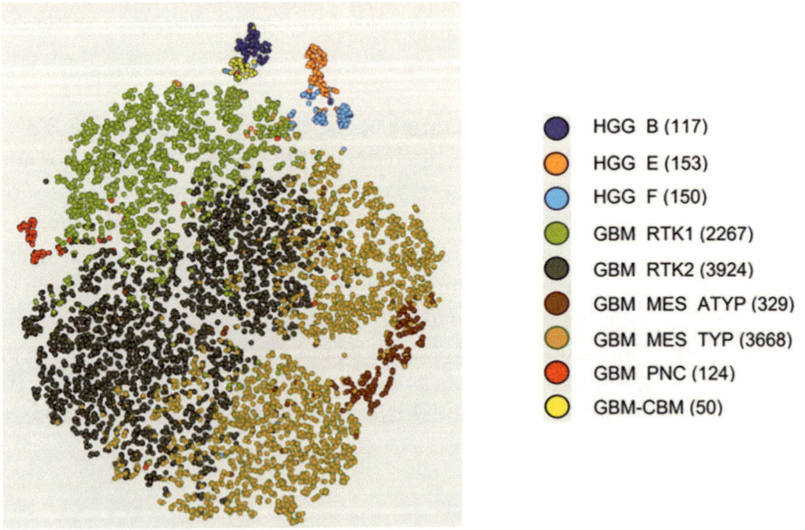

Figure 3.
tSNE showing the distribution of 9 methylation class subsumed within the WHO 2021 diagnosis of glioblastoma, IDH-wildtype. Image reprint from Reuss et al. "Heterogeneity of DNA methylation profiles and copy number alterations in 10,782 adult-type glioblastomas, IDH-wildtype."

(77%), GBM MES TYP (27%), and GBM RTK1 (20%). CDK4 amplification was identified in GBM RTK1 in 26% of cases. MYCN amplification is identified in GBM PNC (10%) most commonly. PDGFRA amplification is identified in GBM CBM (34%), GBM RTK1 (20%), HGG B (16%). The gain of chromosome 7 and loss of chromosome 10 (+7/−10) was identified most commonly is methylation class GBM RTK2 (89%), GBM RTK1 (77%) and GBM MES TYP (73%). Interestingly, groups HGG B and HGG E have only 2% and 3% of their cases that have the +7/−10 signature. The median age of people with the HGG B subgroup was 31.5, while the average age for those with HFF F and GBM RTK1 is 65. This paper also identified differences in glioblastoma cases that were more and less likely to have MGMT methylation, which is important for treatment. The most common groups to be methylated were GBM RTK2 (51%), GBM PNC (50%), and GBM RTK1 (46%). The groups most likely not to be MGMT unmethylated are HGG B (96%), HGG F.

4.3 Correlation with anatomical location

In a separate study by Dumitru et al. [17], GBM methylation classes were correlated with the location of the GBM as a possible explanation of cell origin. They studied a group of 441 glioblastomas in combination with support vector regression-based lesion-symptom mapping to identify the spatial distribution of tumor development, in concordance with prior work by Tejada Neyra et al. [18] who identified IDH-mutated gliomas to cluster around the rostral extension of the lateral ventricles, and Ellingson et al. [19] who found EGFR-amplified and EGFR variant 3 expressing tumors to occur predominantly in the left temporal lobe. The GBM MES subtype was identified to be most common in the left insula (37% of cases), while GBM RTK1 is identified to most commonly be in the right superior frontal gyrus (98% of cases), and RTK2 is found most commonly in left middle frontal gyrus (97%).

The impact of the DNA methylation platform appears significant as it continues to identify subgroups of tumors based on CpG methylation patterns based on cell of origin. This platform has split many diagnostic groups and helps to exemplify the inter-tumoral heterogeneity that exists within the glioblastoma group and many other types of CNS tumors. Time will tell how relevant some of the new classifications are in their translation to clinical treatment.

5. Advancements in spatial biology and transcriptomics

Advancements in technology have led to new platforms such as spatial transcriptomics and spatial proteomics, that can explore the intra-tumoral heterogeneity that exists within one tumor as various regions are compared. This is in contrast to prior "bulk sequencing" methods, where the tissue is homogenized and subsequently run through RNA sequencing or microarray with loss of spatial orientation. Now we can maintain the spatial context, which allows researchers to identify various tumor subtypes on the histologic slide with genetic information available to discern population clusters of cells. A diseased cell can move along a disease specific "trajectory" on T-SNE and UMAP charts, which would make "bulk sequencing" analysis difficult to categorize and might result in unreadable data. With spatial biology we see that diseased cell on the microscopic slide and place it in the proper histological context. Current technologies, such as spatial transcriptomics and spatial proteomics, seek to understand the spatial biology of the tumor's ecosystem in order to derive mechanisms and cell-cell interactions in the tumor microenvironment.

5.1 Classification of cell states

Recent transcriptomic work has tried to categorize cell states in order to understand the tumor biology and this work helps to set the stage for spatial platforms. Neftel et al. [20] used single cell RNA seq techniques on glioblastoma (IDH-wildtype) to reveal the 4 cell states of glioblastoma: neural progenitor-like, oligodendrocyte-progenitor-like, astrocytic-like, and mesenchymal-like states with influences by immune cells. A tumor cell can also express two states at once and is named a "hybrid state." A single tumor can contain many tumor cells in each state, but the overall proportions will vary between tumors. This is thought to be due to spatial and micro-environmental influences. The AC-like state is associated with EGFR amplification, the OPC-like state is associated with PDGFRA, and the NPC-like state is most associated with CDK4 amplification, which all seem to correlate with prior transcriptomics studies by Wang et al. [13]. These associations have been validated in mouse models, demonstrating that the gene alterations lead to the development of a tumor with a cell state dominance. The genetics and cell states seem to work together but can show plasticity as needed for the tumor.

5.2 Capturing intra-tumoral heterogeneity

Later research by Sottoriva et al. [21] helped to further explain the intra-tumoral heterogeneity at the RNA and DNA by analyzing 51 GBM fragments from 10 patients by copy number variations and microarray. They identified that even within the same tumor there were very different copy number variations based on the various regions tested but overall common "early phase mutations" occurred in a majority of cells throughout the tumor. The common "early phase mutations" demonstrated amplifications in EGFR, CDK6, and MET, with losses in CDKN2A/B and PTEN in the tumors sampled. Different regions of the tumor could then branch out and further mutate and then finally culminate in the unique "late phase" gene alterations that are region specific. This study also identified by transcriptomics that 6 out of 10 glioblastomas tested demonstrated genetic signatures for multiple glioblastoma subtypes. For instance, some tumors had regions of coexisting classical and mesenchymal GBM subtypes within the same tumor. Therefore, sampling bias can play a role in the genetic findings identified in a particular patient.

5.3 Spatial transcriptomics

In a study by Greenwald et al. [22], the spatial mapping of 13 GBM's and 6 IDH mutant gliomas sections by spatial transcriptomics identified that one tumor is composed of multiple niche areas of organization. This paper supported a prior spatial transcriptomics paper by Ravi et al. [23] that also identified similar niche areas that composed the glioblastoma tumor. These areas take on specialization and cellular states. It was found that glioblastomas have increased transcription factors that help to synergize the tumor for growth, organization, and overall tumor survival. In the study by Greenwald et al. [22], the IDH mutant gliomas were identified to be relatively disorganized when compared to the glioblastoma group, which is thought to be because of the loss of hypoxic factors in this tumor group.

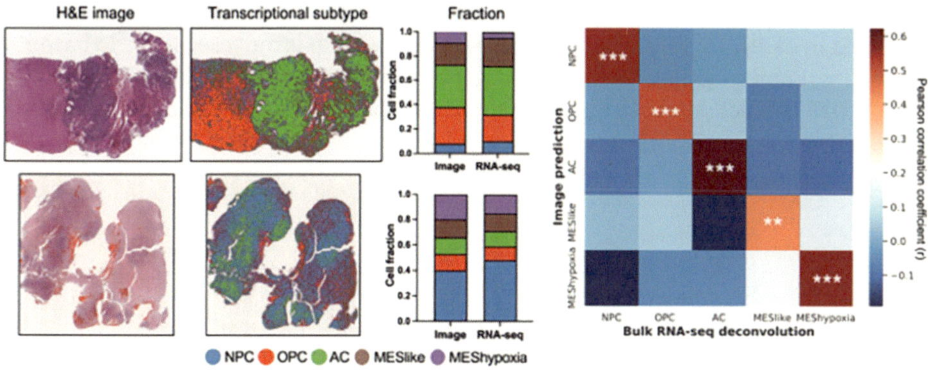

Figure 4.
H&E images and the predicted distribution of transcriptional subtypes in two tumors from the TCGA cohort. Bar graphs depict transcriptional subtype proportions derived from the image prediction versus bulk RNA-seq deconvolution. Heatmap of Pearson correlation coefficient showing the agreement between transcriptional subtype proportions derived from our image predictions versus those estimated from bulk RNA-seq deconvolution (n = 166 *patients).*

5.4 Future directions

The impact of spatial biology on glioblastoma is still in its infancy. These platforms are describing the intra-tumoral heterogeneity of glioblastoma, and aim to identify the underlying mechanism of the tumor. This technique will identify dysregulated networks and derive additional data from spatial contexts. Tumor aggressiveness profiles as well as glioblastoma subtypes for individual tumors are being generated based on the spatial gene profiles of tumor cells as seen in **Figure 4** [21]. Studies in other organ systems have also begun studying the edges of the tumor and have been able to compare the relevant genes to more central regions of the tumor. Overall, these studies hold promise for our understanding of the biology of glioblastoma and the promise for future therapies.

6. Conclusion

The heterogeneity of glioblastoma has been outlined at the histologic, immunohistochemical, molecular, transcriptomic, and methylation levels. The morphologic subtypes are diverse and correlate with underlying genetic findings, which might correlate with longer survivability in some contexts. Technology such as microarray, bulk sequencing and DNA methylation have allowed us to see the inter-tumoral heterogeneity that exists in the category of glioblastoma. Gene-based approaches have separated glioblastoma into 3 groups: Proneural, Classical, and Mesenchymal. Each of these groups correlates with a specific set of genetic mutations and age of onset. DNA methylation now characterizes 9 subclasses of glioblastoma with the most frequently identified groups being: GBM MES TYP, GBM RTK1 and GBM RTK2. As technology has continued to evolve, we now are learning more about the intra-tumoral heterogeneity of glioblastoma. The diversity of niche regions of a single glioblastoma is likely the tumors greatest defense at evading treatment. This will ultimately lead to tumor recurrence and treatment failure, as the heterogeneous groups of surviving tumor cells will then proliferate. The addition of multi-omic approaches that extend to the single cell level with an intact spatial context will allow for personalized medicine to be used in cases, as we learn what each GBM subgroup is most sensitive to based on the tumor composition. More work must be done to integrate all the platforms to characterize clinically relevant groups that encompass all relevant molecular therapeutic targets.

Author details

Samuel Guzman
University of Colorado Anschutz Medical Campus, USA

*Address all correspondence to: samuel.j.guzman@cuanschutz.edu

References

[1] Louis DN, Perry A, Wesseling P, Brat DJ, Cree IA, Figarella-Branger D, et al. The 2021 WHO classification of tumors of the central nervous system: A summary. Neuro-Oncology. 2021;**23**(8):1231-1251

[2] Becker AP, Sells BE, Haque SJ, Chakravarti A. Tumor heterogeneity in glioblastomas: From light microscopy to molecular pathology. Cancers (Basel). 2021;**13**(4)

[3] Sahm F, Korshunov A, Schrimpf D, Stichel D, Jones DT, Capper D, et al. Gain of 12p encompassing CCND2 is associated with gemistocytic histology in IDH mutant astrocytomas. Acta Neuropathologica. 2017;**133**(2):325-327

[4] Watanabe K, Peraud A, Gratas C, Wakai S, Kleihues P, Ohgaki H. p53 and PTEN gene mutations in gemistocytic astrocytomas. Acta Neuropathologica. 1998;**95**(6):559-564

[5] Kozak KR, Moody JS. Giant cell glioblastoma: A glioblastoma subtype with distinct epidemiology and superior prognosis. Neuro-Oncology. 2009;**11**(6):833-841

[6] Oh JE, Ohta T, Nonoguchi N, Satomi K, Capper D, Pierscianek D, et al. Genetic alterations in gliosarcoma and giant cell glioblastoma. Brain Pathology. 2016;**26**(4):517-522

[7] Brat DJ, Scheithauer BW, Medina-Flores R, Rosenblum MK, Burger PC. Infiltrative astrocytomas with granular cell features (granular cell astrocytomas): A study of histopathologic features, grading, and outcome. The American Journal of Surgical Pathology. 2002;**26**(6):750-757

[8] Reis RM, Konu-Lebleblicioglu D, Lopes JM, Kleihues P, Ohgaki H. Genetic profile of gliosarcomas. The American Journal of Pathology. 2000;**156**(2):425-432

[9] Perry A, Aldape KD, George DH, Burger PC. Small cell astrocytoma: An aggressive variant that is clinicopathologically and genetically distinct from anaplastic oligodendroglioma. Cancer. 2004;**101**(10):2318-2326

[10] Kleinschmidt-DeMasters BK, Aisner DL, Birks DK, Foreman NK. Epithelioid GBMs show a high percentage of BRAF V600E mutation. The American Journal of Surgical Pathology. 2013;**37**(5):685-698

[11] Perry A, Miller CR, Gujrati M, Scheithauer BW, Zambrano SC, Jost SC, et al. Malignant gliomas with primitive neuroectodermal tumor-like components: A clinicopathologic and genetic study of 53 cases. Brain Pathology. 2009;**19**(1):81-90

[12] Verhaak RG, Hoadley KA, Purdom E, Wang V, Qi Y, Wilkerson MD, et al. Integrated genomic analysis identifies clinically relevant subtypes of glioblastoma characterized by abnormalities in PDGFRA, IDH1, EGFR, and NF1. Cancer Cell. 2010;**17**(1):98-110

[13] Wang Q, Hu B, Hu X, Kim H, Squatrito M, Scarpace L, et al. Tumor evolution of glioma-intrinsic gene expression subtypes associates with immunological changes in the microenvironment. Cancer Cell. 2017;**32**(1):42-56 e6

[14] Capper D, Jones DTW, Sill M, Hovestadt V, Schrimpf D, Sturm D, et al. DNA methylation-based classification of central nervous system tumours. Nature. 2018;**555**(7697):469-474

[15] Park JW, Lee K, Kim EE, Kim SI, Park SH. Brain tumor classification by methylation profile. Journal of Korean Medical Science. 2023;**38**(43):e356

[16] Reuss DE, Schrimpf D, Cherkezov A, Suwala AK, Lausova T, Snuderl M, et al. Heterogeneity of DNA methylation profiles and copy number alterations in 10782 adult-type glioblastomas, IDH-wildtype. Free Neuropathology. 2024;**5**

[17] Foltyn-Dumitru M, Alzaid H, Rastogi A, Neuberger U, Sahm F, Kessler T, et al. Unraveling glioblastoma diversity: Insights into methylation subtypes and spatial relationships. Neurooncology Advances. 2024;**6**(1):vdae112

[18] Tejada Neyra MA, Neuberger U, Reinhardt A, Brugnara G, Bonekamp D, Sill M, et al. Voxel-wise radiogenomic mapping of tumor location with key molecular alterations in patients with glioma. Neuro-Oncology. 2018;**20**(11):1517-1524

[19] Ellingson BM, Lai A, Harris RJ, Selfridge JM, Yong WH, Das K, et al. Probabilistic radiographic atlas of glioblastoma phenotypes. AJNR. American Journal of Neuroradiology. 2013;**34**(3):533-540

[20] Neftel C, Laffy J, Filbin MG, Hara T, Shore ME, Rahme GJ, et al. An integrative model of cellular states, plasticity, and genetics for glioblastoma. Cell. 2019;**178**(4):835-49 e21

[21] Sottoriva A, Spiteri I, Piccirillo SG, Touloumis A, Collins VP, Marioni JC, et al. Intratumor heterogeneity in human glioblastoma reflects cancer evolutionary dynamics. Proceedings of the National Academy of Sciences of the United States of America. 2013;**110**(10):4009-4014

[22] Greenwald AC, Darnell NG, Hoefflin R, Simkin D, Mount CW, Gonzalez Castro LN, et al. Integrative spatial analysis reveals a multi-layered organization of glioblastoma. Cell. 2024;**187**(10):2485-501 e26

[23] Ravi VM, Will P, Kueckelhaus J, Sun N, Joseph K, Salie H, et al. Spatially resolved multi-omics deciphers bidirectional tumor-host interdependence in glioblastoma. Cancer Cell. 2022;**40**(6):639-55 e13

[24] Zheng Y, Carrillo-Perez F, Pizurica M, Heiland DH, Gevaert O. Spatial cellular architecture predicts prognosis in glioblastoma. Nature Communications. 2023;**14**(1):4122

Chapter 8

Genetic Rearrangements in Brain Tumors: A View from NTRK

Javier A. Jacobo, Nicolle Wagner-Gutiérrez, Jorge H. Aristizabal, Santiago Vallejo, Alejandro González, Iván Bobadilla, Diego Pineda, Oscar Arrieta and Andres F. Cardona

Abstract

There is growing interest in targeted therapies for oncological diseases, with neurotrophic tropomyosin receptor kinase (NTRK) genes emerging as promising targets in various solid tumors. The NTRK genes are essential for central nervous system (CNS) development and have been progressively recognized for their involvement in cancer development. This review explores the physiological role of NTRK genes in CNS development, their involvement in cancer development, and current evidence on the efficacy of NTRK inhibitors in treating CNS tumors. We highlight the prevalence of NTRK gene alterations in CNS tumors and explore the potential of NTRK inhibitors as a treatment option, focusing on recent discoveries and future directions. Additionally, we underscore the need for further research to improve NTRK fusion detection in CNS tumors, elucidate mechanisms of resistance to NTRK inhibitors, and conduct comprehensive clinical trials involving larger cohorts of patients with CNS tumors and brain metastases. This holistic approach, coupled with exploring the synergistic benefits of combining NTRK inhibitors with other therapeutic modalities, holds promise for advancing treatment outcomes in patients with CNS malignancies.

Keywords: NTRK gene fusions, CNS tumors, TRK inhibitors, targeted therapies, neuro-oncology, molecular diagnostics

1. Introduction

To incorporate molecular characteristics as a critical component for accurate diagnosis, the World Health Organization (WHO) updated its classification of central nervous system (CNS) tumors in 2016 [1]. Advancements in molecular profiling methods have enabled the identification of novel tumor entities and improved the stratification of known types through RNA expression analysis, next-generation sequencing, and DNA methylation [1, 2].

Several molecular alterations have gained particular interest given that they could be used as the objective for targeted therapies that have improved prognosis in patients with brain tumors [3]. Genetic alterations in the neurotrophic tropomyosin receptor kinase (NTRK) genes have been identified across various solid tumors, including thyroid, colorectal, salivary gland, and non-small cell lung cancers, as well as in mammary analog secretory carcinoma and secretory breast carcinoma [4, 5]. NTRK gene fusions are present in approximately 1% of all solid tumors and up to 2% of adult primary brain tumors [1]. In pediatric central nervous system tumors, these fusions are more prevalent, occurring in about 5 and 2.5% of high-grade and low-grade gliomas, respectively [6].

Given their significant presence in CNS tumors, NTRK fusions are expected to become essential in diagnostics, requiring specific expertise [1]. Therapeutic results targeting NTRK genes have been promising, and given its close relation with the CNS, this gene alteration has become a target of interest in treating brain tumors. This chapter explores the physiological functions of the NTRK gene, its role in the formation of cancerous lesions, and its potential applications in brain tumor therapies.

2. Gene fusions in brain tumors

Gene fusions are hybrid genes created by joining segments from different genes. These fusions can develop through various mechanisms within cells [7]. Studies indicate that fusion transcripts may emerge from chromosomal rearrangements at the DNA level or through processes such as trans-splicing and cis-splicing involving neighboring genes [8]. Four main types of chromosomal rearrangements can result in gene fusions: (1) deletion of a genomic region between two genes on the same strand, leading to the creation of a fusion gene; (2) duplication of a genomic region on a chromosome, producing tandem duplications; (3) translocation, where genomic regions are exchanged between different chromosomes; and (4) inversion events, in which genes on opposite strands of a chromosome combine to form a fusion gene [8].

2.1 EGFR and FIG-ROS1 fusions

Studies have established that gene fusions are a significant molecular abnormality in glioblastomas. These alterations occur in approximately 30–50% of patients, with most private fusions appearing in only a single patient, though a few recur at low frequencies in high-grade gliomas. Research highlights two major chromosomal hotspots for frequent fusion events: chromosomes 7p and 12q. Other commonly affected chromosomal regions include chromosomes 1, 4, 6, and 19 [9]. In glioblastomas, certain genomic regions frequently undergo amplification, indicating that many gene fusions stem from unbalanced genomic rearrangements. Notably, a significant number of fusion events occur on chromosome 7, particularly near the EGFR locus. Approximately 40% of glioblastoma fusions are attributed to complex genomic rearrangements (CGR), with chromothripsis being a primary mechanism driving these alterations [9, 10].

Chromosomal rearrangements on 12q14–15 are also frequently observed, particularly in CGR-based fusions on chromosome 12 [11]. Certain glioblastoma molecular subtypes show an enrichment of specific fusions. For example, amplifications of EGFR are more common in glioblastoma samples with at least one fusion than in those without (63 versus 38%). Additionally, the classical glioblastoma subtype demonstrates a higher prevalence of fusions (72%) compared to the mesenchymal subtype (39%) [9].

The initial gene fusion identified in glioblastomas was FIG-ROS1, resulting from a 240-kb intra-chromosomal deletion that produces a kinase with continuous activity, contributing to cancer development [12]. Subsequent studies have identified various fusion genes, notably involving growth factor receptors. Among these, EGFR-SEPT14 is the most frequently observed in glioblastomas, with EGFR-PSPH also being documented [13].

2.2 EGFR fusions

Singh et al. first described FGFR-TACC fusions in glioblastomas, demonstrating their oncogenic potential when introduced into astrocytes. These fusion proteins can be targeted with FGFR inhibitors, which have shown efficacy in extending survival in mouse models with FGFR-TACC-driven gliomas [14]. Subsequently, Parker et al. showed that this fusion gene is overexpressed by escaping miR-99a regulation due to losing the 3′ UTR of FGFR3 [15]. FGFR fusions have also been detected in other cancers, such as bladder cancer, cholangiocarcinoma, squamous lung cancer, breast cancer, thyroid cancer, and head and neck squamous cell carcinoma [16]. Several FGFR inhibitors like Dovitinib, BGJ398, and Erdafitinib have been tested in patients with recurrent gliomas [17–20].

2.3 NTRK fusions

The NTRK gene encodes the TRK receptor family, which plays a critical role in neurodevelopment, CNS maintenance, and protection. Rearrangements involving TRK receptors are associated with various solid tumors, including gliomas. RNA sequencing data from TCGA studies revealed NTRK1 fusions with neurofascin (NFASC) and brevican (BCAN), located on 1q32.1 and 1q23.1, respectively [1, 21]. Two other NTRK1 in-frame fusions were recently reported, CHTOP-NTRK1 and ARHGEF2-NTRK1 [22], although their biological implication is unknown now. NTRK1 fusions promote protein expression and the activation of NGF signaling via NGF/TrkA interaction. The role of NTRK1 alterations in high-grade gliomas is unknown. These fusions enhance protein expression and activate NGF signaling through TrkA interaction. While the role of NTRK1 fusions in high-grade gliomas remains uncertain, many NTRK1 fusion partners possess coiled-coil domains, enabling dimerization and activation of the TrkA kinase domain. However, NFASC and BCAN differ in lacking coiled-coil domains, suggesting alternative dimerization mechanisms involving Ig-like domains in TrkA. Additionally, transduction of the NFASC-NTRK1 fusion has been shown to promote cell proliferation in specific models [21]. The therapeutic efficacy of various NTRK inhibitors has already been demonstrated in cases of gliomas and brain metastases originating from lung adenocarcinoma among others.

2.4 MET fusions

MET, a gene coding for a receptor tyrosine kinase, plays a significant role in the development of various cancers, such as gliomas, hepatocellular carcinoma, papillary renal cell carcinoma, head and neck cancers, and non-small cell lung cancer [17]. One notable gene fusion involving MET, identified in gliomas, is the PTPRZ1-MET fusion. This fusion arises due to an intron insertion combined with a tandem duplication involving the protein tyrosine phosphatase receptor type Z1 (PTPRZ1) gene at chromosome 7q31.32 and the MET proto-oncogene at 7q31.2 [13]. Depending on the specific insertion point, the fusion can yield either in-frame or out-of-frame transcripts [18]. Research indicates that MET exon 14 skipping (METex14) frequently

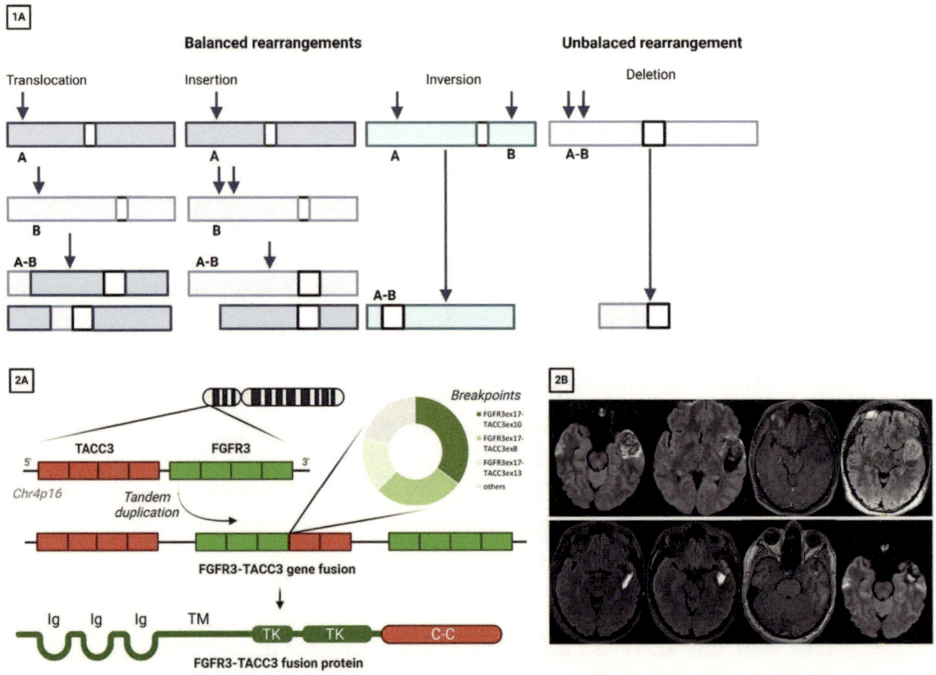

Figure 1.
*A. Chromosomal rearrangements can lead to the reshuffling of coding or regulatory DNA regions between genes. Such rearrangements frequently result in gene fusions, many of which act as key drivers of cancer development. These gene fusions have been instrumental in enhancing our understanding of the molecular mechanisms underpinning tumorigenesis. The specific relationship between gene fusions and tumor phenotypes makes them valuable diagnostic markers, enabling the differentiation of disease subtypes that might otherwise appear indistinguishable. Additionally, gene fusions provide crucial insights for assessing risk, and an increasing number of chimeric proteins generated by these fusions have become highly effective therapeutic targets, significantly improving clinical outcomes for patients. B. Diagram of the human NTRK loci, with exon numbers displayed beneath the corresponding boxes for the NTRK1 transcript variant 1 (NM_001012331.1). C. Imaging sequence of a patient with a diagnosis of left parietotemporal glioblastoma WHO IV IDHR132H-Wt, NTRK1-NFASC fusion, NF1C167fs*10 - subclonal, TERT promoter −124C > T, TMB 0.2 Mt./Mb, MSI(−) treated with gross tumor resection followed by chemoradiation with temozolomide, and larotrectinib, the latter intervention with a profession free survival of 16.2 months.*

co-occurs with PTPRZ1-MET fusions in glioblastomas, present in approximately 14% of cases and this genetic combination is associated with more aggressive tumor behavior and poorer patient survival [13, 19]. In this setting, crizotinib and PLB-1001 (NCT02978261) have been attempted with efficacy, reducing tumor volume, and improving neurological symptoms [20].

These findings support the use of more specific inhibitors for this subgroup of rare gene fusions. Genomic fusions in brain tumors among children and adults have been extensively described in previous studies, highlighting their significance in tumorigenesis [13]. **Figure 1** illustrates structural chromosomal rearrangements that lead to the transfer of coding or regulatory DNA segments between different genes, such as FGFR3-TACC3.

3. NTRK normal physiology in the nervous system

The NTRK complex consists of a family of genes, including NTRK-1, NTRK-2, and NTRK-3, that are in chromosomes 1 (1q22), 9 (9q22), and 15 (15q25). These genes

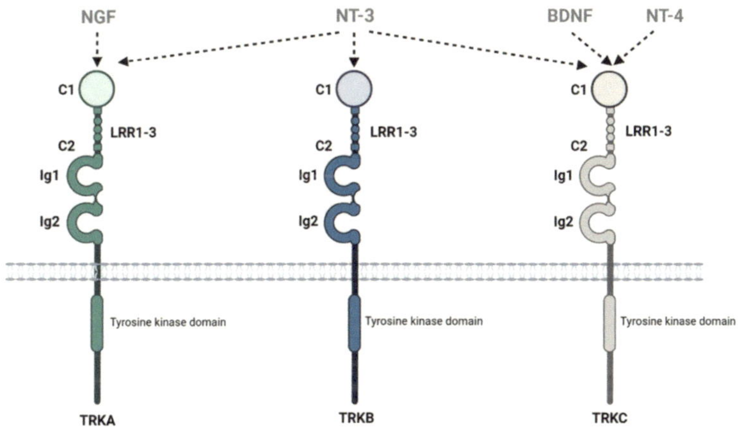

Figure 2.
TRK receptors interact specifically with their corresponding neurotrophins. Neurotrophin receptors, including TRKA, TRKB, and TRKC, exhibit selective binding affinities: nerve growth factor (NGF) binds to TRKA; brain-derived neurotrophic factor (BDNF) and neurotrophin-4 (NT-4) bind to TRKB; and neurotrophin-3 (NT-3) primarily interacts with TRKC. Notably, NT-3 can also bind to TRKA and TRKB under certain conditions. These receptors share a common structural organization, each comprising an extracellular domain, a transmembrane region, and an intracellular tyrosine kinase domain. The extracellular portion includes specific features such as cysteine-rich clusters and immunoglobulin-like domains, characteristic of TRK proteins. The genes encoding these receptors are located on distinct chromosomes: NTRK1 (TRKA) on chromosome 1q21-q22, NTRK2 (TRKB) on 9q22.1, and NTRK3 (TRKC) on 15q25. The intracellular segment includes five critical tyrosine residues: three located in the kinase domain's activation loop, which are crucial for kinase function, and two on the opposite side, which act as docking sites for cytoplasmic adapters and enzymes in a phosphorylation-dependent manner. These structural features facilitate the receptor's role in signal transduction and interaction with neurotrophins.

encode for the tyrosine receptor kinase (TRK) proteins TRK-A, TRK-B, and TRK-C proteins, respectively [21]. These receptors bind specific growth factors as ligands and play essential roles in cell functions, such as promoting growth, differentiation, and apoptosis (**Figure 2**) [22, 23]. Under normal physiological conditions, TRK receptors and their ligands are critical for maintaining the balance between cell survival and cell death, particularly during the development of the central nervous system (CNS) [1]. Studies indicate that NTRK genes are predominantly expressed in the nervous system during both embryogenesis and tissue development. Proper neurotrophin and neurotrophin receptor levels in distinct nervous system regions are essential for maintaining neuronal homeostasis [24]. For instance, in the peripheral nervous system, NTRK signaling is vital for the survival of sensory and sympathetic ganglia. In the CNS, NTRK gene expression is required for neuron migration, growth, and maturation, as well as their successful integration into the cortical layers [25].

4. NTRK fusion in cancer development

The role of NTRK in tumor development is determined by the specific genetic alterations it undergoes. These changes include structural chromosomal rearrangements that result in gene fusions, splice variants, mutations, copy number variations, and increased expression levels. Among these, NTRK fusions are the most prevalent and hold significant clinical relevance due to their responsiveness to currently available targeted therapies [26]. Activation of TRK receptors due to NTRK gene fusions leads to continuous cancer cell growth. This interaction triggers signal transduction

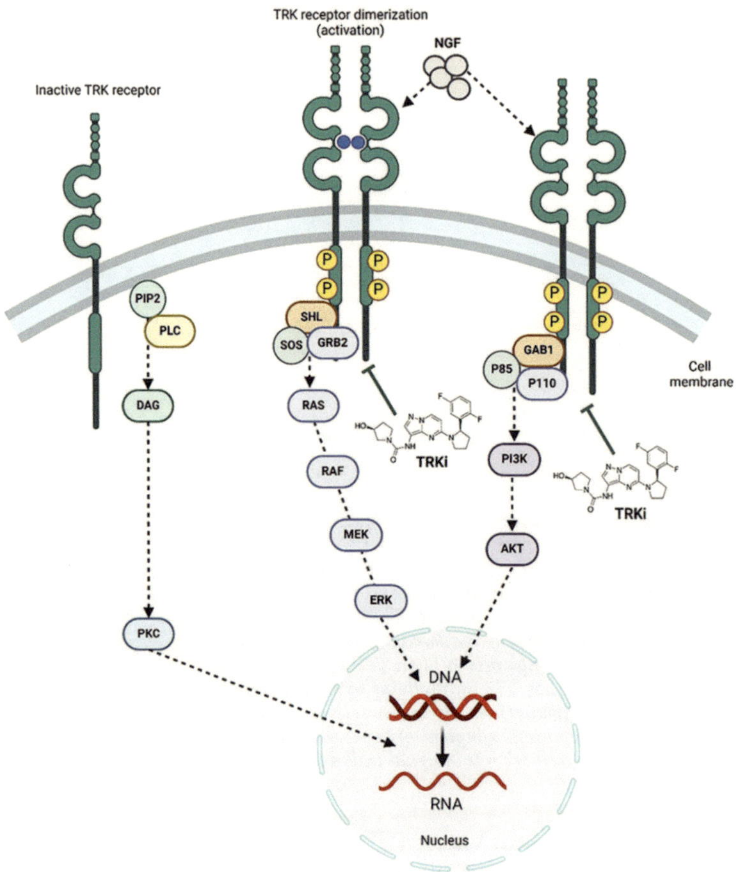

Figure 3.
Activation of TRK receptors and downstream signaling pathways. When neurotrophins bind to TRK receptors, the receptors undergo dimerization followed by autophosphorylation at specific tyrosine residues. This sequence of events is crucial for activating the kinase domain and initiating phosphorylation processes. These modifications enable adaptor proteins to bind, subsequently activating several downstream signaling pathways. For example, nerve growth factor (NGF) binding to TRKA activates the Ras/mitogen-activated protein kinase (MAPK) pathway, driving cellular proliferation and growth. Similarly, neurotrophins binding to TRKB trigger multiple pathways, which are critical for both neuronal survival and differentiation. In contrast, neurotrophin-3 (NT-3) primarily interacts with TRKC, preferentially activating the phosphatidylinositol-3-kinase (PI3K)/AKT pathway, which promotes cell survival and prevents apoptosis.

pathways that promote tumor development, including the Ras/mitogen-activated protein kinase (MAPK), phosphatidylinositol-3-kinase (PI3K)/Akt, and mammalian target of rapamycin (mTOR) pathways [27]. Highlighted in **Figure 3** is an overview of TRK signaling, highlighting the activation of TRKA and the involvement of cysteine-rich clusters.

5. NTRK fusions in CNS tumors

Although NTRK fusions are uncommon in most tumors, they are considered nearly pathognomonic in specific malignancies. Examples include breast secretory carcinomas, mammary analog secretory carcinomas of the salivary glands, infantile fibrosarcomas, and congenital or infantile mesoblastic nephroma, where their prevalence approaches 100% [1, 28, 29]. These fusions are more commonly identified in pediatric cases compared to adults regarding CNS tumors [30, 31]. An extensive analysis of 1465 primary CNS tumors revealed that about 0.6% harbored NTRK fusions. The affected cases included glioblastomas, primary neuroepithelial tumors, and anaplastic astrocytomas [32].

5.1 Gliomas

5.1.1 Pediatric high-grade gliomas (HGG)

HGGs in children represent a heterogeneous group of tumors that frequently lead to poor prognoses. Advances in molecular analyses have identified actionable genetic targets in this population, including NTRK fusions, which are reported in 4–6% of pediatric HGG cases [26, 30, 33]. This relatively high prevalence has made TRK inhibitors an appealing therapeutic approach to investigate for these patients.

5.1.2 Pediatric low-grade gliomas (LGG)

The latest WHO update on pediatric LGG reflects significant advances in the molecular classification of these tumors [2]. Frequent alterations in the MAPK pathway, particularly involving the BRAF gene, such as KIAA1549:BRAF fusions or BRAF V600E mutations, have been widely reported. Therapeutic interventions targeting BRAF mutations have shown significant clinical benefits for affected individuals [34]. Although rare, NTRK fusions have been identified in specific subtypes, including supratentorial low-grade gliomas (LGG) involving the NTRK2 gene [1, 35]. NTRK fusions have also been detected in low-grade and high-grade glioneuronal tumors, highlighting their potential as a therapeutic target in recurrent cases [36, 37].

5.1.3 Adult gliomas

HGGs remain the most prevalent primary brain tumor in adults and are associated with a poor prognosis, despite advancements in surgical and adjuvant treatment approaches [38]. Genetic studies have identified a range of potentially actionable alterations, including NTRK rearrangements, which are observed at varying frequencies, from 1% to as high as 40%, depending on the tumor's molecular and anatomical features [1]. Detecting alterations in NTRK1, NTRK2, or NTRK3 genes could open avenues for innovative therapies targeting NTRK-altered glioblastomas, underscoring the critical need for advanced diagnostic tools and strategies [39]. For LGGs in adults, NTRK1 fusions have been specifically documented in pilocytic astrocytomas [40].

5.2 Detection of NTRK fusions in CNS tumors

NTRK fusions result in the formation of fusion proteins that possess an active tyrosine kinase domain, driving persistent activation of downstream signaling pathways. Although uncommon, these fusions are observed at an average frequency of 0.31% across both pediatric and adult cancers [41]. Nonetheless, given their prevalence in CNS tumors and the lack of effective treatments, NTRK fusion detection is set to become essential in diagnosing these tumors [1]. Since NTRK fusions are now recognized as critical molecular markers in CNS tumors, their detection has the potential to transform patient outcomes through targeted therapies.

Testing for these alterations involves a multi-faceted approach, encompassing a variety of laboratory assays due to the complex nature of oncogenic activation that includes chromosomal rearrangements, gene translation, and protein expression [13]. Key methods involve DNA-centric approaches such as fluorescence in situ hybridization (FISH) and next-generation sequencing (NGS) targeting DNA, which examine chromosomal changes and potential gene rearrangements [1, 42]. Additionally, RNA-based methods like RT-PCR and RNA-NGS assess gene transcription levels, while immunohistochemical staining (IHC) evaluates protein expression, albeit with specificity challenges in CNS tumors due to NTRK's natural expression in neural tissues [4].

Each testing method presents its own advantages and limitations. For example, while IHC is cost-effective and quick, it lacks specificity for fusion variants and may yield false positives in CNS contexts, whereas FISH provides a more specific alternative for confirming NTRK fusions, though it is limited in screening due to the need for multiple independent assays [1]. NGS stands out for its comprehensive profiling capabilities, crucial for precision medicine's demands, but requires significant resources and expertise [32]. As a result, many diagnostic strategies now recommend starting with less specific but rapid IHC screening, followed by more precise but costly tests like NGS or FISH, to refine and confirm initial findings [1]. This tiered approach aligns with the ongoing shift toward integrating extensive molecular profiling, including NTRK fusion assessment, into routine diagnostics for CNS tumors, balancing cost, efficiency, and specificity.

5.3 Treatment for CNS tumors with NTRK gene fusion

The treatment and prognosis of oncological diseases have been profoundly influenced by the discovery of molecular alterations amenable to targeted therapies. While these strategies are now commonplace for cancers such as melanoma, lung, and breast cancer, their routine use in brain tumors remains limited. The identification of NTRK fusions in non-CNS tumors has spurred the development and evaluation of TRK inhibitors over the years. Among these therapies, entrectinib, a tyrosine kinase inhibitor (TKI) targeting TRK receptors (TrkA, TrkB, TrkC) as well as ROS1, was one of the first to be developed. Larotrectinib, a highly selective TRK inhibitor, is another FDA-approved option for treating both adults and children aged 12 years and older with NTRK fusions [43, 44]. However, further evidence is needed to assess the efficacy of these drugs specifically in CNS tumors. A recent review compiled data from four clinical trials that included six CNS tumor patients treated with entrectinib. Of these, four had primary brain tumors—three with HGG and one with an embryonal origin. All demonstrated significant objective responses, with over 50% tumor reduction in some cases and sustained disease control for up to 15 months [45].

For example, the STARTRK-NG trial enrolled 43 patients with a median age of 7 years. Of these, 16 had primary brain tumors, including HGGs, gangliogliomas, and medulloblastomas. Following entrectinib treatment, 50% of patients exhibited either complete or partial responses based on the RANO criteria, with the median duration of response yet to be determined [46]. These results are of great importance since it has been shown that even tumors with little therapeutic options, like diffuse midline gliomas, may harbor NTRK fusions [47], giving these patients additional options for treatment.

Several case studies highlight the potential of using NTRK inhibitors to treat tumors with NTRK or ROS1 fusions. For instance, Papusha et al. described two pediatric cases of supratentorial gliomas with ROS1 fusions. Both patients achieved complete tumor responses following entrectinib treatment [48]. Similarly, Miyachi et al. reported on a pediatric patient with a spinal cord diffuse high-grade glioma harboring an NTRK1 fusion. This patient experienced a durable response to entrectinib [49].

Despite these advances, there remains a significant unmet need for tolerable targeted therapies for children with TRK fusion-positive CNS tumors. Radiotherapy, a common treatment option, often results in long-term neurocognitive challenges [6]. Larotrectinib, a first-in-class, highly selective TRK inhibitor, has demonstrated durable and rapid responses, high disease control rates, and a favorable safety profile in CNS tumors, including both LGG and HGG [6, 50]. For pediatric patients with HGGs, which are associated with limited survival and few treatment options, targeted therapies such as larotrectinib offer an opportunity to improve disease control and delay reliance on more aggressive treatments [1, 51].

5.4 Brain metastases and NTRK fusions

Brain metastases are a common complication in advanced cancers and represent the most prevalent form of brain tumors. These metastases affect 10–26% of patients with a terminal diagnosis [52]. Frequently, they arise from primary malignancies known to exhibit NTRK alterations, including lung, breast, and colorectal cancers [1]. For example, non-small cell lung cancer (NSCLC), one of the leading causes of cancer-related deaths globally, develops brain metastases in as many as 50% of cases [45]. NTRK inhibitors, such as entrectinib and larotrectinib, have shown the ability to penetrate the blood-brain barrier, offering an effective therapeutic option for patients with NTRK fusion-positive brain metastases [1, 53]. Clinical trials have highlighted the significant intracranial efficacy of these inhibitors. Notably, entrectinib has been well-tolerated and effective in phase I and II trials, specifically in TKI-naïve NSCLC patients also diagnosed with brain metastases [44].

6. Conclusion

NTRK alterations, though rare in primary CNS tumors, are more commonly observed in the pediatric population. These genetic changes present a promising target for therapies that have shown encouraging results in improving patient outcomes. This is particularly critical for recurrent or treatment-resistant cases, where few therapeutic options exist.

Future research should prioritize enhancing diagnostic tools for detecting NTRK fusions in CNS tumors and investigating resistance mechanisms to NTRK inhibitors. Expanding clinical trials to include larger cohorts and diverse tumor types will be essential to validate these findings. Additionally, combining NTRK inhibitors with other therapies, such as immunotherapy or chemoradiotherapy, could offer synergistic benefits. Including brain metastases in studies of NTRK-targeted therapies may also provide a new avenue for treatment, offering hope for improved outcomes in these challenging cases.

Author's contributions

All authors contributed to the article and approved the submitted version.

Competing interests

Andrés F. Cardona discloses receiving financial research support from Merck Sharp & Dohme, Boehringer Ingelheim, Roche, Bristol-Myers Squibb, and The Foundation for Clinical and Applied Cancer Research (FICMAC). Additionally, he has served as an advisor, participated in speakers' bureaus, and provided expert testimony for various companies, including Merck Sharp & Dohme, Boehringer Ingelheim, Roche, Bristol-Myers Squibb, Pfizer, Novartis, Celldex Therapeutics, Foundation Medicine, Eli Lilly, and Bayer.

Ethics approval

None.

Author details

Javier A. Jacobo[1*], Nicolle Wagner-Gutiérrez[2], Jorge H. Aristizabal[1], Santiago Vallejo[1], Alejandro González[1], Iván Bobadilla[1], Diego Pineda[1], Oscar Arrieta[3] and Andres F. Cardona[1,4]

1 Neuro-Oncology Unit, Luis Carlos Sarmiento Angulo Cancer Treatment and Research Center – CTIC, Bogotá, Colombia

2 School of Global Public Health, University of North Carolina at Chapel Hill, Chapel Hill, NC, USA

3 General Direction, National Cancer Institute Mexico (INCan), Mexico City, Mexico

4 Institute of Research and Education, Luis Carlos Sarmiento Angulo Cancer Treatment and Research Center – CTIC, Bogotá, Colombia

*Address all correspondence to: jacoboncx@gmail.com

References

[1] Gambella A, Senetta R, Collemi G, Vallero SG, Monticelli M, Cofano F, et al. NTRK fusions in central nervous system tumors: A rare, but worthy target. International Journal of Molecular Sciences. 2020;**21**(3):753

[2] Louis DN, Perry A, Wesseling P, Brat DJ, Cree IA, Figarella-Branger D, et al. The 2021 WHO classification of tumors of the central nervous system: A summary. Neuro-Oncology. 2021;**23**(8):1231-1251

[3] Smolarska A, Pruszynska I, Wasylko W, Godlewska K, Markowska M, Rybak A, et al. Targeted therapies for glioblastoma treatment. Journal of Physiology and Pharmacology. 2023;**74**(3):251-261

[4] Gatalica Z, Xiu J, Swensen J, Vranic S. Molecular characterization of cancers with NTRK gene fusions. Modern Pathology. 2019;**32**(1):147-153

[5] Cocco E, Scaltriti M, Drilon A. NTRK fusion-positive cancers and TRK inhibitor therapy. Nature Reviews. Clinical Oncology. 2018;**15**(12):731-747

[6] Doz F, van Tilburg CM, Geoerger B, Højgaard M, Øra I, Boni V, et al. Efficacy and safety of larotrectinib in TRK fusion-positive primary central nervous system tumors. Neuro-Oncology. 2022;**24**(6):997-1007

[7] Maher CA, Kumar-Sinha C, Cao X, Kalyana-Sundaram S, Han B, Jing X, et al. Transcriptome sequencing to detect gene fusions in cancer. Nature. 2009;**458**(7234):97-101

[8] Annala MJ, Parker BC, Zhang W, Nykter M. Fusion genes and their discovery using high throughput sequencing. Cancer Letters. 2013;**340**(2):192-200

[9] Shah N, Lankerovich M, Lee H, Yoon JG, Schroeder B, Foltz G. Exploration of the gene fusion landscape of glioblastoma using transcriptome sequencing and copy number data. BMC Genomics. 2013;**14**(1):818

[10] Malhotra A, Lindberg M, Faust GG, Leibowitz ML, Clark RA, Layer RM, et al. Breakpoint profiling of 64 cancer genomes reveals numerous complex rearrangements spawned by homology-independent mechanisms. Genome Research. 2013;**23**(5):762-776

[11] Kim T, Lee A, Ahn S, Park JS, Jeun SS, Lee YS. Comprehensive molecular genetic analysis in glioma patients by next generation sequencing. Brain Tumor Research and Treatment. 2024;**12**(1):23-39

[12] Charest A, Lane K, McMahon K, Park J, Preisinger E, Conroy H, et al. Fusion of FIG to the receptor tyrosine kinase ROS in a glioblastoma with an interstitial del(6)(q21q21). Genes, Chromosomes & Cancer. 2003;**37**(1):58-71

[13] You G, Fan X, Hu H, Jiang T, Chen CC. Fusion genes altered in adult malignant gliomas. Frontiers in Neurology [Internet]. 2021;**12**. Available from: https://www.frontiersin.org/journals/neurology/articles/10.3389/fneur.2021.715206/full [Accessed: December 28, 2024]

[14] Singh D, Chan JM, Zoppoli P, Niola F, Sullivan R, Castano A, et al. Transforming fusions of FGFR and TACC genes in human glioblastoma. Science. 2012;**337**(6099):1231-1235

[15] Parker BC, Annala MJ, Cogdell DE, Granberg KJ, Sun Y, Ji P, et al. The tumorigenic FGFR3-TACC3 gene fusion escapes miR-99a regulation in glioblastoma. The Journal of Clinical Investigation. 2013;**123**(2):855-865

[16] Katoh M, Loriot Y, Brandi G, Tavolari S, Wainberg ZA, Katoh M. FGFR-targeted therapeutics: Clinical activity, mechanisms of resistance and new directions. Nature Reviews. Clinical Oncology. 2024;**21**(4):312-329

[17] Zhang J, Babic A. Regulation of the MET oncogene: Molecular mechanisms. Carcinogenesis. 2016;**37**(4):345-355

[18] Bao ZS, Chen HM, Yang MY, Zhang CB, Yu K, Ye WL, et al. RNA-seq of 272 gliomas revealed a novel, recurrent PTPRZ1-MET fusion transcript in secondary glioblastomas. Genome Research. 2014;**24**(11):1765-1773

[19] Hu H, Mu Q, Bao Z, Chen Y, Liu Y, Chen J, et al. Mutational landscape of secondary glioblastoma guides MET-Targeted trial in brain tumor. Cell. 2018;**175**(6):1665-1678.e18

[20] International Cancer Genome Consortium PedBrain Tumor Project. Recurrent MET fusion genes represent a drug target in pediatric glioblastoma. Nature Medicine. 2016;**22**(11):1314-1320

[21] Valent A, Danglot G, Bernheim A. Mapping of the tyrosine kinase receptors trkA (NTRK1), trkB (NTRK2) and trkC(NTRK3) to human chromosomes 1q22, 9q22 and 15q25 by fluorescence in situ hybridization. European Journal of Human Genetics. 1997;**5**(2):102-104

[22] Du Z, Lovly CM. Mechanisms of receptor tyrosine kinase activation in cancer. Molecular Cancer. 2018;**17**(1):58

[23] Marchetti L, Bonsignore F, Gobbo F, Amodeo R, Calvello M, Jacob A, et al. Fast-diffusing p75NTR monomers support apoptosis and growth cone collapse by neurotrophin ligands. Proceedings of the National Academy of Sciences of the United States of America. 2019;**116**(43):21563-21572

[24] Tchetchelnitski V, van den Eijnden M, Schmidt F, Stoker AW. Developmental co-expression and functional redundancy of tyrosine phosphatases with neurotrophin receptors in developing sensory neurons. International Journal of Developmental Neuroscience. 2014;**34**:48-59

[25] Medina DL, Sciarretta C, Calella AM, von Bohlen und Halbach O, Unsicker K, Minichiello L. TrkB regulates neocortex formation through the Shc/PLCγ-mediated control of neuronal migration. The EMBO Journal. 2004;**23**(19):3803-3814

[26] Okamura R, Boichard A, Kato S, Sicklick JK, Bazhenova L, Kurzrock R. Analysis of NTRK alterations in pan-cancer adult and pediatric malignancies: Implications for NTRK-targeted therapeutics. JCO Precision Oncology. 2018;**2018**:PO.18.00183

[27] Liu F, Wei Y, Zhang H, Jiang J, Zhang P, Chu Q. NTRK fusion in non-small cell lung cancer: Diagnosis, therapy, and TRK inhibitor resistance. Frontiers in Oncology. 2022;**12**:864666

[28] Hung YP, Jo VY, Hornick JL. Immunohistochemistry with a pan-TRK antibody distinguishes secretory carcinoma of the salivary gland from acinic cell carcinoma. Histopathology. 2019;**75**(1):54-62

[29] Xu B, Haroon Al Rasheed MR, Antonescu CR, Alex D, Frosina D, Ghossein R, et al. Pan-Trk immunohistochemistry is a sensitive and specific ancillary tool for diagnosing

secretory carcinoma of the salivary gland and detecting ETV6-NTRK3 fusion. Histopathology. 2020;**76**(3):375-382

[30] Lang SS, Kumar NK, Madsen P, Gajjar AA, Gajjar E, Resnick AC, et al. Neurotrophic tyrosine receptor kinase fusion in pediatric central nervous system tumors. Cancer Genetics. 2022;**262-263**:64-70

[31] Zhang Y, Chen F, Donehower LA, Scheurer ME, Creighton CJ. A pediatric brain tumor atlas of genes deregulated by somatic genomic rearrangement. Nature Communications. 2021;**12**(1):937

[32] Solomon JP, Linkov I, Rosado A, Mullaney K, Rosen EY, Frosina D, et al. NTRK fusion detection across multiple assays and 33,997 cases: Diagnostic implications and pitfalls. Modern Pathology. 2020;**33**(1):38-46

[33] Wu G, Diaz AK, Paugh BS, Rankin SL, Ju B, Li Y, et al. The genomic landscape of diffuse intrinsic pontine glioma and pediatric non-brainstem high-grade glioma. Nature Genetics. 2014;**46**(5):444-450

[34] Rosenberg T, Yeo KK, Mauguen A, Alexandrescu S, Prabhu SP, Tsai JW, et al. Upfront molecular targeted therapy for the treatment of BRAF-mutant pediatric high-grade glioma. Neuro-Oncology. 2022;**24**(11):1964-1975

[35] Jones DTW, Hutter B, Jäger N, Korshunov A, Kool M, Warnatz HJ, et al. Recurrent somatic alterations of FGFR1 and NTRK2 in pilocytic astrocytoma. Nature Genetics. 2013;**45**(8):927-932

[36] Deng MY, Sill M, Chiang J, Schittenhelm J, Ebinger M, Schuhmann MU, et al. Molecularly defined diffuse leptomeningeal glioneuronal tumor (DLGNT) comprises two subgroups with distinct clinical and genetic features. Acta Neuropathologica. 2018;**136**(2):239-253

[37] Prabhakaran N, Guzman MA, Navalkele P, Chow-Maneval E, Batanian JR. Novel TLE4-NTRK2 fusion in a ganglioglioma identified by array-CGH and confirmed by NGS: Potential for a gene targeted therapy. Neuropathology. 2018;**38**(4):380-386

[38] Cantrell JN, Waddle MR, Rotman M, Peterson JL, Ruiz-Garcia H, Heckman MG, et al. Progress toward long-term survivors of glioblastoma. Mayo Clinic Proceedings. 2019;**94**(7):1278-1286

[39] Bourhis A, Caumont C, Quintin-Roué I, Magro E, Dissaux G, Remoué A, et al. Detection of *NTRK* fusions in glioblastoma: Fluorescent *in situ* hybridisation is more useful than pan-TRK immunohistochemistry as a screening tool prior to RNA sequencing. Pathology. 2022;**54**(1):55-62

[40] Ferguson SD, Zhou S, Huse JT, de Groot JF, Xiu J, Subramaniam DS, et al. Targetable gene fusions associate with the IDH wild-type astrocytic lineage in adult gliomas. Journal of Neuropathology and Experimental Neurology. 2018;**77**(6):437-442

[41] Wang Y, Long P, Wang Y, Ma W. NTRK fusions and TRK inhibitors: Potential targeted therapies for adult glioblastoma. Frontiers in Oncology. 2020;**10**:593578

[42] Solomon JP, Hechtman JF. Detection of NTRK fusions: Merits and limitations of current diagnostic platforms. Cancer Research. 2019;**79**(13):3163-3168

[43] Drilon A. TRK inhibitors in TRK fusion-positive cancers. Annals of Oncology. 2019;**30** (Suppl. 8):viii23-viii30

[44] Sartore-Bianchi A, Pizzutilo EG, Marrapese G, Tosi F, Cerea G, Siena S. Entrectinib for the treatment of metastatic NSCLC: Safety and efficacy. Expert Review of Anticancer Therapy. 2020;**20**(5):333-341

[45] Tan AC, Itchins M, Khasraw M. Brain metastases in lung cancers with emerging targetable fusion drivers. International Journal of Molecular Sciences. 2020;**21**(4):1416

[46] Desai AV, Robinson GW, Gauvain K, Basu EM, Macy ME, Maese L, et al. Entrectinib in children and young adults with solid or primary CNS tumors harboring NTRK, ROS1, or ALK aberrations (STARTRK-NG). Neuro-Oncology. 2022;**24**(10):1776-1789

[47] Dahl NA, Donson AM, Sanford B, Wang D, Walker FM, Gilani A, et al. NTRK fusions can co-occur with H3K27M mutations and may define druggable subclones within diffuse midline gliomas. Journal of Neuropathology and Experimental Neurology. 2021;**80**(4):345-353

[48] Papusha L, Zaytseva M, Panferova A, Druy A, Valiakhmetova A, Artemov A, et al. Two clinically distinct cases of infant hemispheric glioma carrying ZCCHC8:ROS1 fusion and responding to entrectinib. Neuro-Oncology. 2022;**24**(6):1029-1031

[49] Miyachi M, Sugimoto Y, Sugitatsu Y, Tomida A, Yoshida H, Tsuchiya K, et al. Entrectinib treatment induces a durable response against ARHGEF11::NTRK1 fusion gene-positive spinal cord diffuse pediatric-type high-grade glioma. Pediatric Blood & Cancer. 2023;**70**(10):e30513

[50] Hong DS, DuBois SG, Kummar S, Farago AF, Albert CM, Rohrberg KS, et al. Larotrectinib in patients with TRK fusion-positive solid tumours: A pooled analysis of three phase 1/2 clinical trials. The Lancet Oncology. 2020;**21**(4):531-540

[51] Bornhorst M, Hwang EI. Molecularly targeted agents in the therapy of pediatric brain tumors. Paediatric Drugs. 2020;**22**(1):45-54

[52] Amsbaugh MJ, Kim CS. Brain metastasis. In: StatPearls [Internet]. Treasure Island (FL): StatPearls Publishing; 2024. Available from: http://www.ncbi.nlm.nih.gov/books/NBK470246/ [Accessed: May 29, 2024]

[53] Liu D, Offin M, Harnicar S, Li BT, Drilon A. Entrectinib: An orally available, selective tyrosine kinase inhibitor for the treatment of NTRK, ROS1, and ALK fusion-positive solid tumors. Therapeutics and Clinical Risk Management. 2018;**14**:1247-1252

Chapter 9

Basic Research Advances and Challenges in NF1 and NF2 Related Pediatric Tumors

Qian Dai, Xuan Zhai and Jie Huang

Abstract

This chapter provides a comprehensive overview of the research progress and challenges in neurofibromatosis type 1 (NF1) and neurofibromatosis type 2 (NF2), with a focus on pediatric tumors. First, the chapter discusses the genetic and molecular mechanisms of NF1 and NF2, focusing on the key gene mutations that lead to complex pathologies and different clinical manifestations. Then, the chapter discusses the significant impact of advanced genetic, biochemical, and imaging technologies such as high-throughput sequencing and CRISPR/Cas9 gene editing on advancing the research and treatment of these diseases. The chapter also evaluates the advantages of traditional animal models (including mice, zebrafish, and fruit flies) and their application in studying NF1 and NF2, while analyzing the challenges these models face in modeling the genetic heterogeneity of these diseases. Finally, the chapter discusses emerging therapies such as gene therapy, small molecule drugs, and personalized medicine, which offer hope for more effective treatments. The chapter concludes that continued research and interdisciplinary collaboration are essential to translate scientific discoveries into clinical applications, ultimately improving the treatment outcomes of children with NF1- and NF2-related tumors.

Keywords: NF1 and NF2, pediatric tumors, basic research advances and challenges, cutting-edge technologies, animal models, emerging treatments

1. Introduction

Neurofibromatosis type 1 (NF1) and neurofibromatosis type 2 (NF2) are two autosomal dominant inherited disorders that primarily affect the nervous system, often leading to noncancerous and cancerous tumors, and presenting significant diagnostic and therapeutic challenges, especially for pediatric patients.

NF1, or von Recklinghausen disease, occurs in approximately 1 in 3000 live births and is caused by mutations in the NF1 gene, which encodes the tumor suppressor protein neurofibromin, which regulates the RAS/MAPK signaling pathway [1]. Dysfunction of NF1 leads to uncontrolled cell proliferation and tumor development, manifesting as symptoms such as café-au-lait spots, Lisch nodules, and more severe forms such as plexiform neurofibromas and optic pathway gliomas [2, 3]. Advanced molecular genetic techniques such as high-throughput sequencing have greatly advanced our understanding of NF1 by identifying the various mutations and their effects, guiding the development of targeted therapies such as MEK inhibitors, which have shown promising results in shrinking tumors and improving symptoms in clinical trials [4, 5]. NF2, a disease characterized by bilateral vestibular schwannomas (VS) and meningiomas, affects 1 in 25,000 newborns and is characterized by mutations in the NF2 gene encoding Merlin, a protein that regulates multiple signaling pathways, including the Hippo pathway [6]. Loss of Merlin function leads to conditions such as bilateral vestibular schwannomas and meningiomas, and patients often experience hearing loss, tinnitus, and balance problems [7, 8]. Studies have shown that Merlin interacts with cellular structures to maintain cell integrity and inhibit tumor growth, highlighting potential treatments such as FAK inhibitors that target the pathways activated by Merlin deficiency [9].

Despite advancements, the diversity of clinical presentations complicates early diagnosis and treatment of NF1 and NF2 [10, 11]. For example, some children experiencing minimal symptoms despite severe underlying pathology. Regarding the treatment strategies, especially surgical intervention for symptomatic tumors, carry significant risks for children, and emerging therapies require careful evaluation of their long-term efficacy and safety. Furthermore, reliable biomarkers are urgently needed to track disease progression and assess treatment efficacy, highlighting the need for more personalized and effective management strategies, emphasizing the need for continued research and multidisciplinary collaboration to improve outcomes for pediatric patients with these challenging diseases [12, 13].

In this chapter, we discuss the advances and challenges in basic research on NF1 and NF2-related childhood tumors, focusing on the following key areas: (1) Genetic and molecular basis, which will provide an introduction to the basic genetic and molecular basis of these diseases; (2) Basic research and technological advances, which will highlight some of the latest innovations in research methods and technologies; (3) Challenges in basic research, which will focus on the obstacles encountered in developing treatments for these diseases; and (4) Future directions and emerging areas, which will explore potential research directions and new research areas that may affect future treatment strategies.

2. Genetic and molecular basis

2.1 NF1 gene mutations and tumor development

Neurofibromatosis type 1 (NF1) is associated with mutations in the NF1 gene, which is located on chromosome 17q11.2 and is approximately 350 kb long with 60 exons, making it one of the largest human genes [14]. The gene encodes neurofibromin, an important protein composed of 2818 amino acids that functions as a GTPase-activating protein (GAP) and is critical for regulating the RAS/MAPK signaling pathway [15]. Variants in the NF1 gene, including missense, nonsense, splice site mutations, deletions, and insertions, often result in loss of neurofibromin function. This loss leads to uncontrolled Ras activity, resulting in excessive cell proliferation and reduced apoptosis, which promotes the formation of benign and malignant tumors, such as neurofibromas and malignant peripheral nerve sheath

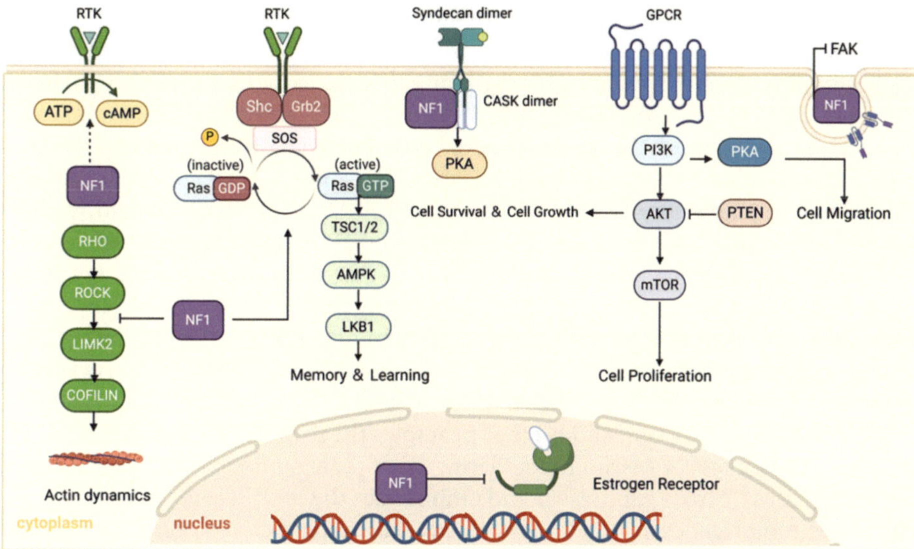

Figure 1.
NF1 signaling pathways. The neurofibromatosis type 1 (NF1) gene plays a crucial role in regulating cellular functions through several key signaling pathways. As a tumor suppressor protein, NF1 controls the RAS/MAPK pathway, which is essential for cell survival and growth. The figure illustrates how the interaction of NF1 with the Ras protein promotes the conversion of Ras from its inactive GDP-bound form to its active GTP-bound form, thereby affecting downstream pathways such as cell survival through the AMPK pathway and cell proliferation through the mTOR pathway. In addition, NF1 interacts with proteins such as syndecan and CASK to regulate cell survival, growth, and migration, as shown by its activation of PKA and its effects on the PI3K pathway. The figure also depicts the role of NF1 in actin dynamics through the Rho and ROCK pathways, thereby affecting cell structure and motility. Moreover, NF1 may be involved in regulating memory and learning through the TSC1/2 and AMPK pathways. Together, this complex signaling network highlights the multifaceted roles of NF1 in cellular processes beyond its tumor suppressor function.

tumors (MPNSTs) [16, 17]. Dysregulation of Schwann cells, fibroblasts, and other cell types underlies the development of a large portion of tumors in NF1 [18]. A key role of neurofibromin is to ensure tight regulation of Ras activity in the RAS/MAPK pathway, which is critical for transmitting signals that affect gene expression and cell cycle progression [19]. Overactivation of this pathway due to NF1 mutations is a major driver of tumorigenesis, often leading to a variety of tumors, including neurofibromas and gliomas [20]. In addition, loss of heterozygosity at the NF1 locus exacerbates tumor progression, making NF1 a complex and challenging disease that requires extensive medical and genetic research to better understand and effectively manage the disease (**Figure 1**) [21].

2.2 NF2 gene mutations and tumor development

The NF2 gene is located on chromosome 22q12.2, is approximately 110 kb long, has 17 exons, and encodes Merlin, a protein from the ezrin-radixin-moesin (ERM) family [22]. This family of proteins links the actin cytoskeleton to the plasma membrane, plays a key role in signal transduction, and is essential for cellular communication and structural integrity [23]. NF2 gene mutations mainly include nonsense mutations and frameshift mutations, resulting in truncated and non-functional Merlin proteins. These deleterious mutations disrupt the ability of Merlin to inhibit key oncogenic pathways, thereby promoting the development of various tumors, especially schwannomas, meningiomas, and ependymomas [24].

The function of Merlin extends to regulating the Hippo pathway, a key regulator of organ size and tissue homeostasis, which regulates cell proliferation and apoptosis. This pathway acts through the transcriptional coactivators YAP and TAZ to promote cell growth and inhibit programmed cell death [25]. Under normal conditions, Merlin activates the Hippo pathway kinases MST1/2 and LATS1/2, which subsequently phosphorylate and inhibit YAP/TAZ activity. Therefore, NF2 gene mutations lead to loss of Merlin function, resulting in uncontrolled YAP/TAZ activity, increased cell proliferation, and improved survival, significantly promoting tumor development [26]. In addition, Merlin's interactions with various cell membrane proteins affect cell adhesion and communication, which are essential for maintaining proper cell structure and preventing tumorigenesis [27]. The loss of these interactions due to NF2 mutations disrupts normal cell function and further promotes the malignant transformation of cells. The complex role of Merlin in regulating multiple signaling pathways highlights its importance as a tumor suppressor and emphasizes the multifaceted nature of NF2-related tumorigenesis [28]. This complex relationship between gene mutations and cell behavior emphasizes the need for targeted therapeutic strategies to correct or compensate for disrupted pathways and restore normal cell function (**Figure 2**).

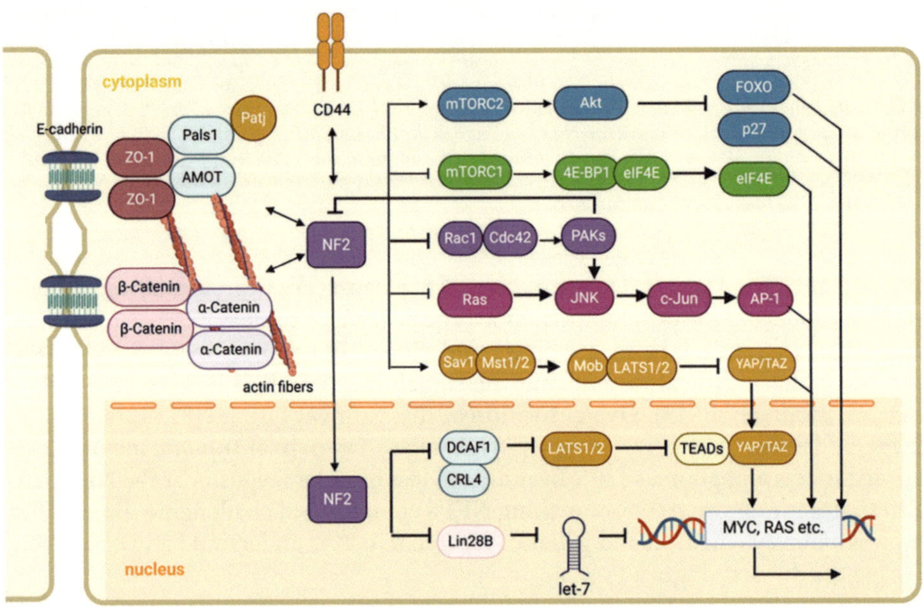

Figure 2.
NF2 signaling pathways. Merlin is a protein encoded by the neurofibromatosis type 2 (NF2) gene that plays a central role in regulating a variety of cellular processes. The figure shows the role of Merlin in cell-cell junctions and its interaction with E-cadherin and catenin attached to actin fibers, highlighting its critical role in maintaining cell adhesion and structural integrity. In addition, the figure details Merlin's effects on the mTOR signaling pathway (mTORC1 and mTORC2), which are key regulators of cell growth and survival through interaction with Akt signaling. Merlin also affects the RAS pathway through Rac1, Cdc42, and PAK, leading to the activation of JNK and transcription factors such as c-Jun and AP-1, which control cell proliferation and apoptosis. In addition, the figure focuses on Merlin's regulation of the Hippo pathway, highlighting its interactions with components such as Sav1 and Mst1/2 to control the activity of YAP/TAZ transcription factors, which are essential for the expression of genes involved in growth and apoptosis. Finally, the pathway outlines Merlin's broader regulatory functions, including control of important oncogenes such as MYC and RAS, highlighting its tumor suppressor role in the pathogenesis of NF2.

3. Basic research and technological advances

3.1 Research innovations in genetic, biochemical, and imaging technologies

In recent years, innovations in genetic, biochemical, and imaging technologies have led to major advances in neurofibromatosis research, enhancing our understanding of NF1 and NF2 and facilitating new diagnostic and therapeutic strategies. High-throughput sequencing, including whole-genome and whole-exome sequencing, has revolutionized the detection of mutations associated with these diseases, revealing a wide range of genetic abnormalities such as point mutations, insertions, deletions, and complex rearrangements [29, 30]. This ability to rapidly and cost-effectively sequence entire genomes has provided key insights into the genetic diversity and complexity of the disease, enabling more precise diagnosis and tailored personalized treatment. The introduction of CRISPR/Cas9 gene editing has further expanded research possibilities, allowing for the creation of precise gene knockouts or the introduction of specific mutations to model the disease in a variety of cell lines and animal models [31]. This capability facilitates detailed studies of the effects of mutations and the exploration of new therapeutic targets, with the potential to directly correct pathological mutations in patients in future gene therapy applications. At the same time, advances in proteomics and metabolomics have deepened our understanding of the molecular pathways altered in NF1 and NF2 [32, 33]. Techniques such as mass spectrometry can exhaustively analyze protein expression and post-translational modifications, revealing key regulators and signaling networks affected by mutations, while metabolomic analysis can identify metabolic changes associated with tumor development and provide biomarkers for early diagnosis and monitoring of treatment response [34, 35]. Imaging technologies are also evolving; MRI, a long-standing tool for diagnosing and monitoring NF-related tumors, now benefits from high-resolution and functional MRI enhancements that allow for better detection and characterization of tumors at an early stage [36]. Detailed imaging data supports precise surgical planning and evaluation of treatment efficacy. In addition, PET imaging, often used in conjunction with MRI or CT, provides functional insights into tumor metabolism and activity through radioactive tracers that can highlight active tumor areas and help assess tumor aggressiveness and treatment response [37]. In addition, emerging optical imaging techniques such as fluorescence and bioluminescence imaging can visualize molecular and cellular processes in living tissue in real time, which is valuable for preclinical studies tracking tumor progression and evaluating experimental treatments in animal models [38]. Together, these technological advances are advancing our understanding and management of neurofibromatosis, with the promise of more effective interventions and improved patient outcomes.

3.2 Advances in animal models

The development and improvement of animal models has greatly improved our understanding of neurofibromatosis type 1 (NF1) and neurofibromatosis type 2 (NF2). Traditional mouse models, including knockout and conditional knockout, have elucidated the role of neurofibromin and Merlin (proteins encoded by the NF1 and NF2 genes) in tumor formation and the specific effects of these mutations on tissue behavior [39]. These models closely resemble aspects of human disease, such as the development of benign and malignant tumors, and have played an important role in studying the tumor microenvironment and revealing key interactions and pathways that promote tumor growth. Other animal models, such as the novel zebrafish model, have the advantages of genetic similarity to humans, rapid development, and high transparency, allowing real-time observation of developmental processes and tumor progression [40]. Zebrafish are valuable for high-throughput screening and genetic interaction studies, and CRISPR/Cas9 technology can be used to create accurate disease models and identify therapeutic targets. In addition, the fruit fly model provides a simplified system with a short life cycle that is well suited for genetic studies, facilitating the discovery of conserved pathways and the regulation of cell proliferation and cytoskeletal dynamics [41]. High-throughput genetic screens in Drosophila have further identified modifiers of NF1 and NF2 phenotypes, enhancing our understanding of the genetic networks involved in tumorigenesis. Collectively, these animal models are essential for advancing the study and development of targeted therapies for NF1 and NF2.

4. Challenges in basic research

4.1 Complexity in the genetic and molecular pathology of NF1 and NF2

Studying NF1 and NF2 presents significant challenges due to the genetic heterogeneity of these diseases. The NF1 gene has 60 exons and is susceptible to a variety of mutations, such as missense, nonsense, splice site mutations, deletions, and insertions, each of which can have different effects on neurofibromin function and lead to different disease manifestations and severity [42]. Similarly, NF2 is also marked by a variety of mutations, including nonsense and frameshift mutations that produce truncated Merlin proteins, which increases the difficulty of a comprehensive understanding of disease mechanisms and the development of universal treatments [43]. Both diseases involve complex pathways; NF1 mutations affect neurofibromin regulation of the key RAS/MAPK pathway, which is essential for cell proliferation and differentiation. Loss of function of neurofibromin leads to overactivity of this pathway, although the specific downstream effects may vary depending on the cellular context [15–17, 19]. Merlin, encoded by NF2, interacts with several signaling pathways, especially the Hippo pathway, to affect cell proliferation and apoptosis [25, 26]. The multifaceted roles of these proteins in different tissues and developmental stages provide additional layers to the understanding of mutation-driven tumorigenesis. In addition, the tumor microenvironment (including the interactions between tumor cells, stromal cells, immune cells, and extracellular matrix components) significantly affects tumor progression and treatment response [44], necessitating a comprehensive understanding of both the intrinsic properties of the tumor and extrinsic environmental factors.

4.2 Difficulties of replicating human disease in model systems

Although mouse models play a key role in studying NF1 and NF2, their genetic and biological differences from humans may influence disease manifestations and drug response. NF1 or NF2 mutant mice often exhibit different tumor types, frequencies, and progression than human patients, and their shorter lifespan and different immune systems limit the study of long-term disease progression and immune interactions [45, 46]. Zebrafish and Drosophila have advantages such as high-throughput screening and real-time imaging, but also face limitations due to significant physiological and anatomical differences from humans, which may hinder their ability to fully replicate human disease pathology [47, 48]. To bridge these gaps, humanized models such as patient-derived xenografts and organoids are being developed by scientists [49]. Although xenografts can improve modeling of human tumor biology, they lack comprehensive human immune system and microenvironmental interactions. Organoids provide a promising platform for exploring human-specific disease mechanisms and therapeutic responses, but improvements are still needed to more accurately model complex tumor cell interactions.

5. Future directions and emerging fields

Gene therapy is a promising approach for treating NF1 and NF2. Advances in CRISPR/Cas9 technology have paved the way for precision gene editing, making it possible to correct disease-causing mutations directly within the genome [50]. For NF1 and NF2, targeted gene editing has the potential to restore the normal function of neurofibromin and merlin, respectively, thereby halting or even reversing tumor progression. Although challenges such as off-target effects and effective delivery systems need to be addressed, ongoing research and clinical trials are making significant progress, making gene therapy a viable treatment option [51, 52]. The development of small molecules and biologics that specifically target aberrant pathways in NF1 and NF2 is another key area of research. For example, MEK inhibitors have shown promise in treating NF1-associated plexiform neurofibromas by inhibiting the overactive RAS/MAPK pathway [53]. Similarly, drugs targeting the Hippo pathway in NF2, such as FAK inhibitors, are under investigation [54]. Personalized medicine approaches that leverage the detailed genetic and molecular profiles of individual patients can improve efficacy and reduce side effects of treatment, thereby providing more targeted and effective treatment options.

6. Conclusion

Significant advances in basic research have not only deepened our understanding of the genetic and molecular basis of NF1 and NF2, but also promoted the development of innovative therapeutic strategies. The application of high-throughput sequencing technology and CRISPR/Cas9 gene editing technology has revolutionized the study of these diseases, and advanced animal models have also provided key insights into the mechanisms of tumorigenesis. Despite significant advances in these technologies, accurately replicating human disease features in model systems and addressing the challenges of genetic complexity remain difficult research problems. Frontier fields such as gene therapy, molecular medicine, and systems biology demonstrate the potential to overcome these obstacles and provide more effective and personalized treatment options. Therefore, continued interdisciplinary research and technological innovation are essential to translate these scientific breakthroughs into clinical applications, which will greatly improve the treatment outcomes and prognosis of pediatric patients with NF1 and NF2.

Acknowledgements

We gratefully acknowledge Yi Liu for the design of figures.

Author contributions

Q.D., X.Z. and J.H. wrote the manuscript. J.H. reread and corrected the manuscript and proposed and drew figures. All authors have read and agreed to the published version of the manuscript.

Funding

None.

Conflicts of interest

The authors declare no conflict of interest.

Author details

Qian Dai[1], Xuan Zhai[2] and Jie Huang[3,4*]

1 Clinical Research Center, The Xinqiao Hospital, Army Medical University, Chongqing, China

2 Department of Neurosurgery, Children's Hospital of Chongqing Medical University, National Clinical Research Center for Child Health and Disorders, Ministry of Education Key Laboratory of Child Development and Disorders, Chongqing Key Laboratory of Child Neurodevelopment and Cognitive Disorders, Chongqing, China

3 International In Vitro Diagnostic Research Institute, Chongqing Medical University and Beituo Qiming Biomedical Research Institute Ltd., Chongqing, China

4 CSTEAM Biotechnology LLC, Dublin, Ohio, USA

*Address all correspondence to: jhuang11_9@hotmail.com

References

[1] Wang W et al. Impacts of NF1 gene mutations and genetic modifiers in neurofibromatosis type 1. Frontiers in Neurology. 2021;**12**:704639. DOI: 10.3389/fneur.2021.704639

[2] Ozarslan B et al. Cutaneous findings in neurofibromatosis type 1. Cancers. 2021;**13**:463. DOI: 10.3390/cancers13030463

[3] Solares I et al. Novel molecular targeted therapies for patients with neurofibromatosis type 1 with inoperable plexiform neurofibromas: A comprehensive review. ESMO Open. 2021;**6**:100223. DOI: 10.1016/j.esmoop.2021.100223

[4] Philpott C et al. The NF1 somatic mutational landscape in sporadic human cancers. Human Genomics. 2017;**11**:13. DOI: 10.1186/s40246-017-0109-3

[5] Pasmant E et al. Neurofibromatosis type 1 molecular diagnosis: What can NGS do for you when you have a large gene with loss of function mutations? European Journal of Human Genetics. 2015;**23**:596-601. DOI: 10.1038/ejhg.2014.145

[6] Gareth Evans D. NF2-related schwannomatosis, synonyms: Neurofibromatosis 2, neurofibromatosis type II. GeneReviews. 1993-2024. ISSN: 2372-0697. Available from: https://www.ncbi.nlm.nih.gov/books/NBK1201/

[7] Bachir S et al. Neurofibromatosis type 2 (NF2) and the implications for vestibular schwannoma and meningioma pathogenesis. International Journal of Molecular Sciences. 2021;**22**:690. DOI: 10.3390/ijms22020690

[8] Moualed D et al. Prevalence and natural history of schwannomas in neurofibromatosis type 2 (NF2): The influence of pathogenic variants. European Journal of Human Genetics. 2022;**30**:458-464. DOI: 10.1038/s41431-021-01029-y

[9] Petrilli A, Fernandez-Valle C. Role of merlin/NF2 inactivation in tumor biology. Oncogene. 2016;**35**:537-548. DOI: 10.1038/onc.2015.125

[10] Choi J et al. Current concepts of neurofibromatosis type 1: Pathophysiology and treatment. Archives of Craniofacial Surgery. 2022;**23**:6-16. DOI: 10.7181/acfs.2022.00633

[11] Gareth Evans D. Neurofibromatosis type 2 (NF2): A clinical and molecular review. Orphanet Journal of Rare Diseases. 2009;**4**:16. DOI: 10.1186/1750-1172-4-16

[12] Park S-J et al. Serum biomarkers for neurofibromatosis type 1 and early detection of malignant peripheral nerve-sheath tumors. BMC Medicine. 2013;**11**:109. DOI: 10.1186/1741-7015-11-109

[13] Oliver Hanemann C et al. Current status and recommendations for biomarkers and biobanking in neurofibromatosis. Neurology. 2016;**87**:S40-S48. DOI: 10.1212/WNL.0000000000002929

[14] Kiuru M, Busam K. The NF1 gene in tumor syndromes and melanoma. Laboratory Investigation. 2017;**97**:146-157. DOI: 10.1038/labinvest.2016.142

[15] Bergoug M et al. Neurofibromin structure, functions and regulation. Cells. 2020;**9**:2365. DOI: 10.3390/cells9112365

[16] Walker J, Upadhyaya M. Emerging therapeutic targets for neurofibromatosis

type 1 (NF1). Expert Opinion on Therapeutic Targets. 2018;**22**:419-437. DOI: 10.1080/14728222.2018.1465931

[17] Long A et al. Analysis of patient-specific NF1 variants leads to functional insights for Ras signaling that can impact personalized medicine. Human Mutation. 2022;**43**:30-41. DOI: 10.1002/humu.24290

[18] Raut NGR et al. Schwann cells modulate nociception in neurofibromatosis 1. JCI Insight. 2024;**9**:e171275. DOI: 10.1172/jci.insight.171275

[19] Kahen EJ et al. Neurofibromin level directs RAS pathway signaling and mediates sensitivity to targeted agents in malignant peripheral nerve sheath tumors. Oncotarget. 2018;**9**:22571-22585. DOI: 10.18632/oncotarget.25181

[20] Lobbous M et al. An update on neurofibromatosis type 1-associated gliomas. Cancers. 2020;**12**:114. DOI: 10.3390/cancers12010114

[21] Garcia-Linares C et al. Dissecting loss of heterozygosity (LOH) in neurofibromatosis type 1-associated neurofibromas: Importance of copy neutral LOH. Human Mutation. 2011;**32**:78-90. DOI: 10.1002/humu.21387

[22] Sato T, Sekido Y. NF2/merlin inactivation and potential therapeutic targets in mesothelioma. International Journal of Molecular Sciences. 2018;**19**:988. DOI: 10.3390/ijms19040988

[23] Beltrami S et al. Neurofibromatosis type 2 protein, NF2: An uncoventional cell cycle regulator. Anticancer Research. 2013;**33**:1-11. Available from: https://www.ncbi.nlm.nih.gov/pmc/articles/PMC3725758

[24] Gareth Evans D. Neurofibromatosis 2 [bilateral acoustic neurofibromatosis, central neurofibromatosis, NF2, neurofibromatosis type II]. Genetics in Medicine. 2009;**11**:599-610. DOI: 10.1097/GIM.0b013e3181ac9a27

[25] Minyang F et al. The hippo signalling pathway and its implications in human health and diseases. Signal Transduction and Targeted Therapy. 2022;**7**:376. DOI: 10.1038/s41392-022-01191-9

[26] Fa-Xing Y et al. Hippo pathway in organ size control, tissue homeostasis, and cancer. Cell. 2015;**163**:811-828. DOI: 10.1016/j.cell.2015.10.044

[27] Ramesh V. Merlin and the ERM proteins in Schwann cells, neurons and growth cones. Nature Reviews Neuroscience. 2004;**5**:462-470. DOI: 10.1038/nrn1407

[28] McClatchey A, Fehon R. Merlin and the ERM proteins – regulators of receptor distribution and signaling at the cell cortex. Trends in Cell Biology. 2009;**19**:198-206. DOI: 10.1016/j.tcb.2009.02.006

[29] Tamura R. Current understanding of neurofibromatosis type 1, 2, and schwannomatosis. International Journal of Molecular Sciences. 2021;**22**:5850. DOI: 10.3390/ijms22115850

[30] Pemov A et al. Comparative clinical and genomic analysis of neurofibromatosis type 2-associated cranial and spinal meningiomas. Scientific Reports. 2020;**10**:12563. DOI: 10.1038/s41598-020-69074-z

[31] Pacesa M et al. Past, present, and future of CRISPR genome editing technologies. Cell. 2024;**187**:1076-1100. DOI: 10.1016/j.cell.2024.01.042

[32] Duo X et al. NF2: An underestimated player in cancer metabolic

reprogramming and tumor immunity. NPJ Precision Oncology. 2024;**8**:133. DOI: 10.1038/s41698-024-00627-5

[33] Botero V et al. Neurofibromin regulates metabolic rate via neuronal mechanisms in drosophila. Nature Communications. 2021;**12**:4285. DOI: 10.1038/s41467-021-24505-x

[34] Yang G et al. Serum-derived exosomes from neurofibromatosis type 1 congenital tibial pseudarthrosis impaired bone by promoting osteoclastogenesis and inhibiting osteogenesis. Experimental Biology and Medicine. 2021;**246**:130-141. DOI: 10.1177/1535370220962737

[35] Bian Z et al. TRIM65/NF2/YAP1 signaling coordinately orchestrates metabolic and immune advantages in hepatocellular carcinoma. Advanced Science. 2024;**15**:e2402578. DOI: 10.1002/advs.202402578

[36] Ahlawat S et al. Current whole-body MRI applications in the neurofibromatosis. Neurology. 2016;**87**:S31-S39. DOI: 10.1212/WNL.0000000000002929)

[37] Liu J et al. Image-based differentiation of benign and malignant peripheral nerve sheath tumors in neurofibromatosis type 1. Frontiers in Oncology. 2022;**12**:898971. DOI: 10.3389/fonc.2022.898971

[38] Li Y et al. Current and emerging imaging techniques for neurofibromatosis type 1–associated cutaneous neurofibromas. Journal of Investigative Dermatology. 2023;**143**:1397-1405. DOI: 10.1016/j.jid.2023.03.1681

[39] Gutmann D, Giovannini M. Mouse models of neurofibromatosis 1 and 2. Neoplasia. 2002;**4**:279-290. DOI: 10.1038/sj.neo.7900249

[40] Rajan ARD et al. Generation of a zebrafish neurofibromatosis model via inducible knockout of nf2. bioRxiv. 2024:2024.04.23.590787. DOI: 10.1101/2024.04.23.590787

[41] Durkin J et al. Neurofibromin 1 regulates early developmental sleep in drosophila. Neurobiology of Sleep and Circadian Rhythms. 2023;**15**:100101. DOI: 10.1016/j.nbscr.2023.100101

[42] Mo J et al. Neurofibromin and suppression of tumorigenesis: Beyond the GAP. Oncogene. 2022;**41**:1235-1251. DOI: 10.1038/s41388-021-02156-y

[43] Petrilli AM, Fernandez-Valle C. Role of merlin/NF2 inactivation in tumor biology. Oncogene. 2016;**35**:537-548. DOI: 10.1038/onc.2015.125

[44] Le LQ, Parada LF. Tumor microenvironment and neuro-fibromatosis type I: Connecting the GAPs. Oncogene. 2007;**26**:4609-4616. DOI: 10.1038/sj.onc.1210261

[45] Brossier N, Carroll S. Genetically engineered mouse models shed new light on the pathogenesis of neurofibromatosis type I-related neoplasms of the peripheral nervous system. Brain Research Bulletin. 2012;**88**:58-71. DOI: 10.1016/j.brainresbull.2011.08.005

[46] Osum S et al. Spontaneous and engineered large animal models of neurofibromatosis type 1. International Journal of Molecular Sciences. 2021;**22**:1954. DOI: 10.3390/ijms22041954

[47] Wolman M et al. Modulation of cAMP and Ras signaling pathways improves distinct behavioral deficits in a zebrafish model of neurofibromatosis type 1. Cell Reports. 2014;**8**:1265-1270. DOI: 10.1016/j.celrep.2014.07.054

[48] Williams JA et al. A circadian output in drosophila mediated by neurofibromatosis-1 and Ras/MAPK. Science. 2001;**293**:2251-2256. DOI: 10.1126/science.1063097

[49] Nguyen HTL et al. A platform for rapid patient-derived cutaneous neurofibroma organoid establishment and screening. Cell Reports Methods. 2024;**4**:100772. DOI: 10.1016/j.crmeth.2024.100772

[50] Leier A et al. Mutation-directed therapeutics for neurofibromatosis type I. Molecular Therapy Nucleic Acids. 2020;**20**:739-753. DOI: 10.1016/j.omtn.2020.04.012

[51] Yuan R et al. Gene therapy for neurofibromatosis type 2-related schwannomatosis: Recent progress, challenges, and future directions. Oncology and Therapy. 2024;**12**:257-276. DOI: 10.1007/s40487-024-00279-2

[52] Staedtke V et al. Gene-targeted therapy for neurofibromatosis and schwannomatosis: The path to clinical trials. Sage Journals. 2024;**21**:51-66. DOI: 10.1177/174077452312079

[53] Vasudevan H et al. Functional interactions between neurofibromatosis tumor suppressors underlie Schwann cell tumor de-differentiation and treatment resistance. Nature Communications. 2024;**15**:477. DOI: 10.1038/s41467-024-44755-9

[54] Lv L, Zhou X. Targeting hippo signaling in cancer: Novel perspectives and therapeutic potential. MedComm. 2023;**4**:e375. DOI: 10.1002/mco2.375

Section 4

Therapeutics

Chapter 10

Craniopharyngioma: Contemporary Management and Emerging Treatments

Abdullah Alobaid, Razan Almufarriji, Sarah Binabdulqader and Yazeed Alotaibi

Abstract

Craniopharyngioma management presents significant challenges due to its complex location and potential impact on critical structures. This comprehensive chapter offers a detailed review of contemporary management approaches, highlighting advancements in microscopic and endoscopic surgeries, radiotherapy, and innovative medical treatments. Emphasis is placed on the importance of a multidisciplinary strategy, aiming to enhance patient outcomes by balancing effective tumor control with the preservation of quality of life. Additionally, we explore diagnostic improvements, full treatment plans, and the potential of emerging therapies. This chapter explores these topics and provides valuable insights into current practices and future paths in the management of craniopharyngioma.

Keywords: craniopharyngioma, surgery, management, endocrine, radiation

1. Introduction

Craniopharyngiomas (CPs) are uncommon, benign tumors that originate from residual cells of Rathke's pouch and are typically found in the sellar/parasellar region. These tumors are classified by the World Health Organization (WHO) as grade I, reflecting their generally non-malignant nature, though rare instances of malignant transformation have been noted. CPs are histologically categorized into two types: adamantinomatous (ACP) and squamous papillary (PCP). ACP is more frequently diagnosed in children under the age of 14, constituting 5–10% of central nervous system (CNS) tumors in this age group, whereas PCP is more prevalent in adults [1, 2].

A study by Momin et al., using data from the Central Brain Tumor Registry of the United States, reported an incidence rate of 0.16 confirmed Craniopharyngioma cases per 100,000 people. The study identified a bimodal distribution pattern, with incidence peaks in children aged 5–9 years and adults aged 55–69 years. Furthermore, the highest incidence rates were observed among Black individuals, followed by

White individuals, with Black ethnicity being linked to a lower survival rate. These findings corroborate previous research by Zacharia et al., which highlighted Black ethnicity as an age-adjusted relative risk factor for craniopharyngioma compared to White ethnicity [3].

CPs can exert pressure on surrounding neural structures and the pituitary gland, often resulting in growth hormone deficiency due to the tumor's compressive nature, surgical treatments, or radiation therapy. Consequently, growth hormone deficiency is the most common endocrine disorder associated with these tumors. Additionally, adamantinomatous craniopharyngiomas are significantly more prevalent across all age groups compared to papillary tumors. Recent discoveries in the molecular pathology of these tumors suggest the potential for targeted therapies, which may reduce the rate of morbidity [4].

2. History

Craniopharyngioma was first described by Friedrich Albert von Zenker in 1857 and further histologically described by Jakob Erdheim. Surgical intervention was first successfully done in 1909 by A. E. Halstead of Chicago [5].

In 1937, Carpenter's group examined the radiosensitivity of craniopharyngiomas by treating four cases with cyst aspiration and radiation. Although these tumors were formerly deemed radio-resistant, research revealed that external beam radiation diminished their progression and symptom severity [6].

3. Pathophysiology

3.1 Tumor characteristics

Craniopharyngiomas are primarily divided into two histological types: adamantinomatous craniopharyngioma (ACP) and papillary craniopharyngioma (PCP). ACPs are the more common subtype, diagnosed across all age groups but predominantly in children. The age distribution for ACP diagnosis is asymmetrically bimodal, with a significant peak between ages 5 and 14 and a smaller peak between ages 50 and 74. Structurally, ACPs tend to attach to surrounding tissues and consist of a combination of cysts and nodules, often exhibiting fibrosis, calcifications, and hemorrhages. ACPs can be challenging to treat due to their invasive nature, which makes complete surgical resection difficult. These tumors are also associated with a higher rate of recurrence and can cause significant endocrine and neurological deficits due to their location near the pituitary gland and hypothalamus. Conversely, PCPs constitute 11–14% of craniopharyngiomas and primarily occur in adults, with an average age of diagnosis around 44 ± 15 years. PCPs are linked with higher 5-year survival rates and exhibit a less aggressive progression compared to ACPs. Structurally, PCPs are solid and well-defined, making them more amenable to complete surgical removal. They tend to be less invasive and have a lower recurrence rate. Despite these advantages, PCPs can still cause substantial morbidity due to their proximity to critical brain structures, potentially leading to visual disturbances and hormonal imbalances. Overall, PCPs have a better prognosis and are generally easier to manage than ACPs [7, 8].

3.2 Genetic and molecular review

Significant strides have been made recently in understanding the genetic mechanisms driving craniopharyngiomas, which could have substantial implications for treatment approaches.

3.2.1 Adamantinomatous craniopharyngioma (ACP)

ACP is largely driven by activating mutations in the CTNNB1 gene, which encodes β-catenin. These mutations, identified in more than two-thirds of ACP cases, make β-catenin resistant to proteasomal degradation, leading to its accumulation in the nucleus and the activation of the WNT signaling pathway. This is pathologically unique to ACP and not observed in other pituitary tumors. In about one-third of ACP cases, CTNNB1 mutations are absent, indicating that other genetic or epigenetic factors might also activate the WNT pathway. Additionally, recent findings have highlighted the involvement of the MAPK/ERK pathway in ACP, opening new therapeutic possibilities. For example, MEK inhibitors like trametinib show promise in targeting this pathway [7, 9].

3.2.2 Papillary craniopharyngioma (PCP)

In PCP, the critical pathogenic event is the B-Rapidly Accelerated Fibrosarcoma (BRAF) V600E mutation, present in about 90% of cases. This mutation, which occurs in approximately 7% of all human cancers, results in a constitutively active BRAF protein that drives cell proliferation and tumor growth. Though rare, there are instances where both CTNNB1 and BRAF mutations coexist. Previous research has not shown significant chromosomal abnormalities in any craniopharyngioma subtype. The availability of BRAF inhibitors, such as vemurafenib and dabrafenib, suggests that PCP patients could benefit from these targeted therapies. Studies, including those by Himes BT et al., have demonstrated that dabrafenib monotherapy can significantly reduce tumor size in recurrent PCP cases, with patients remaining symptom-free for up to a year and showing no radiographic signs of tumor progression. Moreover, combination therapy with dabrafenib and trametinib has been effective in reducing PCP in patients with BRAF V600E mutations [7, 9].

4. Clinical presentation

4.1 Signs and symptoms

Although benign, craniopharyngiomas can cause a variety of symptoms due to their proximity to essential brain structures. These symptoms typically arise from the tumor's pressure on nearby areas such as the pituitary gland, optic nerves, and hypothalamus.

Endocrine symptoms:

Craniopharyngiomas often disrupt the function of the pituitary gland, leading to multiple hormonal deficiencies. Common endocrine symptoms include:

- Growth and puberty issues: Delayed growth and puberty, caused by reduced secretion of growth hormone and gonadotropins.

- Hypothyroidism: Symptoms such as weight gain, fatigue, irritability, and cognitive delays due to a decrease in thyroid-stimulating hormone (TSH).

- Adrenal insufficiency: Symptoms like altered blood sugar and blood pressure, fatigue, and weakness due to reduced adrenocorticotropic hormone (ACTH) levels.

Neurological symptoms:
The growth of craniopharyngiomas can compress the optic chiasm and optic nerves, leading to visual impairments. These include:

- Visual field defects: Loss of peripheral vision that can progress to more severe visual impairment.

- Headaches: Often due to increased intracranial pressure.

- Hydrocephalus: Tumor growth can block cerebrospinal fluid flow, causing headaches, nausea, vomiting, and balance issues.

Hypothalamic dysfunction:
Craniopharyngiomas can also impact the hypothalamus, leading to:

- Hypothalamic obesity: Rapid weight gain that is resistant to diet and exercise.

- Thermoregulation issues: Problems with body temperature regulation, excessive thirst, and imbalances in heart rate and blood pressure.

- Behavioral changes: Including alterations in sleep patterns and personality changes [10–14].

5. Diagnostic evaluation

5.1 Imaging

Computed tomography (CT) and magnetic resonance imaging (MRI) are important diagnostic tools for the characterization of these tumors. The size of the lesion as well as its relationship to important adjacent structures, such as the pituitary gland, optic apparatus, third ventricle, and major intracranial vessels can be detected by CT and MRI. CT scan detects calcifications precisely in craniopharyngioma tissue, which is a finding in approximately 90% of these tumors [15].

5.2 CT of adamantinomatous craniopharyngioma

Adamantinomatous craniopharyngiomas typically present with several distinctive features on computed tomography (CT) scans. These tumors frequently exhibit large cystic components with densities similar to cerebrospinal fluid (CSF), which are a prominent characteristic and present in about 90% of cases. Additionally, the solid components of these tumors often demonstrate soft tissue density and show enhancement with contrast in approximately 90% of cases. Calcifications are another significant feature observed in around 90% of cases, and these are usually stippled and located peripherally within the tumor. These imaging characteristics are crucial for the accurate diagnosis and assessment of adamantinomatous craniopharyngiomas (**Figure 1**) [16, 17].

5.3 CT of papillary craniopharyngioma

Papillary craniopharyngiomas are distinct from their adamantinomatous counterparts, typically presenting as predominantly solid masses with occasional cystic components. On computed tomography (CT) scans, these tumors often exhibit a solid, non-calcified structure, which differentiates them from the adamantinomatous type that commonly shows calcifications. Papillary craniopharyngiomas are usually located in the suprasellar region and tend to enhance homogeneously with contrast. The lack of significant calcification and the presence of solid enhancement are key imaging characteristics that aid in distinguishing papillary craniopharyngiomas from other types of craniopharyngiomas and suprasellar tumors (**Figure 2**) [18–20].

5.4 MRI of adamantinomatous craniopharyngioma

These tumors typically present with a combination of cystic and solid components. The cystic areas often appear hyperintense on T2-weighted images and variable on T1-weighted images, depending on the cyst contents (which may include protein, blood, or cholesterol). The solid components generally enhance with contrast. Calcifications, a hallmark of adamantinomatous craniopharyngiomas, are better seen on CT but can influence the MRI signal (**Figure 3**).

5.5 MRI of papillary craniopharyngioma

Papillary Craniopharyngioma are more likely to appear as predominantly solid masses with less frequent cystic components. On MRI, these tumors usually enhance

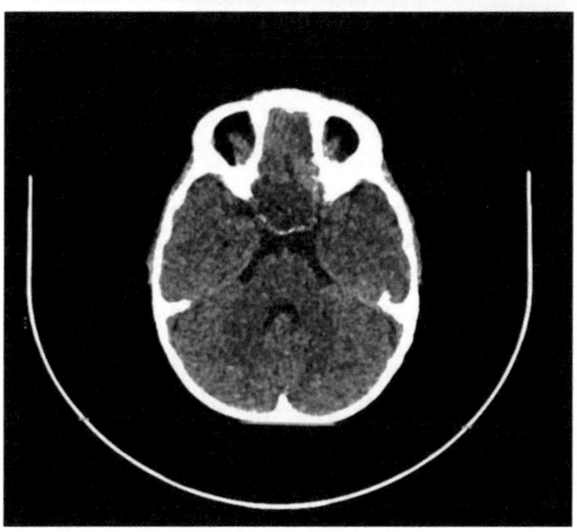

Figure 1.
CT brain of a patient with confirmed pathology of Adamantinomatous craniopharyngioma.

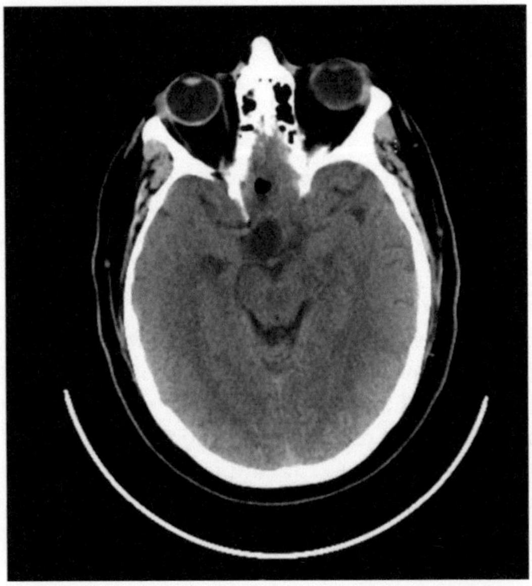

Figure 2.
Ct brain of a patient with confirmed papillary craniopharyngioma.

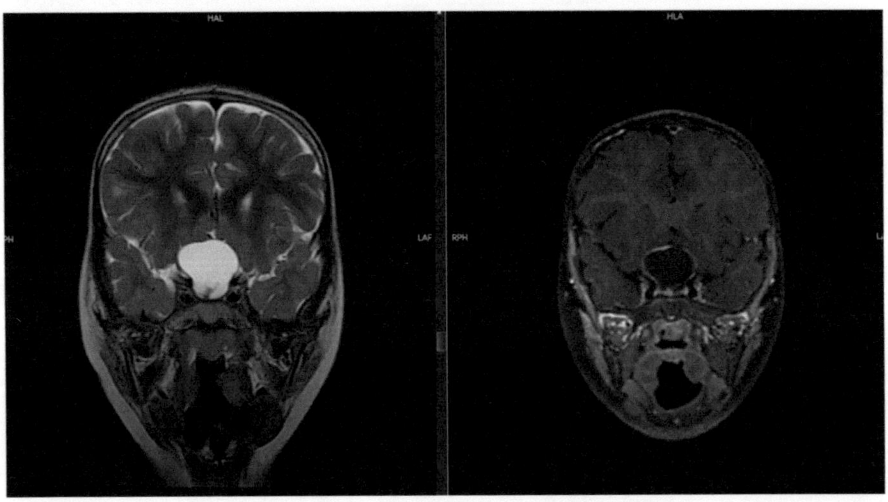

Figure 3.
T1 post-contrast and T2 coronal MRI of a patient with confirmed Adamantinomatous craniopharyngioma.

homogeneously with contrast and lack the significant calcifications seen in the adamantinomatous subtype. They often occupy the suprasellar region and can cause compression of adjacent structures such as the optic chiasm and hypothalamus. MRI is invaluable for assessing the tumor's relationship to critical brain structures, which is essential for surgical planning. Features such as the tumor's impact on the pituitary stalk, hypothalamus, and optic pathways are meticulously evaluated to determine the best approach for treatment and to predict potential postoperative complications (**Figure 4**) [21, 22].

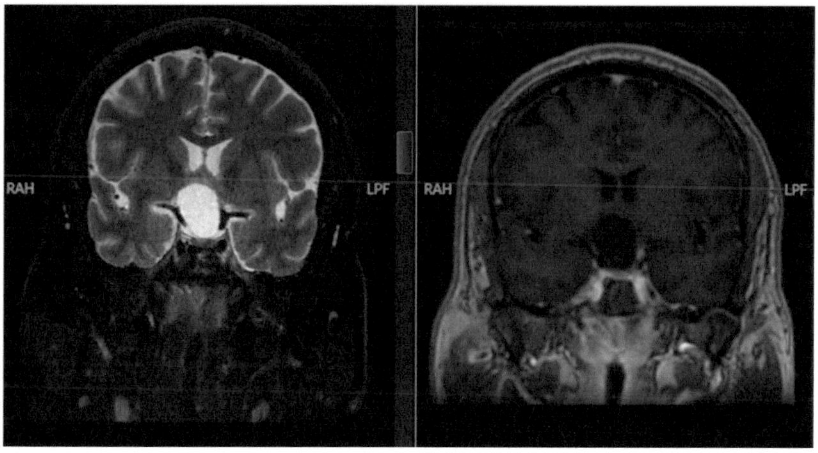

Figure 4.
T1 post-contrast and T2 coronal MRI of a patient with confirmed papillary craniopharyngioma.

6. Management strategies

6.1 Surgical approaches

Surgical treatment remains the mainstay of treatment for craniopharyngioma (CP), given its benign histopathological grading and its proximity to vital neurovascular structures (hypothalamus and optic chiasm) [3]. The primary goal of surgery is to achieve tumor control while minimizing tumor and treatment-related morbidity and preserving neuropsychological, visual, and endocrine function. Therefore, a conservative approach constituting subtotal resection followed by radiation therapy became the most acceptable line of management for CP (**Figure 5**) [24, 25].

The rapid advancement in microscopic and endoscopic skull base techniques led to significant improvement in surgical outcomes and tumor control. Various transcranial surgical approaches have been applied to craniopharyngioma resection utilizing different surgical corridors including anterior (subfrontal), anterolateral (orbitozygomatic, pterional, and transpetrosal), and interhemispheric approaches. The endoscopic endonasal approach has evolved and gained wide acceptance among neurosurgeons for the treatment of CP [26].

Some authors have used a tailored surgical approach based on anatomical characteristics to guide the selection of the surgical approach. The relationship between the tumor and structures such as the diaphragma sellae, third ventricle, optic chiasm, and pituitary stalk is often considered [27].

Purely intrasellar and intrasellar/suprasellar tumors are best approached through the endoscopic endonasal route. The endoscopic endonasal approach allows clear visualization of the pituitary gland and optic chiasm, the inferior surface of the chiasm and hypothalamus. However, lateral extension of the tumor beyond the carotid will limit the utilization of this approach, and transcranial routes will be more favorable in those cases [26].

Transcranial approaches are preferred for suprasellar tumors, especially in cases with hypothalamic and third ventricle extension [28]. The subfrontal approach is ideal for midline craniopharyngioma with anterior skull base extension. It allows

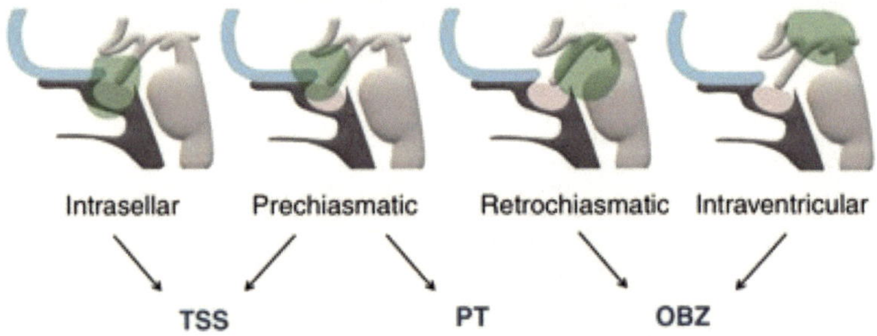

Figure 5.
Illustration showing different locations of craniopharyngioma with suggested suitable approach. Adopted from: Ref. [23].

good visualization of the optic nerve and chiasm as well as the ipsilateral carotid artery. However, this approach does not allow for good visualization of tumors extending into the third ventricle and is not feasible for patients with a prefixed chiasm. The pterional approach, a unilateral surgical technique, offers a short trajectory to retrochiasmatic craniopharyngioma and is primarily used for tumors located in the suprasellar cistern. The transpetrosal approach has been advocated by few authors for retrochiasmatic tumors. However, their true utilization is limited due to the risk of temporal lobe retraction and vein Labbe injury [26, 29].

Surgical treatment of craniopharyngioma is associated with significant morbidity related to hypothalamic and pituitary axis involvement. The overall risk of panhypopituitarism following surgical treatment of craniopharyngioma can reach up to 59% [30]. Diabetes insipidus (DI) is observed in 8–35% of patients preoperatively, and the risk of postoperative DI ranges between 50 and 90% in some series [30–33]. Comparing endoscopic versus transcranial resection of CP, there was no significant difference between both groups in terms of the risk of Panhypopituitarism and DI [34]. The risk of CSF leak is significantly higher following endoscopic resection of craniopharyngioma, with an overall incidence of 9% in a recent meta-analysis [34].

6.2 Radiation therapy

Surgical resection, followed by radiation therapy, became a widely accepted modality of treatment for most CPs. Various radiation modalities are applied to treat CPs given their heterogeneous nature. External beam radiation therapy is delivered to most CPs in two forms: three-dimensional conformal radiotherapy (3DCRT) and intensity-modulated photon radiotherapy (IMRT). 3DCRT is used for most CPs and delivers a homogenous dose to the whole tumor. IMRT, on the other hand, changes the strength of beams in certain areas, allowing stronger doses in particular tumor areas while lessening the damage to nearby normal tissues [3, 35, 36].

Proton beam therapy is a valuable and safe option especially in children with craniopharyngioma given its advantage of depositing energy at a defined point along their path, reducing the harmful effects on normal tissues around the tumor [3, 37]. Proton therapy has shown improved cognitive outcomes as compared to photon therapy in children with craniopharyngioma [38, 39].

Stereotactic radiosurgery (gamma knife), which delivers a single large dose of radiation to the target from multiple angles, is a valid alternative for patients with small CPs. However, its theoretical risk of introducing optic neuropathy for lesions close to the optic chiasm limits its utilization [40, 41].

Brachytherapy is a valid treatment option for cystic CPs. Intracavitary brachytherapy irradiation with β-emitting sources such as phosphorus-32 (P-32) or yttrium-90 has shown excellent results with minimal morbidity and progression-free survival rates at 5 and 10 years of 95.5 and 84.4%, respectively [3, 42–44].

6.3 Medical management

6.3.1 Bleomycin

It is a polypeptide antibiotic (bleomycin A2 and B2) secreted by Streptomyces verticillus, inhibiting RNA and DNA synthesis. It was first reported in the treatment of craniopharyngioma in 1985 [45, 46]. A dose of 1 to 15 mg of bleomycin is delivered through the Ommaya reservoir, often with stereotactic guidance. Intracystic administration of bleomycin resulted in a 50% reduction of cyst volume in a single case series [47]. However, the risk of cerebral edema, infarction, and death has been reported with the use of bleomycin therapy [47–49].

6.3.2 Interferon alpha (IFN)

It has been viewed as a valid alternative to bleomycin therapy. Its antitumoral properties and relatively low neurotoxic effects made it superior to bleomycin in the treatment of craniopharyngioma, with a 90% reduction in the cyst volume in one series [50, 51].

6.3.3 BRAF and MEK inhibitors

Targeted therapy for papillary craniopharyngioma has gained increased attention recently. The use of vemurafenib, dabrafenib, and trametinib, either as monotherapies or in combination, has been studied extensively. Vemurafenib has shown limited efficacy and disease progression, while dabrafenib and trametinib showed more promising results [52–55]. However, their long-term efficacy remains to be determined.

7. Follow-up and long-term care

7.1 Surveillance protocols

There is no consensus regarding post-treatment imaging surveillance of craniopharyngioma and the duration of imaging follow-up should be guided by patient symptoms, the extent of resection, and the treatment provided. Immediate postoperative MRI +/− CT within 48–72 hours with fat-saturated post-contrast imaging to assess for residual and surgery-related complications [56]. The general expert recommendation is to follow with MRI every 3 months for 1 year, then every 6 months for 1 year then annual for 5 years if no residual or radiation given, if patient received radiation or there is a residual then every 1–2 year for life [57, 58]. Regular ophthalmological assessment, interval neuropsychological assessment, and long-term endocrinological follow-up are strongly recommended [56, 59].

7.2 Recurrence management

Approximately 20 to 30% of patients will experience a recurrence/progression within 5 years after the initial treatment. Recurrent craniopharyngioma is challenging, as the majority of patients present with asymptomatic radiological recurrence/progression, and there exists no high-quality evidence for the optimal management of recurrent craniopharyngioma [60, 61]. The rate of tumor recurrence is highly dependent on RT administration regardless of whether surgery was performed and the extent of resection when surgery was performed. Subtotal resection with no radiation was significantly associated with recurrence/progression [60, 61]. Factors associated with recurrence rates include the following: pediatric cases compared to adult cases, delayed or non-use of radiotherapy (RT), large tumor size (>5 cm), suprasellar location, adherence to neurovascular structures, cystic craniopharyngioma, histological presence of whorl-like arrays, and highly calcified tumors. Growth hormone (GH) presents little or no risk in this context. Other studies have explored the molecular diagnostics of craniopharyngiomas (CP), including markers such as Ki-67, p53 gene, vascular endothelial growth factor (VEGF), and cathepsins. These molecular markers may have significant value in understanding increased recurrence rates [1]. Ectopic craniopharyngioma is a very rare phenomenon, there are 63 reported cases that are believed to be secondary to seeding through either a surgical approach or CSF. Most are adamantinomatous subtype [62].

To date, there is no consensus on the optimal treatment for the recurrence of craniopharyngioma. Treatment options include reoperation, adjuvant radiation, stereotactic radiosurgery (SRS), and intracystic therapy. Hoong Wei Gan et al. wrote guidelines for pediatric craniopharyngioma and provided the following strong recommendations for managing recurrence:

1. Offer further surgery to avoid or reduce the radiation field before radiotherapy in children and young people with cystic or solid recurrences after a radiologically complete resection without previous irradiation.

2. Offer further cyst drainage before radiotherapy in children and young people with progressive, primarily cystic recurrences following initial incomplete resection without previous irradiation.

3. Offer radiotherapy with further surgery to reduce the radiation field in children and young people with progressive, primarily solid recurrences following initial incomplete resection without previous irradiation.

4. Offer a repeat course of conventional radiotherapy for the treatment of disease progression or recurrence after previous irradiation only in exceptional cases and only after all other therapeutic modalities have been explored, given its high morbidity [63].

7.3 Multidisciplinary approach

7.3.1 Endocrinology

Hormonal disturbances are present in approximately 65–90% of cases, reflecting injury to the hypothalamus-pituitary axis. These disturbances can be exacerbated by treatment, contributing to high morbidity and mortality. Baseline endocrine hormones, including AFP, β-hCG (to rule out germ cell tumor), and prolactin, should be evaluated before any definitive surgery, as well as IGF-1, TSH, free T4, LH, FSH, testosterone/estradiol, paired early morning plasma/urine osmolalities and electrolytes, and, if dexamethasone has not been administered, morning cortisol +/− ACTH levels. Most patients will require hormonal replacement therapy and need close endocrinological follow-up [56, 64–66].

7.3.2 Neuropsychology

The anatomical location and treatment of craniopharyngioma significantly influence visual, endocrine, and neuropsychological functions, impacting the overall quality of life [67]. Psychological issues are linked to diminished quality of life, disrupted social relationships, extended rehabilitation periods, poor treatment adherence, and the emergence of "abnormal illness behavior" [68, 69]. Risk factors include large tumors (>7 cm^3), extension into the third ventricle, and hypothalamic invasion [68, 70]. Studies have found that irritability is the most prevalent symptom, followed by agitation and delusions. Other symptoms include memory deficits, emotional impairments, mood disturbances, attention issues, and sleep disorders [68]. Therefore, a baseline neurocognitive assessment is highly recommended [56]. Comprehensive patient care should include support from psychology and social work, coaching, monitoring of school performance and family life, and diagnostic neurocognitive testing.

7.3.3 Ophthalmology

At diagnosis, 62–84% of craniopharyngioma (CP) patients exhibit visual impairment. The visual prognosis depends significantly on the initial visual status, with 32% of patients showing improvement [59]. Pre-treatment evaluations should include assessments of visual acuity, visual fields, optic nerves, and ocular motility, taking into account age-specific standards for visual acuity. Visually evoked potentials may be considered for infants and disabled children, but not for routine surveillance. Consistent post-surgical follow-up is crucial to monitor improvements and manage the risk of recurrence [56, 60].

7.3.4 Physiotherapy and dietitian

Most patients with craniopharyngioma experience metabolic disturbances, either due to the disease itself or as a consequence of its treatment. Hypothalamic obesity syndrome is particularly common among craniopharyngioma patients, with an incidence reported between 38 and 58%. Due to hyperphagia, reduced metabolic rate, and decreased physical activity, the risk of cardiovascular mortality is significantly elevated [71, 72]. Weight management through lifestyle interventions, including a low-calorie diet and daily physical activity, is strongly recommended for these patients [72, 73].

7.3.5 Rehabilitation

Patients with craniopharyngioma often suffer from fatigue and sleep disorders, which are observed in 70% of cases. These issues are linked to neuroendocrine dysfunction affecting the sleep-wake cycle and necessitate comprehensive neuroendocrine and sleep management [74].

8. Emerging treatments

8.1 Immunotherapy

Elevated inflammatory markers are involved in the pathogenesis of craniopharyngioma, with some studies linking high levels of M2 macrophages to tumor angiogenesis, progression, and a poorer prognosis [75, 76]. Although many potential markers are under investigation, none have yet entered clinical trials [58].

8.2 Nivolumab and tovorafenib for treatment of craniopharyngioma in children and young adults: Phase 2 clinical trial (NCT04006667)

The current study assesses the tolerability and efficacy of combination therapy with PD-1 (nivolumab) and pan-RAF-kinase (Tovorafenib) inhibition for the treatment of children and young adults with craniopharyngioma. The study started in September 12, 2022, and completion in March 1, 2028 [60].

8.3 MEKTOVI (binimetinib): Phase 2 clinical trial (NCT02703464)

This study focuses on an oral, highly selective reversible inhibitor of mitogen-activated extracellular signal-regulated kinase 1 (MEK1) and MEK2 for pediatric patients diagnosed with recurrent Adamantinomatous Craniopharyngioma, including those who have undergone surgery and/or radiation therapy. The trial commenced on April 10, 2023, and is expected to be completed by April 10, 2027 [60].

8.4 A phase II trial of intensity-modulated proton therapy for incompletely resected craniopharyngioma and observation for craniopharyngioma after radical resection: Phase 2 clinical trial (NCT02727453)

This Phase II clinical trial investigates the efficacy of intensity-modulated proton therapy (IMPT) for patients with incompletely resected craniopharyngioma and the outcomes of observation for patients who have undergone radical resection. The trial aims to evaluate the therapeutic potential and safety of IMPT in controlling tumor growth while minimizing damage to surrounding healthy tissues. Additionally, the study will observe the progression and recurrence rates in patients who have had radical resection without further immediate treatment. The goal is to provide comprehensive data on both treatment approaches to inform future therapeutic strategies for craniopharyngioma. The study started on June 22, 2016, and was completed in July 2027 [60].

8.5 Treatment of BRAF (B-rapidly accelerated fibrosarcoma) mutated papillary craniopharyngioma (Swecranio): Phase 2 clinical trial (NCT04615810)

Papillary craniopharyngioma harbors a BRAF mutation in 90% of cases. Treatment with BRAF and MEK inhibitors (dabrafenib and trametinib) offers a potential alternative to high-risk surgery, either by preventing the need for surgery with significant side effects or by providing an additional option when further surgery is not recommended. The study began on September 1, 2023, and is scheduled for completion on April 10, 2028 [60].

8.6 ACTEMRA® for the treatment of pediatric adamantinomatous craniopharyngioma: Phase 2 clinical trial (NCT04663320)

ACTEMRA (tocilizumab), produced by Genentech, a biotechnology company in South San Francisco, California, is an IL-6 receptor antagonist. This drug is being used to treat pediatric patients with recurrent Adamantinomatous Craniopharyngioma, including those who have undergone surgery and/or radiation therapy. The study commenced on December 16, 2022, and is expected to be completed by December 2026 [60].

9. Conclusion

The management of craniopharyngioma has advanced considerably with improvements in surgical techniques, targeted therapies, and radiotherapy. Modern approaches now emphasize a multidisciplinary strategy to balance effective tumor management with the preservation of quality of life.

Ongoing clinical trials continue to explore innovative treatments, including immunotherapy, aiming to further improve patient outcomes.

In summary, contemporary management of craniopharyngioma integrates cutting-edge technology and personalized care, aiming to optimize survival and quality of life while addressing the complexities of this challenging tumor.

Conflict of interest

The authors declare no conflict of interest.

Author details

Abdullah Alobaid[1*], Razan Almufarriji[1], Sarah Binabdulqader[1] and Yazeed Alotaibi[2]

1 King Fahad Medical City, Riyadh, Saudi Arabia

2 Alnoor Specialist Hospital, Mecca, Saudi Arabia

*Address all correspondence to: abdullah.alobaid@medportal.ca

References

[1] Serbis A, Tsinopoulou VR, Papadopoulou A, et al. Predictive factors for pediatric craniopharyngioma recurrence: An extensive narrative review. Diagnostics (Basel). 2023;**13**(9):1588. DOI: 10.3390/diagnostics13091588

[2] Alboqami MN, Khalid S, Albaiahy A, Bukhari BH, et al. Craniopharyngioma: A comprehensive review of the clinical presentation, radiological findings, management, and future perspective. Heliyon. 2024;**10**(11):e32112. DOI: 10.1016/j.heliyon.2024.e32112

[3] Diaz MJ, Kwak SH, Root KT, Fadil A, Nguyen A, Ladehoff L, et al. Current approaches to craniopharyngioma management. Frontiers in Bioscience (Landmark Ed). 2022;**27**(12):328

[4] Müller HL. The diagnosis and treatment of craniopharyngioma. Neuroendocrinology. 2020;**110**(9-10):753-766

[5] Barkhoudarian G, Laws ER. Craniopharyngioma: History. Pituitary. 2013;**16**(1):1-8. DOI: 10.1007/s11102-012-0402-z

[6] Roderick E, Karavitaki N, Wass JA. Craniopharyngiomas: Historical aspects of their management. Hormones (Athens, Greece). 2008;**7**(3):271-274. DOI: 10.14310/horm.2002.1208

[7] Jensterle M, Jazbinsek S, Bosnjak R, et al. Advances in the management of craniopharyngioma in children and adults. Radiology and Oncology. 2019;**53**(4):388-396. DOI: 10.2478/raon-2019-0036

[8] Coury JR, Davis BN, Koumas CP, et al. Histopathological and molecular predictors of growth patterns and recurrence in craniopharyngiomas: A systematic review. Neurosurgical Review. 2020;**43**(1):41-48. DOI: 10.1007/s10143-018-0978-5

[9] Lithgow K, Hamblin R, Pohl U, et al. . In: Feingold KR, Anawalt B, Blackman MR, et al., editors. Craniopharyngiomas [Internet]. South Dartmouth (MA): MDText.com, Inc.; 2000. Available from: https://www.ncbi.nlm.nih.gov/books/NBK538819/ [Accessed: February 26, 2022]

[10] Mayo Clinic Staff. Craniopharyngioma - Overview. Rochester, Minnesota, USA: Mayo Clinic; 2023. Available from: https://www.mayoclinic.org/diseases-conditions/craniopharyngioma/symptoms-causes/syc-20350231

[11] Verywell Health. Craniopharyngioma: Symptoms, Treatment, and Outlook. Available from: https://www.verywellhealth.com/craniopharyngioma-overview-5183035

[12] National Organization for Rare Disorders (NORD). Craniopharyngioma - Symptoms, Causes, Treatment. Available from: https://rarediseases.org/rare-diseases/craniopharyngioma/

[13] Stanford Medicine. Craniopharyngioma. Brain Tumor Center. Available from: https://med.stanford.edu/brain-tumor/conditions/craniopharyngioma.html

[14] Society for Endocrinology. Craniopharyngioma. You and Your Hormones. Available from: https://www.yourhormones.info/endocrine-conditions/craniopharyngioma/

[15] Mushtaq A, Fayaz M, Bhat AR, et al. Comprehensive analysis of craniopharyngioma: Epidemiology, clinical characteristics, management strategies, and role of radiotherapy. Cancer Diagnosis & Prognosis. 2024;**4**(4):521-528. DOI: 10.21873/cdp.10358

[16] Jastania R, Saeed M, Al-Khalidi H, et al. Adamantinomatous craniopharyngioma in an adult: A case report with NGS analysis. International Medical Case Reports Journal. 2020;**13**:123-137. DOI: 10.2147/imcrj.s243405

[17] Radiopaedia. Adamantinomatous Craniopharyngioma. Radiology Reference Article. Available from: https://radiopaedia.org/articles/adamantinomatous-craniopharyngioma [Accessed: July 9, 2024]

[18] Radiopaedia. Papillary craniopharyngioma. Radiology Reference Article. Available from: https://radiopaedia.org/articles/papillary-craniopharyngioma

[19] SpringerLink. Neuroradiological Diagnosis of Craniopharyngiomas. Available from : https://link.springer.com/article/10.1007/s10143-020-01320-7

[20] Crotty TB et al. Papillary craniopharyngioma: A clinicopathological study of 48 cases. Journal of Neurosurgery. 1995;**83**(2):206-214. Available from: https://thejns.org/view/journals/j-neurosurg/83/2/article-p206.xml

[21] Prieto R, Pascual JM, Barrios L. Topographic diagnosis of craniopharyngiomas: The accuracy of MRI findings observed on conventional T1 and T2 images. American Journal of Neuroradiology. 2017;**38**(11):2073-2080. Available from: https://www.ajnr.org/content/38/11/2073

[22] Neurosurgical Review. Preoperative MRI Diagnosis of Papillary Craniopharyngiomas: The Revealing Clues. Available from: https://link.springer.com/article/10.1007/s10143-021-01615-0

[23] Massa D, Glerean M, Rasmussen J, Altszul M, Fainstein-Day P, Ajler P. Craniopharyngiomas: Experience and results. Neurocirugia (Astur: Engl Ed). 2021;**32**(3):105-113. English Spanish. DOI: 10.1016/j.neucir.2020.03.008. Epub 2020 May 21

[24] Sainte-Rose C, Puget S, Wray A, Zerah M, Grill J, Brauner R, et al. Craniopharyngioma: The pendulum of surgical management. Child's Nervous System. 2005;**21**:691-695

[25] Puget S, Garnett M, Wray A, Grill J, Habrand JL, Bodaert N, et al. Pediatric craniopharyngiomas: Classification and treatment according to the degree of hypothalamic involvement. Journal of Neurosurgery: Pediatrics. 2007;**106**(1):3-12

[26] Lei C, Chuzhong L, Chunhui L, Peng Z, Jiwei B, Xinsheng W, et al. Approach selection and outcomes of craniopharyngioma resection: A single-institute study. Neurosurgical Review. 2021;**44**:1737-1746

[27] Morisako H, Goto T, Goto H, Bohoun CA, Tamrakar S, Ohata K. Aggressive surgery based on an anatomical subclassification of craniopharyngiomas. Neurosurgical Focus. 2016;**41**(6):E10

[28] Mortini P, Gagliardi F, Bailo M, Losa M. Surgical approach to craniopharyngiomas: Transcranial routes. In: Diagnosis and Management of Craniopharyngiomas: Key Current Topics. Berlin, Germany: Springer; 2016. pp. 85-99

[29] Kunihiro N, Goto T, Ishibashi K, Ohata K. Surgical outcomes of the minimum anterior and posterior combined transpetrosal approach for resection of retrochiasmatic craniopharyngiomas with complicated conditions. Journal of Neurosurgery. 2014;**120**(1):1-1

[30] Frič R, König M, Due-Tønnessen BJ, Ramm-Pettersen J, Berg-Johnsen J. Long-term outcome of patients treated for craniopharyngioma: A single center experience. British Journal of Neurosurgery. 2023:1-9. DOI: 10.1080/02688697.2023.2179600 [In press]

[31] Honegger J, Buchfelder M, Fahlbusch R. Surgical treatment of craniopharyngiomas: Endocrinological results. Journal of Neurosurgery. 1999;**90**(2):251-257

[32] Ghirardello S, Hopper N, Albanese A, Maghnie M. Diabetes insipidus in craniopharyngioma: Postoperative management of water and electrolyte disorders. Journal of Pediatric Endocrinology and Metabolism. 2006;**19**:413

[33] Shi XE, Wu B, Fan T, Zhou ZQ, Zhang YL. Craniopharyngioma: Surgical experience of 309 cases in China. Clinical Neurology and Neurosurgery. 2008;**110**(2):151-159

[34] Na MK, Jang B, Choi KS, Lim TH, Kim W, Cho Y, et al. Craniopharyngioma resection by endoscopic endonasal approach versus transcranial approach: A systematic review and meta-analysis of comparative studies. Frontiers in Oncology. 2022;**12**:1058329

[35] Aggarwal A, Fersht N, Brada M. Radiotherapy for craniopharyngioma. Pituitary. 2013;**16**:26-33

[36] O'steen L, Indelicato DJ. Advances in the management of craniopharyngioma. F1000Research. 2018;**7**

[37] Jimenez RB, Ahmed S, Johnson A, Thomas H, Depauw N, Horick N, et al. Proton radiation therapy for pediatric craniopharyngioma. International Journal of Radiation Oncology* Biology* Physics. 2021;**110**(5):1480-1487

[38] Friedman DL, Whitton J, Leisenring W, Mertens AC, Hammond S, Stovall M, et al. Subsequent neoplasms in 5-year survivors of childhood cancer: The childhood cancer survivor study. JNCI: Journal of the National Cancer Institute. 2010;**102**(14):1083-1095

[39] Merchant T, Indelicato D, Hua CH, Wu S, Conklin H. Comparison of academic achievement scores after proton and photon therapy in children and young adults with craniopharyngioma. In: Pediatric Blood & Cancer. Vol. 64. NJ, USA: Wiley; 2017. pp. S15-S15

[40] Leber KA, Berglöff J, Pendl G. Dose—Response tolerance of the visual pathways and cranial nerves of the cavernous sinus to stereotactic radiosurgery. Journal of Neurosurgery. 1998;**88**(1):43-50

[41] Chung WY, Pan DH, Shiau CY, Guo WY, Wang LW. Gamma knife radiosurgery for craniopharyngiomas. Journal of Neurosurgery. 2000;**93**(supplement. 3):47-56

[42] Voges J, Sturm V, Lehrke R, Treuer H, Gauss C, Berthold F. Cystic craniopharyngioma: Long-term results after intracavitary irradiation with stereotactically applied colloidal β-emitting radioactive sources. Neurosurgery. 1997;**40**(2):263-270

[43] Hasegawa T, Kondziolka D, Hadjipanayis CG, Lunsford LD. Management of cystic craniopharyngiomas with phosphorus-32 intracavitary irradiation. Neurosurgery. 2004;**54**(4):813-822

[44] Yu X, Christ SM, Liu R, Wang Y, Hu C, Feng B, et al. Evaluation of long-term outcomes and toxicity after stereotactic phosphorus-32–based intracavitary brachytherapy in patients with cystic craniopharyngioma. International Journal of Radiation Oncology* Biology* Physics. 2021;**111**(3):773-784

[45] Takahashi H, Nakazawa S, Shimura T. Evaluation of postoperative intratumoral injection of bleomycin for craniopharyngioma in children. Journal of Neurosurgery. 1985;**62**(1):120-127

[46] Zhang S, Fang Y, Cai BW, Xu JG, You C. Intracystic bleomycin for cystic craniopharyngiomas in children. Cochrane Database of Systematic Reviews. 2016;**2016**:CD008890

[47] Hukin J, Steinbok P, Lafay-Cousin L, Hendson G, Strother D, Mercier C, et al. Intracystic bleomycin therapy for craniopharyngioma in children: The Canadian experience. Cancer: Interdisciplinary International Journal of the American Cancer Society. 2007;**109**(10):2124-2131

[48] Broggi G, Giorgi C, Franzini A, Leocata F, Riva D. Therapeutic role of intracavitary bleomycin administration in cystic craniopharyngioma. In: Craniopharyngioma: Surgical Treatment. Milano: Springer Milan; 1995. pp. 113-119

[49] Bartels U, Laperriere N, Bouffet E, Drake J. Intracystic therapies for cystic craniopharyngioma in childhood. Frontiers in Endocrinology. 2012;**3**:39

[50] Cavalheiro S, Dastoli PA, Silva NS, Toledo S, Lederman H, Da Silva MC. Use of interferon alpha in intratumoral chemotherapy for cystic craniopharyngioma. Child's Nervous System. 2005;**21**:719-724

[51] Ferrantini M, Capone I, Belardelli F. Interferon-α and cancer: Mechanisms of action and new perspectives of clinical use. Biochimie. 2007;**89**(6-7):884-893

[52] Ganau M, Foroni RI, Gerosa M, Ricciardi GK, Longhi M, Nicolato A. Radiosurgical options in neuro-oncology: A review on current tenets and future opportunities. Part II: Adjuvant radiobiological tools. Tumori Journal. 2015;**101**(1):57-63

[53] Gopal M, Thakur G, Puduvalli V. Initial presentation of papillary craniopharyngioma with BRAF mutation treated with adjuvant chemotherapy (867). Neurology. 2020;**94**(supplement. 15):867

[54] Khaddour K, Chicoine MR, Huang J, Dahiya S, Ansstas G. Successful use of BRAF/MEK inhibitors as a neoadjuvant approach in the definitive treatment of papillary craniopharyngioma. Journal of the National Comprehensive Cancer Network. 2020;**18**(12):1590-1595

[55] Nussbaum PE, Nussbaum LA, Torok CM, Patel PD, Yesavage TA, Nussbaum ES. Case report and literature review of BRAF-V600 inhibitors for treatment of papillary craniopharyngiomas: A potential treatment paradigm shift. Journal of Clinical Pharmacy & Therapeutics. 2022;**47**(6):826-831

[56] Children's Cancer and Leukaemia Group (CCLG). Craniopharyngioma: Guideline for the Management of Children and Young People (CYP) Aged <19 Years. UK: CCLG; 2021

[57] Bowers DC, Verbruggen LC, Kremer LC, Hudson MM, Skinner R, Constine LS, et al. Surveillance for subsequent neoplasms of the CNS for childhood, adolescent, and young adult cancer survivors: A systematic review and recommendations from the international late effects of childhood cancer guideline harmonization group. The Lancet Oncology. 2021;**22**(5):e196-e206

[58] Lara-Velazquez M, Mehkri Y, Panther E, Hernandez J, Rao D, Fiester P, et al. Current advances in the management of adult craniopharyngiomas. Current Oncology. 2022;**29**(3):1645-1671

[59] Sowithayasakul P, Beckhaus J, Boekhoff S, Friedrich C, Calaminus G, Müller HL. Vision-related quality of life in patients with childhood-onset craniopharyngioma. Scientific Reports. 2023;**13**(1):19599

[60] Zheng Y, Ong SH, Vellayappan B, Nga VD. Management of first recurrence or progression of craniopharyngioma after resection alone: A systematic review and individual-participant data meta-analysis. Journal of Clinical Neuroscience. 2023;**118**:123-131

[61] Fouda MA, Karsten M, Staffa SJ, Scott RM, Marcus KJ, Baird LC. Management strategies for recurrent pediatric craniopharyngioma: New recommendations. Journal of Neurosurgery. Pediatrics. 2021;**27**(5):548-555

[62] Ji C, Cheng H, Zhou X, Cao X, Qiao N, Shi C, et al. Ectopic recurrence craniopharyngioma: Series report and literature review. Chinese Neurosurgical Journal. 2023;**9**(1):13. DOI: 10.1186/s41016-023-00326-3

[63] Gan HW, Morillon P, Albanese A, Aquilina K, Chandler C, Chang YC, et al. National UK guidelines for the management of paediatric craniopharyngioma. The Lancet Diabetes & Endocrinology. 2023;**11**(9):694-706

[64] Del Baldo G, Vennarini S, Cacchione A, Amelio D, De Ioris MA, Fabozzi F, et al. Multidisciplinary management of craniopharyngiomas in children: A single center experience. Diagnostics (Basel). 2022;**12**(11):2745

[65] Cheng L, Zhu H, Wang J, Wu S, Zhang S, Wang J, et al. Risk factor and replacement therapy analysis of pre- and postoperative endocrine deficiencies for craniopharyngioma. Cancers (Basel). 2023;**15**(2):340

[66] Sklar CA. Craniopharyngioma: Endocrine abnormalities at presentation. Pediatric Neurosurgery. 1994;**21**(Suppl. 1):18-20

[67] Müller HL. Craniopharyngioma: Long-term consequences of a chronic disease. Expert Review of Neurotherapeutics. 2015;**15**(11):1241-1244

[68] Zhao R, Lu P, Fan Y, Li C, Liu C, Zhao P, et al. Clinical analysis of risk factors of postoperative psychiatric disorders in patients with adult craniopharyngioma. Frontiers in Neurology. 2021;**12**:754349

[69] Grassi L. Psychiatric and psychosocial implications in cancer care: The agenda of psycho-oncology. Epidemiology and Psychiatric Sciences. 2020;**29**:e89

[70] Giese H, Haenig B, Unterberg A, Zweckberger K. Neurological and neuropsychological outcome after resection of craniopharyngiomas. Journal of Neurosurgery. 2019;**132**(6):1425-1434

[71] Roth CL. Hypothalamic obesity in craniopharyngioma patients: Disturbed

energy homeostasis related to extent of hypothalamic damage and its implication for obesity intervention. Journal of Clinical Medicine. 2015;**4**(9):1774-1797

[72] Lamas OC. Consecuencias metabólicas del craneofaringioma y su tratamiento. Endocrinología y Nutrición. 2013;**60**:529-534

[73] European Society of Paediatric Oncology. Craniopharyngioma: Standard Clinical Practice Recommendations. Version 2. Brussels, Belgium: European Society of Paediatric Oncology; 2021

[74] Romigi A, Feola T, Cappellano S, De Angelis M, Pio G, Caccamo M, et al. Sleep disorders in patients with Craniopharyngioma: A physiopathological and practical update. Frontiers in Neurology. 2022;**12**:817257

[75] Mori M, Takeshima H, Kuratsu J. Expression of interleukin-6 in human craniopharyngiomas: A possible inducer of tumor-associated inflammation. International Journal of Molecular Medicine. 2004;**14**:505-509

[76] Lin D, Wang Y, Zhou Z, Lin Z. Immune microenvironment of primary and recurrent craniopharyngiomas: A study of the differences and clinical significance. World Neurosurgery. 2019;**127**:e212-e220

Chapter 11

Perspective Chapter: Theory and Application of Tumor Treating Fields in Brain Tumor Treatment

Dongjiang Chen, Johnny Odeh and Ping Shi

Abstract

Glioblastoma (GBM) is the most common primary brain tumor in adults and continues to portend poor survival, despite multimodal treatment using surgery and chemoradiotherapy. The addition of Tumor Treating Fields (TTFields) to standard therapy has been shown to extend survival for patients, leading to the clinical approval of this approach by the FDA. TTFields represent a non-invasive anticancer modality consisting of low-intensity, intermediate-frequency alternating electric fields. It exhibits a broad mechanism of action by disrupting a multitude of biological processes, including cell proliferation, DNA repair, cell permeability, and immunological responses, to elicit therapeutic effects. This chapter describes advances in our current understanding of the mechanisms by which TTFields mediate anticancer effects. Additionally, we summarize the landscape of TTFields clinical trials across brain tumors and consider how emerging data might inform future clinical applications for TTFields.

Keywords: glioblastoma, GBM, tumor treating fields, TTFields, brain tumor, clinical trials

1. Introduction

GBM is the most common and aggressive type of primary brain tumor. It is responsible for most of the roughly 200,000 deaths worldwide from central nervous system tumors each year [1]. Even with maximum surgical removal of the tumor followed by radiation therapy and chemotherapy with temozolomide (TMZ), the average survival time is about 15 months [2]. This situation has not improved significantly in recent decades, highlighting the urgent need for more effective treatments for this devastating disease.

TTFields, with the market name of Optune Gio by Novocure, are a new non-invasive cancer treatment that uses low-intensity (1–3 V/cm), intermediate-frequency (100–300 kHz) alternating electric fields. These electric fields apply physical forces on charged and polar molecules in the body. The effectiveness of TTFields therapy depends on the duration of treatment, with evidence showing that using TTFields for more than 18 hours a day improves survival [3]. The frequency of the electric field also matters and varies by cancer type. For glioma cells, TTFields are most effective at an optimal frequency of 200 kHz [4].

Two key clinical trials, EF-11 and EF-14, have been instrumental in the FDA's approval of TTFields for treating recurrent and newly diagnosed GBM (ndGBM) [5, 6]. The EF-11 trial showed that TTFields are effective for patients with recurrent GBM, while the EF-14 trial demonstrated that adding TTFields to the standard TMZ treatment significantly increased the median overall survival (mOS) by 4.9 months and median progression-free survival (mPFS) by 2.7 months in patients with ndGBM, without adding significant side effects. These results led to the FDA's approval of TTFields for ndGBM in 2015, marking a significant advancement in GBM treatment.

TTFields work by affecting several critical processes within cancer cells, such as cell division, DNA repair, autophagy, immune responses, and cell membrane permeability. Early data suggest that combining TTFields with other treatments, like radiotherapy, chemotherapy, and immunotherapy, may improve their effectiveness. Ongoing research and clinical trials are exploring its use in brain metastases and various extracranial tumors.

In summary, TTFields represent a significant advance in the treatment of GBM and potentially other brain tumors. Ongoing research into mechanisms of action and optimization of clinical use holds great promise for improving outcomes for patients facing these challenging diagnoses.

2. Mechanism of action using TTFields to treat brain tumors

2.1 TTFields disrupt mitotic processes

Mitosis disruption is one of the first anti-tumoral mechanisms identified. Studies have shown that the proliferation rate of the cells is more sensitive to TTFields-induced cell death [7]. Specifically, TTFields interact with key components involved in cell division, particularly proteins with high dipole moments such as tubulin and septin, disrupting critical stages of mitosis.

During metaphase, tubulin dimers in cancer cells align to form microtubules, essential for the mitotic spindle. TTFields cause these tubulin molecules to oscillate and spin due to the alternating electric fields, leading to instability in microtubule polymerization. This results in errors in spindle assembly and abnormal geometric shapes, causing delays in mitosis and the formation of cells with incorrect numbers of chromosomes (aneuploidy) [7, 8]. As mitosis progresses to anaphase, TTFields continue their disruptive action. Septin proteins, which help form the contractile ring necessary for cell division, are affected by the electric fields. TTFields interfere with the proper localization and function of septin, causing disorganized contraction of the cell membrane. This leads to membrane blebbing (bubbling) and ultimately disrupts cell division, leading to cell death [9].

In telophase, TTFields generate concentrated electric fields at the cleavage furrow, where the cell division is set to occur. This creates a dielectrophoretic effect, pushing charged macromolecules and organelles toward the narrowest part of the dividing cell. The increased pressure and disrupted organization lead to cell rupture and death [10]. Beyond these direct effects on mitotic structures, TTFields also influence the broader cellular environment. They reduce the stability and expression of CDK2-associated RNA (CDK2-AS1), which is crucial for cell cycle progression, leading to cell cycle arrest in the G1 phase and further preventing tumor cell proliferation [11].

2.2 TTFields impair DNA damage repair

Impaired DNA damage repair is another hallmark of TTFields. DNA repair is a crucial process that allows cells to fix damage caused by various factors, including radiation and chemotherapy. By interfering with this process, TTFields enhance the susceptibility of cancer cells to these treatments, leading to increased cell death and improved treatment outcomes.

One of the primary ways TTFields impair DNA repair is by inducing replication stress. The electric fields generated by TTFields create physical forces that interfere with the normal progression of DNA replication, leading to the formation of R-loops. These R-loops, which are RNA-DNA hybrid structures, act as markers of replication stress and hinder the proper repair of DNA double-strand breaks. This disruption of DNA replication increases the accumulation of DNA damage in cancer cells, making them more vulnerable to additional stressors [12].

Moreover, TTFields downregulate the expression of crucial DNA repair genes, such as BRCA1 and BRCA2 [13]. These genes play an essential role in homologous recombination, a process that accurately repairs DNA double-strand breaks. The reduction in BRCA1 and BRCA2 expression compromises the ability of cancer cells to repair damaged DNA effectively. This impairment is particularly significant because it makes cancer cells more sensitive to treatments that induce DNA damage, such as radiation therapy and certain chemotherapeutic agents like temozolomide [14, 15]. Poly ADP-ribose polymerase (PARP) is a protein involved in single-strand DNA break repair. While TTFields robustly activate PARP-mediated DNA repair in glioma stem cells (GSCs), concomitant exposure to PARP inhibitors leads to the accumulation of DNA damage and ultimately cell death, especially in cells already deficient in other DNA repair pathways [16].

Studies have shown that cancer cells treated with TTFields exhibit more significant and prolonged DNA damage when combined with ionizing radiation [17, 18]. This combination results in a higher number of γH2AX foci, markers of DNA double-strand breaks, indicating increased DNA damage. Preliminary data suggest that applying TTFields prior to or concurrently with radiotherapy shows increased sensitivity compared to TTFields administered after radiation therapy *in vitro* [13]. Whether this holds true clinically is currently undergoing validation.

2.3 TTFields increase permeability of cell membranes

TTFields create mechanical stresses and forces on the cell membrane, causing disruptions in its integrity. The electric fields can alter the arrangement and function of membrane proteins and lipids, leading to the formation of transient pores. These pores increase the permeability of the cell membrane, allowing for greater influx of multiple agents such as Dextran-FITC, ethidium D, or 5-aminolevulinic acid (5-ALA) by measuring increased bioluminescence or scanning augmented number (53.5 ± 19.1 vs. 23.9 ± 11.0) and size (240.6 ± 91.7 nm^2 vs. 129.8 ± 31.9 nm^2) of holes on the cellular membrane [19]. Additionally, there is a significant increase in the uptake of membrane-associating reagents with a size of 20 kDa, and no larger than 50 kDa, into glioma cells with TTFields. These changes are reversible and return to normal within 24 h of ceasing TTFields treatment [19].

One significant effect of increased cell membrane permeability is the enhanced uptake of chemotherapeutic drugs. Cancer cells exposed to TTFields show higher intracellular concentrations of drugs like Withaferin A. This increased drug concentration within the cancer cells enhances the efficacy of chemotherapy, leading to synergistic treatment outcomes [20].

Additionally, TTFields can also affect the transport of ions and other small molecules across the cell membrane. The electric fields can modulate the activity of ion channels and transporters, altering the intracellular ionic environment. This disruption can lead to changes in cell signaling pathways, further sensitizing cancer cells to therapeutic interventions. For example, increased calcium influx due to TTFields can activate Ca_v 1.2 channels that promote GBM cell death providing the rationale to combine TTFields therapy with Ca^{2+} antagonists that are already in clinical use [21].

Moreover, the increased permeability of the cell membrane caused by TTFields may enhance the delivery of other therapeutic agents, such as targeted drugs and nanoparticles [22]. The ability of TTFields to create transient pores in the cell membrane can facilitate the entry of these agents into the cancer cells, improving their therapeutic efficacy. This has significant implications for the development of combination therapies that utilize TTFields to enhance the delivery and effectiveness of novel anticancer agents.

2.4 TTFields disrupt the blood brain barrier (BBB)

The BBB is a selective barrier that protects the brain from harmful substances in the bloodstream while allowing essential nutrients to pass through. However, this protective function can also hinder the delivery of therapeutic agents to brain tumors, posing a challenge for effective treatment [23]. TTFields have been shown to disrupt the integrity of the BBB in several ways, thereby enhancing the delivery of chemotherapeutic drugs and other therapeutic agents to the central nerve system (CNS).

The concept was first tested by a group using low-voltage pulses (5–100 V) to an external human BBB model. Although the exact mechanism was unclear, the paracellular pathway was affected, leading to a brief breach of the BBB [24]. Salvador et al. explored the effects of TTFields on the BBB and found that TTFields resulted in a reversible opening of the BBB. In their *in vitro* experiments using mouse cerebellar microvascular endothelial cells, immunofluorescence analysis showed that the tight junction (TJ) protein claudin-5 delocalized from the cell membrane to the cytoplasm when treated with TTFields. This relocation was mediated through the activation of the Rho/Rho kinase pathway, which phosphorylates claudin-5, disrupting its binding to other TJ-anchored proteins and increasing BBB permeability. Further *in vivo* experiments demonstrated that TTFields allowed paclitaxel, a chemotherapeutic agent normally restricted by the BBB, to exert its effects, reducing both tumor volume and tumor cell proliferation in rats [25].

Additionally, an *in vitro* 3D coculture model of the human BBB, constructed using human brain microvascular endothelial cells (HBMVECs) and immortalized human pericytes, showed that TTFields increased BBB permeability by altering the location of intracellular TJ proteins in HBMVECs [26]. However, in both pre-clinical studies, only the 100 kHz frequency has been proven to affect the BBB, which is not the approved frequency for clinical GBM treatment. A future strategy that involves combining two TTFields frequencies (i.e., 100 and 200 kHz) might be worth exploring for GBM and other brain tumor treatments. The lower 100 kHz frequency could be used to open the BBB for enhanced drug delivery, followed by a switch to 200 kHz to target the proliferating GBM cells.

2.5 TTFields and anti-tumoral immunity

Over the past decade, the field of cancer immunotherapy has witnessed remarkable advancements, prompting a reevaluation of traditional cancer treatments like radiotherapy, chemotherapy, and surgical therapy. The critical question is whether these methods are immunogenic and can be effectively combined with immunotherapy. As a relatively recent entrant in this domain, TTFields also need to establish their value. Fortunately, an increasing body of evidence suggests that TTFields can effectively activate the immune system through unique mechanisms, making them a promising candidate within the current immunotherapy landscape.

TTFields are believed to cause tumor cell death by disrupting the mitotic spindle, resulting in chromosome missegregation and eventually apoptosis. This process triggers immunogenic cell death (ICD), where tumor cell death generates an endoplasmic reticulum stress response, producing reactive oxygen species and releasing immune signaling molecules. These events increase the immunogenicity of tumor cells and enhance the immune functions of dendritic cells (DCs) [27].

In vitro studies have shown that TTFields-treated cells exhibit increased secretion of high-mobility group box 1 (HMGB1) protein, a key ICD marker. Additionally, TTFields treatment leads to the translocation of calreticulin (CRT) to the cell surface, signaling DCs to engulf the dying cells. These ICD markers were also observed in mouse models, where TTFields treatment resulted in significant elevations of circulating HMGB1 and phosphorylated eukaryotic translation initiation factor 2 (p-eIF2), reinforcing the idea that TTFields induce ICD [28].

Furthermore, TTFields activate innate immunity through the release of large micronuclei clusters and nuclear protrusions, which are often not encapsulated by the nuclear envelope. This disruption activates DNA sensors like cyclic GMP-AMP synthase (cGAS) and absent in melanoma 2 (AIM2), leading to the formation of inflammasomes. The cGAS-STING pathway, predominant in many cell types, activates proinflammatory cytokines and type 1 interferons (T1IFNs), while the AIM2 pathway activates inflammasomes leading to cell death. These pathways collectively enhance the immune response against tumors [29].

The potential association between TTFields and the adaptive immune system is becoming evident through DC activation. TTFields-prepared cells enhance phagocytosis by bone marrow-derived DCs (BMDCs) and stimulate BMDC maturation [27]. *In vivo* models have demonstrated that TTFields enhance cytotoxic T cells recruitment within mouse GBM tumors [29]. Clinical settings further affirm these findings, with some patients showing substantial T cell influx and signs of T cell activation toward memory development after TTFields therapy [29, 30].

Additionally, TTFields do not hinder the maturation or functionality of T cells. Studies have shown that T cells retain their pivotal anti-tumoral functions, including IFN-γ secretion and cytotoxic degranulation, under TTFields exposure [30]. This indicates that TTFields can be combined with immunotherapies like immune checkpoint inhibitors (ICIs) or CAR-T cell therapy to enhance therapeutic efficacy.

2.6 Other cancer biology functions impaired by TTFields

Studies have shown that TTFields significantly decrease the migration and invasion capabilities of various glioma cell lines, including U87, U373, A172, LN18, and LN229, as well as glioma stem cells T325 and ZH161 [31, 32]. TTFields can destroy primary cilia, which are abundant on the surface of glioma cell membranes, by disrupting SHH pathway activity and interfering with glioma cell invasion and migration ability [33].

TTFields have also been shown to inhibit vascular endothelial cell growth [32], downregulate the expression of HIF1α, VEGF, and MMP2/9, and inhibit both neovascularization and epithelial-mesenchymal transition (EMT). These effects are mediated through the downregulation of the PI3K/AKT/NF-κB signaling pathway [34].

TTFields reduce the expression of the glycolytic biomarker pyruvate kinase M2 (PKM2) in human GBM. This reduction can be non-invasively detected using a novel radiotracer, [^{18}F] DASA-23 [35]. Additionally, TTFields, when combined with the CUSP9v3 drug repurposing approach (which includes nine repurposed drugs plus metronomic temozolomide), induce metabolic reprogramming and exhibit synergistic anti-glioblastoma activity *in vitro* [36].

2.7 Resistant mechanism of TTFields

Although TTFields significantly impact tumor cell behavior in many aspects and lead to prolonged survival in ndGBM patients, resistance to TTFields eventually develops, leading to treatment failure and disease progression. Autophagy is a hallmark of TTFields treatment effects and is believed to be linked with the resistance mechanism of glioma cells. Specifically, depletion of AMP-activated protein kinase (AMPK) or autophagy-related protein 7 (ATG7) inhibited the upregulation of autophagy in response to TTFields, as well as sensitized cells to the treatment, suggesting that cancer cells utilize autophagy as a resistance mechanism to TTFields [37].

Utilizing a machine learning algorithm combined with rigorous experimental validation, prostaglandin E2 receptor 3 (PTGER3) has been identified as another key mediator responsible for the resistance mechanism by regulating the stemness of GBM cells [38]. This resistance mechanism mediated by PTGER3 is particularly linked to long-term resistance, in contrast to the more immediate effects of autophagy.

3. Current and future use of TTFields for brain tumors

3.1 Current GBM regimen with TTFields

Prior to the EF-14 trial, the standard treatment for GBM involved maximum surgical resection followed by radiation and chemotherapy. The EF-14 trial introduced TTFields to this regimen, significantly improving patient outcomes. The median PFS increased from 4.0 months to 6.7 months, while the mOS improved from 16.0 months to 20.9 months [5].

Further subgroup analysis revealed a more pronounced benefit in the Asian population, with mOS increasing from 15.2 to 27.2 months [39]. Elderly patients with ndGBM typically have a poorer prognosis than younger patients, but the addition of TTFields to the treatment regimen was well tolerated in elderly patients. This new regimen increased PFS from 3.9 months to 6.5 months and OS from 13.7 months to 17.4 months in this cohort [40].

Moreover, patients with high compliance to TTFields treatment (daily usage of more than 22 hours) experienced a greater survival benefit: HR = 0.78; $p = 0.031$; OS at compliance ≥75% vs. < 75% [3]. Thus, the current recommendation is to use the device for at least 18 hours a day.

Based on previous validation, several directions are currently being explored to further enhance the efficacy of TTFields in treating GBM with ongoing trials summarized in **Table 1**.

3.2 Adjusted treatment regimen under exploration

The current regimen based on the EF-14 clinical trial applies TTFields post-concomitant radiation and chemotherapy. The concept of initiating TTFields prior to and concurrently with radiation was first tested in pre-clinical models [13]. Following the confirmation of safety in a phase I study [41], subsequent trials, such as PriCoTTF and EF-32, have been conducted to investigate this approach further.

The PriCoTTF is a phase I/II study that enrolled 33 patients with ndGBM. In this study, TTFields were initiated immediately after surgery and continued concurrently with chemoradiation and adjuvant chemotherapy for a total of approximately 9 months. Radiation therapy was conducted with the TTFields arrays present on the patients' scalps and TTFields rechallenge was permitted upon GBM recurrence. As of the 2023 ASCO Annual Meeting, the mOS had not yet been reached (48% of events had occurred). Multivariable Cox regression analysis found that OS was independently associated with the number of days patients received more than 23 hours of TTFields therapy (HR 0.96, 95% CI 0.93–0.99, P = 0.008) [42].

The randomized, prospective, open-label phase III trial (TRIDENT, EF-32, NCT04471844) aims to evaluate whether the concurrent initiation of TTFields and postoperative radiation therapy improves clinical outcomes compared to the standard treatment regimen. This trial is set to enroll 950 patients at 129 sites worldwide, with the primary endpoint being patient OS. The estimated primary completion date for this study is August 2024 [43].

3.3 TTFields leverage immune therapies

Previous phase III trials that added only ICIs to standard therapy failed to improve survival in GBM patients, likely because ICIs require pre-existing infiltration of immune cells within tumors [44, 45]. A growing body of evidence suggests that TTFields can effectively induce ICD, stimulate innate immunity, and drive immune cell infiltration, thereby "heating up" immunologically cold tumors, making TTFields a good candidate combining with ICIs.

The 2-THE-TOP trial (NCT03405792) is a phase II prospective single-arm open-label clinical trial in which 26 ndGBM patients were treated with pembrolizumab, TTFields, and TMZ after completing concurrent chemoradiotherapy. The triple therapy was well tolerated by the patients. The final analysis showed that patients in the 2-THE-TOP study had a median PFS of 12.0 months compared to 5.8 months for the historical EF-14 cohort. The mOS was 24.8 months versus 14.6 months, respectively [46]. This promising pilot study has led to the announcement of a phase III trial (EF-41/Keynote D58) to further confirm the therapeutic benefits of this combination.

TTFields could also enhance DC activation and antigen uptake, improving the efficacy of cancer vaccines. One approach being explored is personalized neoantigen vaccines (PNVs), as in the NCT03223103 trial for GBM. The combined treatment is well tolerated with the induction of robust epitope-specific T cell responses [47]. Other immunotherapy approaches that could benefit from combining with TTFields include CAR-T cell therapy. TTFields may create a more favorable tumor microenvironment to attract CAR-T cells and enhance their cytotoxicity.

Trial number	ND/R	Phase	Arm(s)	Enrollment	Primary outcome measures	Current status
NCT06353360	ND	II	Experimental: TTFields + TMZ + Tislelizumab	30	Progression-Free Survival	Not Yet Recruiting
NCT06222138	ND	N/A	TTFields	80	Overall Survival, Time to Progression	Not Yet Recruiting
NCT06136611	ND	I	Experimental: TTFields Before/After Surgery No Intervention: Routine GBM Care	42	Incidence of Treatment-Emergent Adverse Events	Not Yet Recruiting
NCT06017063	ND	N/A	Experimental: Intervention Arm - TTFields + Psychological intervention No Intervention: Control Arm - TTFields alone	275	Efficacy of Intervention	Not Yet Recruiting
NCT05973903	R	I/II	Pembrolizumab + Lenvatinib + TTFields	47	Progression-Free Survival (6 months)	Not Yet Recruiting
NCT05086497	ND	N/A	Arm 1: TTFields + "standard array mapping" Arm 2: TTFields + "Alternative (more precise) array mapping"	155	Time to progression	Recruiting
NCT04902586	ND	II	Experimental: Chemoradiotherapy + TMZ + TTFields + RT No Intervention: Chemoradiotherapy + TMZ + RT	30	Disease-Free Survival	Unknown
NCT04717739	ND	N/A	TTFields	500	Time of TTFields Usage, TTFields Adverse Events, Lifestyle Changes, Changes in Sleep Quality et al.	Recruiting
NCT04689087	R	N/A	Experimental: TTFields + BPC chemotherapy used after relapse surgery	40	Overall Survival at 6 Months	Unknown
NCT04671459	Both	II	SRS + TTFields	40	One-Year Survival Rate	Active, Not Recruiting
NCT04492163	R	II	TTFields	25	Progression-Free Survival	Unknown

DOI: http://dx.doi.org/10.5772/intechopen.1007376

Trial number	ND/R	Phase	Arm(s)	Enrollment	Primary outcome measures	Current status
NCT04474353	ND	I	Gadolinium, TMZ, Stereotactic Radiosurgery (SRS), TTFields	12	Dose-Limiting Toxicity (DLT)	Active
NCT04471844	ND	III	Arm 1: TMZ + RT + TTFields Arm 2: TMZ + RT + TTFields (after 6 weeks)	950	Overall Survival	Active
NCT04469075	Both	II	Topical Clindamycin Phosphate and Triamcinolone Acetonide, TTFields	58	Grade 2 or Higher Skin Toxicity	Recruiting
NCT04397679	ND	I	RT + TMZ + Chloroquine + TTFields	2	Rate of Grade 3 or Higher Dermatitis	Active
NCT04223999	R	II	Experimental: Intervention Skull remodeling Surgery + TTFields + Best Practice Treatment Active Comparator: TTFields + Best Practice Treatment	70	Overall Survival (12 months)	Recruiting
NCT04221503	R	II	Experimental (Cohort A): Niraparib + TTFields Active Comparator (Cohort B): Surgical Resection + Niraparib + TTFields	30	Disease Control: Complete Response, Partial Response, Stable Disease	Active, Not Recruiting
NCT03780569	ND	N/A	RT + TMZ + TTFields	10	Safety of Combined Radiotherapy/TMZ and TTFields	Unknown
NCT03687034	N/A	I	BRCX014 + TMZ + TTFields	21	Number of Treatment-Related Adverse Events	Unknown
NCT03405792	ND	II	Experimental: TMZ + TTFields + Pembrolizumab Control: TMZ + TTFields	40	Progression-Free Survival	Active, Not Recruiting
NCT03258021	ND	N/A	TTFields	710	Overall Survival, TTFields-Related Serious Adverse Events, TTFields Treatment Compliance, Time to First GBM Progression, Changes in Quality of Life et al.	Unknown
NCT03194971	Both	II	TTFields	20	Pathological Assessment	Recruiting
NCT03223103	ND	I	MTA-Vaccine: Mutation-derived tumor vaccine (Peptides. + Poly-ICLC + TTFields)	13	Dose-Limiting Toxicity (DLT)	Active

Trial number	ND/R	Phase	Arm(s)	Enrollment	Primary outcome measures	Current status
NCT05030298	ND	I/II A	TMZ, TTFields Arm 1: Stereotactic Biopsy, Radiosurgery, Surgery Arm 2: Surgery, Radiation Therapy, Chemotherapy	40	Adverse Events	Recruiting
NCT03642080	Both	N/A	TTFields	48	Progression of Disease	Unknown

ND: newly diagnosed GBM, R: recurrent GBM, TMZ: temozolomide, RT: radiotherapy, SRS: Stereotactic radiosurgery.

Table 1.
Current clinical trials exploring the efficacy of TTFields in treating glioblastoma.

DOI: http://dx.doi.org/10.5772/intechopen.1007376

NCT number	Disease	Phase	Arm(s)	Enrollment	Primary outcome measures	Current status
NCT05746325	Leptomeningeal Metastases Within the Spine	I	MRI + Lumbar Puncture + TTFields	5	Incidence of Significant Toxicity of TTFields, Feasibility of TTFields to complete 30-day trial	Recruiting
NCT05310448	Glioma with at least partial involvement of the thalamus, cerebral peduncles, midbrain, pons, or medulla	I	RT + TTFields	10	Incidence of Adverse Events	Recruiting
NCT05341349	Melanoma Brain Metastases	I	Arm 1: SRS + Pembrolizumab + TTFields Arm 2: SRS + Nivolumab and Ipilimumab + TTFields	10	Percentage of Patients Developing Grade 3 CNS Toxicity	Recruiting
NCT04967027	Brain Metastases	I	Resistant to Drug/RT TTFields Treatment	5	Adverse Events, Time to Progression, Overall Survival Rate	Unknown
NCT03033992	Supratentorial High-Grade Glioma (HGG) Ependymoma (Stratum 1) Newly Diagnosed Diffuse Intrinsic Pontine Glioma (Stratum 2)	N/A	Arm 1: TTFields Arm 2: RT + TTFields	80	Pediatric Device Usage Compliance, Pediatric Device-Related Toxicity, Feasibility of Concurrent TTFields/RT, Device-Limiting Toxicities, Overall Survival	Recruiting
NCT02831959	NSCLC Brain Metastases	III	Arm 1: SRS + TTFields Treatment Arm 2: SRS + Best Standard of Care	270	Time to Intracranial Progression	Active, not recruiting
NCT01755624	NSCLC Brain Metastases	II	Arm 1 TTFields Arm 2: Best Standard of Care	18	Time to Local/Distant Progression in Brain	Unknown

Table 2.
Ongoing clinical trials utilizing TTFields for the treatment of non-GBM brain tumors

3.4 Combination therapies with specific targets

Several other trials are exploring different aspects of TTFields therapy based on preliminary studies. One direction involves combining TTFields with the PARP inhibitor niraparib. A phase II study (NCT04221503) is investigating this combination in patients with recurrent high-grade glioma (HGG). Although the combination therapy has been found to be safe, it has not yet demonstrated a significant signal of efficacy [48].

Another focus is on overcoming the resistance mechanisms associated with TTFields. Since autophagy is linked to cancer cell survival under TTFields treatment, chloroquine, an autophagy inhibitor, is being tested in combination with TTFields in a clinical trial (NCT04397679) to determine its potential to enhance treatment efficacy. Additionally, a retrospective study evaluated the effect of celecoxib, a cyclooxygenase-2 (COX-2) inhibitor, when combined with TTFields. The study found that patients not receiving celecoxib (n = 14) had a mOS of 8.1 months, while those receiving celecoxib (n = 28) had a mOS of 12.9 months (chi-square 5.42, p = 0.002, HR = 2.1, 95% CI = 1.19–5.59) [49]. Since COX-2 is upstream of PTGER3, another potential target to overcome TTFields resistance, it may be worthwhile to conduct a prospective clinical trial to confirm the benefits of combining celecoxib with TTFields.

3.5 Clinical trials to treat other brain tumors

Since TTFields treatment to the brain has been shown to be safe and to extend OS in GBM patients, there is an acute need to test its efficacy in brain metastases, which are more common than GBM, or lower-grade gliomas (**Table 2**). In the recently completed phase III trial (METIS, EF-25, NCT02831959), 298 mutation-negative non-small cell lung cancer (NSCLC) patients with 1–10 brain metastases were enrolled and randomized to receive either TTFields therapy with supportive care or supportive care alone following stereotactic radiosurgery (SRS). The primary endpoint, time to intracranial progression from SRS, was significantly prolonged in the group receiving SRS followed by TTFields therapy with best supportive care (BSC) compared to the group receiving SRS plus BSC alone (median of 21.9 vs. 11.3 months; HR = 0.67 [0.48–0.93], p = 0.02) [50]. In addition to NSCLC, another ongoing phase I trial (NCT05341349) is studying the combination of SRS, ICIs, and TTFields for the treatment of melanoma brain metastases.

4. Conclusion

TTFields have emerged as a revolutionary non-invasive treatment modality, offering new hope for patients with GBM and potentially other challenging brain malignancies. By leveraging low-intensity, intermediate-frequency alternating electric fields, TTFields disrupt crucial cellular processes, including mitosis, DNA repair, cell membrane permeability, and immune responses, thereby exerting multifaceted anticancer effects. Pilot studies such as 2-THE-TOP have raised hope to further improvements in patient survival.

As research advances, the potential of TTFields continues to expand. Ongoing studies are exploring the efficacy of TTFields in combination with ICIs, PARP inhibitors, autophagy inhibitors, and other novel therapies to enhance therapeutic outcomes and overcome resistance mechanisms. Furthermore, the promising results from trials investigating TTFields in brain metastases highlight the versatility and broad applicability of this treatment. By continuing to unravel the underlying mechanisms and optimizing clinical protocols, TTFields may become a revolutionize cancer care, especially for brain tumors that have very limited treatment options with traditional methods.

Acknowledgements

JO was a fellow in the USC/CHLA Summer Oncology Research Fellowship (SORF) Program, supported in part by the National Cancer Institute of the National Institutes of Health under Award Number R25CA225513 and by the Norris Comprehensive Cancer Center in Los Angeles, Children's Hospital Los Angeles, Concern Foundation for Cancer Research, Curing Kids Cancer, and Tri Delta. The content is solely the responsibility of the authors and does not necessarily represent the official views of the National Institutes of Health.

Conflict of interest

Dongjiang Chen has received personal honoraria from Novocure for consultant work. The book chapter preparation was performed by the authors independently of Novocure. Dongjiang Chen is the inventor of three patent applications related to the work reported in this book chapter. However, royalty-free commercialization rights were transferred to Novocure per the funding agreement. Other co-authors declare no conflict of interest.

Author details

Dongjiang Chen[1*], Johnny Odeh[2] and Ping Shi[3]

1 Division of Neuro-Oncology, Brain Tumor Center, Keck School of Medicine of University of Southern California, Los Angeles, CA, United States of America

2 Paul L. Foster School of Medicine, Texas Tech Health Sciences Center of El Paso, El Paso, TX, United States of America

3 Department of Pathology, Penn State Health Hershey Medical Center, Penn State College of Medicine, Hershey, PA, United States of America

*Address all correspondence to: dongjiang.chen@med.usc.edu

References

[1] Brain, G.B.D. and C.N.S.C.C. Other. Global, regional, and national burden of brain and other CNS cancer, 1990-2016: A systematic analysis for the global burden of disease study 2016. Lancet Neurology. 2019;**18**(4):376-393

[2] Stupp R et al. Radiotherapy plus concomitant and adjuvant temozolomide for glioblastoma. The New England Journal of Medicine. 2005;**352**(10):987-996

[3] Toms SA et al. Increased compliance with tumor treating fields therapy is prognostic for improved survival in the treatment of glioblastoma: A subgroup analysis of the EF-14 phase III trial. Journal of Neuro-Oncology. 2019;**141**(2):467-473

[4] Kirson ED et al. Disruption of cancer cell replication by alternating electric fields. Cancer Research. 2004;**64**(9):3288-3295

[5] Stupp R et al. Effect of tumor-treating fields plus maintenance temozolomide vs maintenance temozolomide alone on survival in patients with glioblastoma: A randomized clinical trial. JAMA. 2017;**318**(23):2306-2316

[6] Stupp R et al. NovoTTF-100A versus physician's choice chemotherapy in recurrent glioblastoma: A randomised phase III trial of a novel treatment modality. European Journal of Cancer. 2012;**48**(14):2192-2202

[7] Giladi M et al. Mitotic spindle disruption by alternating electric fields leads to improper chromosome segregation and mitotic catastrophe in cancer cells. Scientific Reports. 2015;**5**:18046

[8] Timmons JJ et al. Tubulin's response to external electric fields by molecular dynamics simulations. PLoS One. 2018;**13**(9):e0202141

[9] Gera N et al. Tumor treating fields perturb the localization of septins and cause aberrant mitotic exit. PLoS One. 2015;**10**(5):e0125269

[10] Kirson ED et al. Alternating electric fields arrest cell proliferation in animal tumor models and human brain tumors. Proceedings of the National Academy of Sciences of the United States of America. 2007;**104**(24):10152-10157

[11] Xu S et al. Whole transcriptome and proteome analyses identify potential targets and mechanisms underlying tumor treating fields against glioblastoma. Cell Death & Disease. 2022;**13**(8):721

[12] Karanam NK et al. Tumor treating fields cause replication stress and interfere with DNA replication fork maintenance: Implications for cancer therapy. Translational Research. 2020;**217**:33-46

[13] Karanam NK et al. Tumor-treating fields elicit a conditional vulnerability to ionizing radiation via the downregulation of BRCA1 signaling and reduced DNA double-strand break repair capacity in non-small cell lung cancer cell lines. Cell Death & Disease. 2017;**8**(3):e2711

[14] Fishman H et al. Tumor treating fields (TTFields) increase the effectiveness of temozolomide and lomustine in glioblastoma cell lines. Journal of Neuro-Oncology. 2023;**163**(1):83-94

[15] Mumblat H et al. Tumor treating fields (TTFields) downregulate the Fanconi Anemia-BRCA pathway and

increase the efficacy of chemotherapy in malignant pleural mesothelioma preclinical models. Lung Cancer. 2021;**160**:99-110

[16] Vanderlinden A et al. DNA damage response inhibitors enhance tumour treating fields (TTFields) potency in glioma stem-like cells. British Journal of Cancer. 2023;**129**(11):1829-1840

[17] Kim EH et al. Biological effect of an alternating electric field on cell proliferation and synergistic antimitotic effect in combination with ionizing radiation. Oncotarget. 2016;**7**(38):62267-62279

[18] Giladi M et al. Tumor treating fields (TTFields) delay DNA damage repair following radiation treatment of glioma cells. Radiation Oncology. 2017;**12**(1):206

[19] Chang E et al. Tumor treating fields increases membrane permeability in glioblastoma cells. Cell Death Discovery. 2018;**4**:113

[20] Chang E et al. Synergistic inhibition of glioma cell proliferation by Withaferin a and tumor treating fields. Journal of Neuro-Oncology. 2017;**134**(2):259-268

[21] Neuhaus E et al. Alternating electric fields (TTFields) activate Ca(v)1.2 channels in human glioblastoma cells. Cancers (Basel). 2019;**11**(1):1-21

[22] Desai PP, Prabhu S. Tumor treating fields (TTFields) targeted self assembling nanoparticles for pancreatic cancer treatment: In vitro and in vivo assessment. Cancer Research. 2024;**84**(6_Supplement):477-477

[23] Arvanitis CD, Ferraro GB, Jain RK. The blood-brain barrier and blood-tumour barrier in brain tumours and metastases. Nature Reviews Cancer. 2020;**20**(1):26-41

[24] Sharabi S et al. Transient blood-brain barrier disruption is induced by low pulsed electrical fields in vitro: An analysis of permeability and trans-endothelial electric resistivity. Drug Delivery. 2019;**26**(1):459-469

[25] Salvador E et al. Tumor treating fields (TTFields) reversibly permeabilize the blood-brain barrier In vitro and In vivo. Biomolecules. 2022;**12**(10):1-20

[26] Salvador E et al. Tumor treating fields (TTFields) induce cell junction alterations in a human 3D In vitro model of the blood-brain barrier. Pharmaceutics. 2023;**15**(1):1-12

[27] Voloshin T et al. Tumor-treating fields (TTFields) induce immunogenic cell death resulting in enhanced antitumor efficacy when combined with anti-PD-1 therapy. Cancer Immunology, Immunotherapy. 2020;**69**(7):1191-1204

[28] Barsheshet Y et al. Tumor treating fields (TTFields) concomitant with immune checkpoint inhibitors are therapeutically effective in non-small cell lung cancer (NSCLC) In vivo model. International Journal of Molecular Sciences. 2022;**23**(22):1-15

[29] Chen D et al. Tumor treating fields dually activate STING and AIM2 inflammasomes to induce adjuvant immunity in glioblastoma. The Journal of Clinical Investigation. 2022;**132**(8):1-21

[30] Diamant G et al. T cells retain pivotal antitumoral functions under tumor-treating electric fields. Journal of Immunology. 2021;**207**(2):709-719

[31] Silginer M et al. Biological activity of tumor-treating fields in preclinical glioma models. Cell Death & Disease. 2017;**8**(4):e2753

[32] Kim EH et al. Tumor treating fields inhibit glioblastoma cell migration,

invasion and angiogenesis. Oncotarget. 2016;**7**(40):65125-65136

[33] Shi P et al. Tumor treating fields suppression of ciliogenesis enhances temozolomide toxicity. Frontiers in Oncology. 2022;**12**:837589

[34] Chen H et al. Growth inhibition of malignant melanoma by intermediate frequency alternating electric fields, and the underlying mechanisms. The Journal of International Medical Research. 2012;**40**(1):85-94

[35] Patel CB et al. Tumor treating fields (TTFields) impairs aberrant glycolysis in glioblastoma as evaluated by [(18) F]DASA-23, a non-invasive probe of pyruvate kinase M2 (PKM2) expression. Neoplasia. 2021;**23**(1):58-67

[36] Cao Q et al. Tumor treating fields (TTFields) combined with the drug repurposing approach CUSP9v3 induce metabolic reprogramming and synergistic anti-glioblastoma activity in vitro. British Journal of Cancer. 2024;**130**(8):1365-1376

[37] Shteingauz A et al. AMPK-dependent autophagy upregulation serves as a survival mechanism in response to tumor treating fields (TTFields). Cell Death & Disease. 2018;**9**(11):1074

[38] Tran DD, Le SB, Chen D. Methods for Restoring Sensitivity to TTFields in TTFields-Resistant Cancer Cells with PTGER3 Inhibitors. Novocure GmbH: Novocure Israel Ltd; 2024

[39] Kim CY et al. Tumor treating fields plus temozolomide for newly diagnosed glioblastoma: A sub-group analysis of Korean patients in the EF-14 phase 3 trial. Journal of Neuro-Oncology. 2020;**146**(3):399-406

[40] Ram Z et al. Efficacy and safety of tumor treating fields (TTFields) in elderly patients with newly diagnosed glioblastoma: Subgroup analysis of the phase 3 EF-14 clinical trial. Frontiers in Oncology. 2021;**11**:671972

[41] Bokstein F et al. Concurrent tumor treating fields (TTFields) and radiation therapy for newly diagnosed glioblastoma: A prospective safety and feasibility study. Frontiers in Oncology. 2020;**10**:411

[42] Kebir S et al. Safety and efficacy of tumor treating fields (TTFields) prior and concomitant to radiotherapy in patients with newly diagnosed glioblastoma: Results from PriCoTTF. Journal of Clinical Oncology. 2023;**41**(16_Suppl.):2050-2050

[43] Shi W et al. Phase 3 TRIDENT study (EF-32): Tumor treating fields (TTFields; 200 kHz) concomitant with chemoradiation, and maintenance TTFields therapy/temozolomide in newly diagnosed glioblastoma. Journal of Clinical Oncology. 2023;**41**(16_Suppl.):TPS2083-TPS2083

[44] Lim M et al. Phase III trial of chemoradiotherapy with temozolomide plus nivolumab or placebo for newly diagnosed glioblastoma with methylated MGMT promoter. Neuro-Oncology. 2022;**24**(11):1935-1949

[45] Omuro A et al. Radiotherapy combined with nivolumab or temozolomide for newly diagnosed glioblastoma with unmethylated MGMT promoter: An international randomized phase III trial. Neuro-Oncology. 2023;**25**(1):123-134

[46] Tran D et al. 581 final analysis of 2-THE-TOP: A phase 2 study of TTFields (Optune) plus pembrolizumab plus maintenance temozolomide (TMZ) in patients with newly diagnosed glioblastoma. Journal for Immunotherapy of Cancer. 2023;**11**(Suppl. 1):A661-A661

[47] Kodysh J et al. 334 phase I study of safety and activity of personalized neoantigen-based vaccines in combination with tumor treating fields for newly diagnosed glioblastoma patients. Journal for Immunotherapy of Cancer. 2021;**9**(Suppl. 2):A360-A360

[48] Bagley SJ et al. P17.04.B a phase 2 study of NIRAPARIB concomitant with tumor treating fields (TTFIELDS) IN patients with recurrent high-grade glioma (HGG). Neuro-Oncology. 2023;**25**(Supplement_2):ii117-ii117

[49] Wong E et al. EXTH-61. Celecoxib improves OUTCOME of patients treated with tumor treating fields. Neuro-Oncology. 2019;**21**(Supplement_6):vi95

[50] Mehta MP et al. Results from METIS (EF-25), an international, multicenter phase III randomized study evaluating the efficacy and safety of tumor treating fields (TTFields) therapy in NSCLC patients with brain metastases. Journal of Clinical Oncology. 2024;**42**(16_Suppl.):2008-2008

Chapter 12

Enhancing the Efficacy of Chemotherapeutic Drugs *Via* Encapsulation within Nanocomplexes Designed to Cross the Blood-Brain Barrier and Target Tumors

Joe B. Harford, Sang-Soo Kim, Kathleen F. Pirollo, Antonina S. Rait and Esther H. Chang

Abstract

The blood-brain barrier (BBB) blocks ~98% of drugs, so brain tumors tend to be refractory to chemotherapy. Transferrin receptors (TfRs) are expressed on the endothelial cell that comprise the BBB and mediate the movement of transferrin into the brain *via* transcytosis. Tumor cells overexpress TfRs, so encapsulating drugs within nanocomplexes that bind to TfRs has the potential to enhance both entry into the brain and delivery to tumor cells. Here, we present data on the use of TfR-targeted platform nanotechnology termed scL (for single-chain Liposome) to encapsulate five different chemotherapeutic agents. Data are provided showing that scL nanoformulations of these drugs were more effective in killing cancer cells than their unencapsulated counterparts. It is not our intention to study any one of these nanoformulations in detail but rather to highlight the general versatility of this drug delivery system. The scL formulation of TMZ (scL-TMZ) was more effective than unencapsulated TMZ against TMZ-resistant glioblastoma (GBM) and displayed improved efficacy in impeding tumor growth and extending lifespan in mice bearing intracranial GBM tumors. The scL formulation of irinotecan displayed both enhanced potency in killing lung cancer cells in culture and improved *in vivo* efficacy in a murine lung cancer xenograft model.

Keywords: nanomedicine, tumor-targeted delivery, temozolomide, imatinib, sunitinib, erlotinib, irinotecan, transferrin receptor, blood-brain barrier

1. Introduction

Worldwide, there are approximately 20 million new cancer cases and 10 million cancer-caused deaths annually with the risk of having cancer before age 75 being about 1 in 5 [1]. Treatments for cancers can involve surgery, radiotherapy, chemotherapy,

IntechOpen

hormone therapy, and immunotherapy with therapeutic strategies for individual patients often encompassing some combination of these modalities. Chemotherapy remains a mainstay of cancer treatment, and evidence-based treatment guidelines together with global site-specific cancer incidence rates suggest that nearly 60% of all cancer patients would benefit from chemotherapy. This means that in the year 2040, 15 million cancer patients worldwide will be candidates for chemotherapy [2].

The term *chemotherapy* and the first concerted efforts in this field are ascribed to Paul Ehrlich who over a century ago sought to identify anticancer drugs [3]. Ehrlich's goal remains the goal in chemotherapy today *i.e.*, to distinguish between cancer cells and normal cells with the aim of killing the former while sparing the latter. This aspirational goal is particularly challenging when chemotherapies are administered intravenously with the intention of reaching not only the primary tumor but also those cancer cells that have migrated to other sites. By its very nature, systemic administration of chemotherapeutic drugs exposes non-cancer cells to the toxic chemicals and brings into play the risk of adverse side-effects. The history of the clinical use of anticancer drugs has involved many distinct chemical entities many of which kill cancer cells because the tumor cells are dividing more rapidly than most normal cells. The toxic side-effects of chemotherapies often have their origins in the off-target effects on normal cells, particularly normal cells that themselves undergo more rapid division (*e.g.*, cells of the mouth, gut, or bone marrow).

The packaging of drugs into intelligently designed nano-sized delivery vehicles has long been envisioned as having the potential to both improve efficacy and reduce toxicity of chemotherapeutic agents. A variety of nanocarriers including liposomes, polymeric micelles, dendrimers, magnetic nanoparticles, mesoporous nanoparticles, gold nanoparticles, silver nanoparticles, carbon nanotubes, quantum dots, solid lipid nanoparticles, nanowafers and nanorods have been explored in this context [4–6]. Among the most promising uses of nanotechnology in drug delivery are those that are designed to achieve some degree of preferential accumulation of the chemotherapeutic drug in tumors. This accumulation may be passive as described for the enhanced permeability and retention (EPR) effect wherein features of the blood vessels feeding tumors result in nanoparticles preferentially permeating and being retained by tumors [7]. The EPR effect leads to somewhat higher concentrations of the nanoparticles (and their contents) in the tumors than in surrounding normal tissues even if the nanoparticles lack any active targeting mechanism. In contrast to the passive EPR effect, nanoparticles can actively accumulate in tumors if, for example, they possess a targeting moiety that interacts with some molecular entity that is overexpressed on the tumor cells (*e.g.*, hormone receptors, folate receptors, TfRs, tumor-specific surface antigen, *etc.*) [8, 9]. More active targeting of tumors involves designing drug delivery vehicles that selectively "home" to tumor cells in analogy to a "smart bomb". Any success in targeting tumor cells preferentially would tend to move a drug's therapeutic index in a favorable direction on both fronts *i.e.*, making it more effective in killing tumor cells while making it less toxic to normal cells.

Every potential chemotherapeutic drug has its inherent chemistry that influences its biodistribution and pharmacokinetic properties. Nanotechnology has been seen as a way of altering biodistribution and pharmacokinetics in a way that might render chemotherapeutic drugs more efficacious. Chemical entities when formulated as nanomedicines will almost certainly have pharmacokinetic and biodistribution properties distinct from those of the "free" drug reflecting the nature of the nanoformulation. For example, most of the chemistries of chemotherapeutic agents turn out to be incompatible with efficient crossing of biological barriers of the body with the

BBB being the most often discussed example. The BBB is a physical barrier formed by brain capillary endothelial cells with tight junctions between them that impede simple diffusion of drugs into the brain [10]. It has been estimated that ~98% of small molecule drugs do not appreciably cross the BBB by simple diffusion making the BBB a "bottleneck in brain drug development" [11]. Extensive discussions of the nature of the BBB, the challenges of drug delivery to the brain and the various technologies employed to aid delivery of pharmaceuticals to the brain are beyond the scope of this article, but these topics have been recently covered in an excellent review [12]. Nanotechnology has been envisioned as a possible means of moving chemotherapeutic drugs across the BBB to treat brain tumors, and the various strategies to enhance brain tumor drug delivery have been reviewed [13, 14]. One of the more promising approaches involves "Trojan Horse Liposomes" that cross the BBB *via* transcytosis of brain capillary endothelial cells mediated by the TfR [12, 15].

It has been stated that "The main challenges in drug delivery systems are to protect, transport and release biologically active compounds at the right time in a safe and reproducible manner, usually at a specific target site" [16]. Clearly, it is far easier to articulate these lofty goals than to achieve them in practice. We are developing several products that utilize a platform technology for targeted delivery termed scL (for single chain Liposome). The scL nanocomplex has three components: a cationic liposome capable of encapsulating a variety of therapeutic entities; a targeting moiety in the form of a single chain monoclonal antibody fragment (scFv) that recognizes the TfR; and the therapeutic payload itself (see **Figure 1A**). Multiple types of cancer

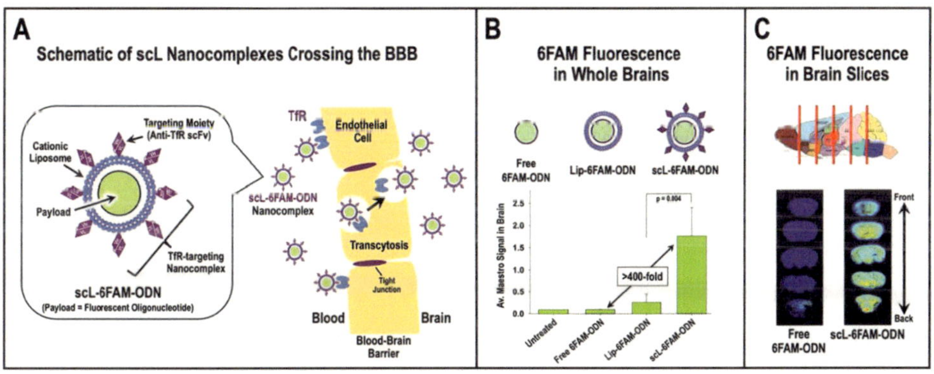

Figure 1.
The scL platform technology for drug delivery. (A) Schematic representation of the scL nanocomplexes and their being ferried across the BBB via TfR-mediated transcytosis, a process that normally supplies the brain with iron by transcytosis of diferric transferrin. The scL nanocomplexes have three components i.e., *a cationic liposome; a chemotherapeutic payload; and a targeting moiety (single-chain antibody fragment recognizing the TfR). Under appropriate conditions, the scL nanocomplexes carrying their payloads self-assembles with all molecular interactions being noncovalent. (B) Schematic of the various forms of a 6-FAM-labeled oligonucleotide (ODN) and their ability to deliver payloads into the brain. Lip-6FAM-ODN (shown in the middle) lacks the TfRscFv targeting moiety represented by the diamond-shaped objects on the scL-6FAM-ODN (shown on the right). At 24 hr. after IV injection of 100 μg of the indicated form of the 6-FAM-ODN, brains were removed and the fluorescent signal quantified in the whole excised brain using a Maestro imaging system with signal intensity expressed in units of 10^6 photons/cm^2/sec. Shown are mean signals ±SD (n = 2–7 mice per group). The small signal in the untreated lane (*i.e., *from the brains from naive mice that received no 6-FAM-ODN) represents background autofluorescence in the brain. The 6FAM fluorescence signal in brains of mice receiving scL-6-FAM-ODN was estimated to be ~400x that seen with free 6-FAM-ODN after subtracting the autofluorescence in the untreated lane. (C) When brains are sliced as shown and the payload visualized using a Maestro imaging system, the fluorescent signal emanating from scL-6FAM-ODN is seen throughout the brain and is markedly higher than that seen in slices of the brain from a mouse receiving free 6FAM-ODN.*

cells have elevated levels of the TfR on their surface when compared to their normal cell counterparts [17]. Indeed, the TfR has been designated as a universal cancer biomarker candidate [18], and the TfR pathway has long been recognized for its potential to target cancer cells in drug delivery [19, 20]. Our scL nanocomplexes are designed to be taken up by cells through the physiological pathway of TfR-mediated endocytosis. We have previously shown that after intravenous administration, both primary and metastatic tumors take up and express reporter gene payloads carried by scL nanocomplexes while normal tissues adjacent to the tumors do not [21]. The scL nanodelivery system has proven to be quite versatile in that it is capable of encapsulating a variety of types of payloads including plasmid DNAs for gene therapy [22], antisense oligonucleotides and siRNAs for downmodulation of gene expression [23–25], and small molecules (<1000 Daltons) having applications to either cancer treatment or cancer imaging [21, 26, 27]. Readers are directed to these prior publications for more detailed characterization of the physical properties of scL nanocomplexes and to the data demonstrating that their uptake by cells is TfR-mediated (*i.e.*, requiring the TfRscFv targeting moiety on the nanocomplexes).

Significantly, two investigational agents (SGT-94 and SGT-53) using the scL delivery vehicle have entered human trials as gene therapies for cancers [28–30], and one (SGT-53) is now in Phase II for patients with advanced pancreatic cancers with promising interim results [31]. The ability of intravenously administered SGT-53 to target tumors and to spare normal tissue was confirmed using biopsies of tumors and normal skin derived from patients in an SGT-53 clinical trial [29]. The liposomes (without cargo), the empty scL nanocomplex (with the targeting moiety but without a payload) and the full SGT-53 complexes have been characterized in terms of size by dynamic light scattering techniques and electron microscopy [22]. While all scL nanocomplexes are nanosized (<300 nm) irrespective of their payload, those nanocomplexes carrying smaller molecular payloads generally tend to have an average size somewhat smaller than those carrying plasmid DNAs. Using an scL nanocomplex carrying a plasmid expression vector encoding β-galactosidase and mice with widely disseminated metastatic pancreatic cancer, we have demonstrated that both the primary tumor and foci of metastatic tumor cells are selectively targeted and express β-galactosidase with minimal expression of this reporter gene in adjacent normal tissues [21].

All mammalian cells acquire iron used in metabolism *via* TfR-mediated endocytosis of diferric transferrin, an abundant serum protein. Like other serum proteins, transferrin has a molecular weight (~80 kDa) that prevents its simple diffusion into the brain from the blood. For the brain to acquire iron, TfRs on the brain capillary endothelial cells are employed to shuttle transferrin across the BBB. In this process, referred to as receptor-mediated transcytosis, TfRs bind their ligand on the blood side and release it on the brain side of the BBB (shown schematically in **Figure 1A**). Once on the brain side of the BBB, the ligand can be taken into brain cells *via* TfR-mediated endocytosis in a manner comparable to its uptake in peripheral tissues. To demonstrate that scL nanocomplexes can effectively hijack this physiological pathway, we intravenously administered scL-6FAM-ODN, a nanocomplexes carrying as its cargo a fluorescently labeled oligonucleotide (6FAM-ODN) to mice. Other groups of mice were given either free 6FAM-ODN or a liposomal formulation of 6FAM-ODN lacking the TfRscFv targeting moiety of the scL delivery vehicle. At 24 hr. after a single tail vein injection, brains were excised, and their level of 6-FAM fluorescence quantified using a Maestro® imaging system. After subtracting the small amount autofluorescence in the brains, it was estimated that the uptake of the payload from scL-6FAM-ODN was approximately 400-fold higher than that seen with when unencapsulated 6FAM-ODN was similarly injected (**Figure 1B**). The fluorescent payload's delivery into the brain was highly dependent upon the targeting moiety of the scL nanocomplexes as the signal in the brain after intravenous administration of Lip-6FAM-ODN (which lacks the scL targeting moiety) was significantly lower. When brain slices were examined after intravenous administration of either free 6FAM-ODN or scL-6FAM-ODN, the markedly higher fluorescent signal that derives from the scL nanocomplex was seen throughout the brain (**Figure 1C**). In mice with intracranial brain tumors, TfR-mediated transcytosis to cross the BBB is followed by TfR-mediated endocytosis by tumor cells that results in accumulation of the fluorescent payload (Cy5-ODN) in the tumors (**Figure 2**). Collectively, the data in **Figures 1** and **2** indicate that scL nanocomplexes can carry their payloads across the BBB *via* TfR-mediated transcytosis, and once on the brain side, deliver their cargo payloads with a high degree of selectivity into intracranial tumor cells that overexpress TfRs.

By encapsulating chemotherapeutic agents in scL nanocomplexes that facilitate TfR-mediated uptake by tumors, it may be possible to achieve higher levels of the drug within the cancer cells and thereby improve their efficacy in blocking tumor growth. In this article, the focus will be on using scL nanocomplexes to deliver a number of older chemotherapeutic drugs namely TMZ, imatinib, sunitinib, erlotinib, and irinotecan. Rather than providing a detailed study of any single chemotherapeutic agents, our intention here is to showcase at a higher level the capability and versatility of nanotechnology in general and the scL platform technology in particular as a means for creating new and improved formulations of previously approved chemotherapeutic drugs. With cells derived from several tumor types, our data indicate that an scL nanoformulation of each drug examined is more effective in killing cancer cells (i.e., display lower IC_{50} values) than its unencapsulated counterpart (termed "free drug"). For example, the nanoformulation of TMZ has been shown to be superior to free TMZ in treating mice with intracranial GBM tumors that are notoriously refractory to treatment. Lung cancers often metastizize to the brain. Because lung cancer remains the most common and lethal of cancers and novel therapeutic approaches are urgently needed, we also assessed a nanoformulation of irinotecan (scL-Irinotecan)

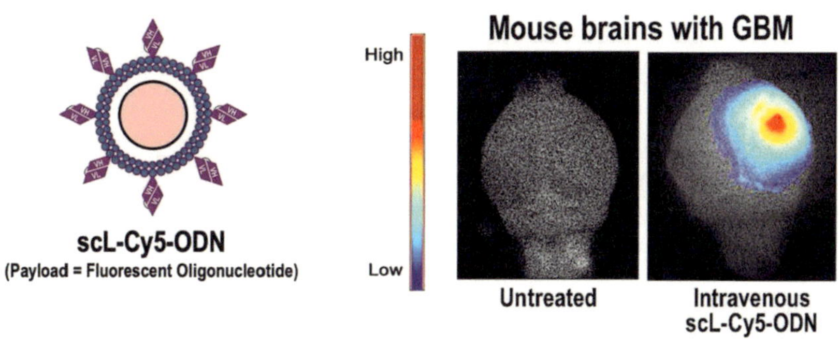

Figure 2.
Schematic of an scL nanocomplex carrying as payload oligonucleotide (ODN) fluorescently labeled with Cyanine5 (Cy5). At 24 hr. after a single intravenous injection of 25 μg of Cy5-ODN as scL-Cy5-ODN into mice bearing intracranial U97 glioblastoma (GBM), brains were excised, and the fluorescent signal visualized in the whole brain using a Maestro imaging system. An untreated tumor-bearing brain is shown (left panel) for comparison to the high fluorescence signal seen in the brain tumor (right panel).

and found it to be more effective than free irinotecan in treating athymic mice with subcutaneously established lung cancer xenografts. It is suggested that the scL nanocomplex delivery vehicle might be useful in creating novel formulations of additional chemotherapeutic drugs beyond those examined here and could also aid in delivering to the brain drugs for other neurological diseases or conditions.

2. Materials and methods

Drugs: Temozolomide (TMZ) was purchased from Sigma (St. Louis, MO). Irinotecan hydrochloride was obtained from ScinoPharm Taiwan, Ltd. (Tainan, Taiwan). Imatinib (Gleevec®), sunitinib (Sutent®), and erlotinib (Tarceva®) were acquired from the pharmacy at Georgetown University Hospital (Washington, DC).

Cell lines: All human cancer cell lines except U87-luc2 and U87R were obtained from American Type Culture Collection (ATCC; Manassas, VA). Each cell line was maintained at 37°C in a 5% CO_2 atmosphere using the culture media recommended for each line by ATCC. All media were supplemented with 10% heat-inactivated fetal bovine serum (Omega Scientific, Los Angeles, CA), 2 mM L-glutamine (Mediatech, Manassas, VA), and 50 μg/mL each of penicillin, streptomycin, and neomycin (Gibco, Waltham, MA). U87-luc2, a luciferase expressing GBM line, was purchased from Caliper Life Sciences (Hopkinton, MA). U87R, a TMZ-resistant subclone of U87, was established as previously described [32] by growing U87 cells for three weeks in medium containing 100 μM TMZ. U87-luc2 and U87R, once established, were used under culture conditions identical to those used for their parental cell line U87. The cell lines utilized in the experiments shown in this article represent GBM (U87, U87-luc2, and U87R), melanoma (MDA-MB-435), as well as lung (A549), prostate (DU145), pancreas (PANC-1), breast (MDA-MB-231), and colon (HT-29) cancers. All experiments were performed with mycoplasma-free cells.

Preparation of the scL nanocomplexes encapsulating chemotherapeutic agents: The scL delivery vehicle has been utilized to encapsulate a variety of payload types [21–27]. These prior publications contain more detailed characterization of the physical properties of scL nanocomplexes including their size distribution, charge (zeta potential) and appearance in electron microscopy as well as data demonstrating that the uptake of scL nanocomplexes by cells is TfR-mediated (*i.e.*, requiring the TfRscFv targeting moiety on the nanocomplexes). Incorporation of the chemotherapeutic agents (molecular weights ranging from 194 to 587 Daltons) into cationic liposome was performed using the ethanol injection method as described previously [33] with chemical payloads added to the lipids at a molar ratio of drug to total lipid of 1:1. In all cases, the liposomes were comprised of a 1:1 molar ratio of 1,2-dioleoyl-3-trimethylammonium propane (DOTAP) and dioleoylphosphatidyl ethanolamine (DOPE) (Avanti Polar Lipids, Alabaster, AL). Before the addition of a targeting moiety, the liposomal formulation of a drug is termed "Lip-drug name". In some cases, empty liposomes (designated simply "Lip") were included to assess lipid toxicity in culture-based assays or non-specific anti-tumor efficacy in animal models. For all scL nanocomplexes in this article, the targeting moiety (TfRscFv) is a recombinant single-chain antibody fragment that recognizes both the human and murine TfRs [22]. The scL-drug nanocomplexes were formed by merely mixing TfRscFv with preformed Lip-drug complexes as described previously [34]. The TfRscFv is not covalently associated with the nanocomplexes. For animal injections, 50% dextrose was added to each sample to achieve a final concentration of 5% dextrose in the injected material. The size and zeta potential of scL-drug nanocomplexes were confirmed using a Zetasizer Nano ZS System (Malvern Panalytical, Malvern, UK). All scL-drug formulations were nanosized (<300 nm by number average) and had a positive zeta potential of (+30 to +50 mV). The positive zeta potential discourages the aggregation of the nanocomplexes via charge-charge repulsion. In the experiments represented in the current article, freshly prepared nanocomplexes were employed in each case. When scL-drug nanocomplexes were compared head-to-head to either untargeted Lip-drug nanocomplexes or unencapsulated drug, these comparisons involved equimolar amounts of the chemotherapeutic agent.

Tumor cell survival assays via XTT assays: Cell viability was measured using an XTT assay (Polysciences, Warrington, PA) in triplicate as previously described [26]. Cells were treated as described in each figure legend, and cell viability was determined 96 h post-treatment. The IC_{50} values represent the drug concentration that resulted in 50% cell death and were interpolated from the graphs of drug concentration versus percent cells surviving using SigmaPlot (Systat Software Inc., San Jose, CA).

Animal models: All animal experiments were approved by the Georgetown University Institutional Animal Care and Use Committee. All animal experiments were performed in the AAALAC-accredited, USDA-registered animal facility of Georgetown University adhering to the Guide for the Care and Use of Laboratory Animals as required by the Office of Laboratory Animal Welfare (OLAW). After a single tail vein injection of scL-Cy5-ODN, the payload of which is an oligonucleotide fluorescently labeled with Cyanine 5 (Cy5-ODN), brains of mice bearing intracranial U87 GBM tumors were removed and imaged via the Maestro® imaging system (Caliper Life Sciences, Hopkinton, MA). For the orthotopic intracranial U87-luc2 tumor model used in **Figure 3**, female athymic nude mice (Harlan, Indianapolis, IN) that were 5 to 6 weeks old were stereotactically inoculated with U87-luc2 cells (5.0×10^5 cells per mouse) as described previously [26]. After 7–10 days, the intracranial tumors were visualized by magnetic resonance imaging (MRI) and the tumor volume at the time of treatment quantified. To measure intracranial U87-luc2 tumor growth and to assess therapeutic efficacy, non-invasive bioluminescence imaging was performed with the Xenogen IVIS® in vivo imaging system (Caliper Life Sciences, Hopkinton, MA). To assess the impact of chemotherapeutic formulations on survival of mice with brain tumors, animals with established intracranial U87-luc2 tumor xenografts were systemically injected (via tail vein) with the indicated formulation following the treatment schedule shown in **Figure 3B**. All mice were euthanized when they became moribund. Survival was monitored and plotted using the Kaplan-Meier method. For the subcutaneous xenograft tumor model employing A549 lung cancer cells, female athymic nude mice were inoculated at 5 to 6 weeks of age with A549 cells suspended in Matrigel (BD Biosciences, San Diego, CA) on bilateral flanks ($3x10^6$ cells/injection site). Mice were distributed into treatment groups (n = 10 for scL-Irinotecan and n = 5 for all other treatment groups) such that each group began with tumors of similar average size (~$50mm^3$). Treatment was started 2 weeks after tumor cell inoculation and involved twice per week tail vein injections of 0.25 mL of 5% dextrose containing 200 μg of either free irinotecan or an equivalent amount of irinotecan as untargeted Lip-Irinotecan or TfR-targeting scL-Irinotecan.

Immunofluorescence imaging for γH2AX, an indicator of DNA damage: U87 cells seeded at $5x10^4$ cells/chamber of Falcon culture slides were treated with either

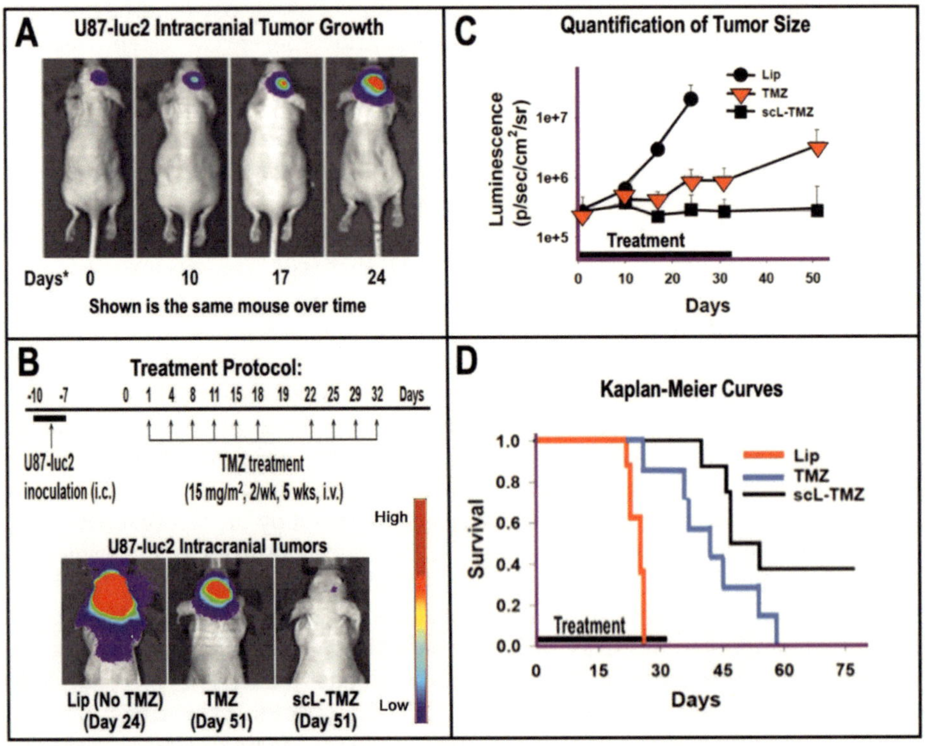

Figure 3.
*The nanocomplex formulation scL-TMZ is more effective than free TMZ in treating mice bearing intracranial U87-luc2 GBM tumors as detected and quantified in living animals using IVIS® imaging system. (A) Growth of intracranial U87-luc2 tumors over time. *Day 0 is 7–10 days after innoculaiton of tumor cells and the start of the treatment protocol depicted in Panel B. Imaging based on the luciferase produced by the tumors was via an IVIS® imaging system, IVIS® images of a single mouse without any treatments on the indicated days are shown. The increasing luminescence signal indicates that the intracranial U87-luc2 tumor in this mouse is increasing in size over time (red color corresponds to a higher signal than blue color). (B) Shown are the treatment schedule and IVIS® images of mice from the indicated groups* i.e., *mice treated either with Lip* i.e., *liposomes with no TMZ (at Day 24) and with free TMZ or with scL-TMZ (both at Day 51). (C) Quantification of luminescence signal in the various treatment groups (n = 7–8) are shown as means with error bars indicating standard deviations. The luminescence signals indicate that scL-2PAM impedes tumor growth more effectively than does free TMZ. (D) Kaplan–Meier survival curves for mice treated with either Lip or free TMZ or scL-TMZ as shown in Panel B. A log-rank statistical analysis showed statistical significance (P < 0.001).*

scL-TMZ or unencapsulated TMZ at 100 μM for 3 h, after which the media was replaced with fresh drug-free media. At 48 h post-transfection, cells were fixed, permeabilized, and incubated with rabbit polyclonal anti-γH2A histone family, member X (γH2AX) (phospho-S139) antibody (Abcam, Cambridge, MA) followed by DyLight 488-conjugated donkey anti-rabbit antibody (BioLegend, San Diego, CA). Slides were mounted with VECTASHIELD antifade mounting medium with DAPI (Vector Laboratories, Newark, CA) and imaged with an Olympus IX71 inverted fluorescent microscope at 400X magnification.

Statistical analysis: In the figures, results are presented as means ±SD (shown as error bars). Statistical significance was determined using the analysis of variance (ANOVA) (SigmaPlot, Systat Software Inc., San Jose, CA). P values of <0.05 were considered significant. Survival curves were compared using a log-rank test (SigmaPlot).

3. Results

3.1 Comparing nano-encapsulated scL-TMZ with free TMZ against GBM cells in culture

We have encapsulated TMZ using scL nanodelivery platform as depicted schematically in **Figure 4**. TMZ (Temodar® or Temodal®) is an alkylating agent of 194 Da that was initially approved for refractory astrocytoma in 1999 with subsequent approval as first-line therapy for GBM that represent the most common primary malignant brain tumor in adults [35]. Initial treatment for GBM generally consists of maximal surgical resection and radiation therapy with concurrent TMZ chemotherapy that is then often followed by adjuvant TMZ chemotherapy [36–38]. Damaging GBM cell DNA to push the cells into apoptosis is the objective of TMZ treatment, and GBM resistance to TMZ correlates with elevated levels of the DNA repair enzyme O6-methylguanine-DNA methyltransferase (MGMT) [37, 38]. Even with a very aggressive treatment regimen, five-year relative survival for GBM patients is low ranging from 3% in adults over age 65 to 27% among those aged 20 to 39 [35]. These grim survival statistics clearly indicate that there is room for improvement in the current treatment of GBM. Among the features of TMZ that contribute to less-than-optimal effectiveness is its limited ability to diffuse across the BBB.

We and others have sought to address this issue by encapsulating TMZ in various ways aimed at improving its ability to cross the BBB [39]. Our approach has been to use the scL delivery system designed to traverse the BBB *via* TfR-mediated transcytosis as shown schematically in **Figure 1A** with the scL nanocomplex effectively serving as a "Trojan horse" for payload delivery into the brain. As shown in **Figures 1** and **2**, fluorescently-tagged oligonucleotides (6FAM-ODN) can be visualized in the brain after intravenous administration of these molecules as payloads within scL nanocomplexes [22, 24]. The delivery of these payloads into the brain is clearly dependent upon the TfRscFv targeting moiety i.e., uptake of comparable liposomal formulations lacking the TfRscFv are markedly lower (**Figure 1B**). Accumulation of a fluorescently tagged payload in a GBM tumor growing in the mouse brain is shown as **Figure 2** with ~400-times more fluorescence in brain with s In mice without tumors, the TfRscFv

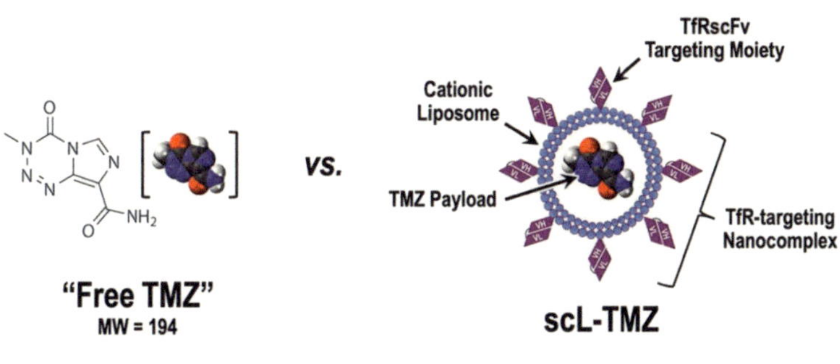

Figure 4.
*Schematic representation of unencapsulated TMZ (*a.k.a. *"Free TMZ") and scL-TMZ, the scL nanocomplex carrying TMZ as its payload. TMZ within scL-TMZ is depicted using a space-filling calotte model. Here, scL-TMZ serves as a representative example of scL-encapsulated chemotherapeutic agents. All scL formulations carrying the various chemotherapeutic drugs employ the same nanodelivery system. In efficacy experiments against tumor cells* in vitro *or* in vivo, *the scL formulation of a given chemotherapeutic drug was always compared head-to-head with the unencapsulated version of that same drug at equimolar concentrations.*

targeting moiety of the scL nanocomplex was also shown to be crucial in the delivery of an siRNA that was detected within neurons, astrocytes, and microglial cells isolated from the brains of mice that had received nano-encapsulated siRNA [24].

We compared the ability of free TMZ and scL-TMZ (both schematically depicted in **Figure 4**) to damage DNA in human GBM (U87) cell line. U87 cells in tissue culture were treated with TMZ or scL-TMZ at 100 μM for 3 h, and DNA damage was assessed using an antibody against γH2AX at 48 h post-treatment (**Figure 5A**). Phosphorylation of the Ser-139 residue of the histone variant H2AX, yields γH2AX considered to be an early cellular response to double-strand DNA breaks [40]. Detection of this phosphorylation event has emerged as a highly specific and sensitive molecular marker for monitoring DNA damage initiation. As can be seen in **Figure 5A**, the markedly higher level of γH2AX in cells treated with scL-TMZ indicates that is nanoformulation is markedly more effective at inducing the DNA damage than an equimolar amount of free TMZ. Because producing DNA damage is central to the mechanism of action of TMZ in cancer chemotherapy, these results in cell culture suggested that scL-TMZ would be more effective than free TMZ in killing GBM cells and more efficacious in treating GBM.

The development of TMZ-resistance in patients with GBM is quite common, and this chemoresistance is often associated to higher levels of a DNA repair enzyme MGMT that reverses TMZ-induced DNA alkylation. Because many patients develop TMZ-resistance, we were interested in assessing the ability of scL-TMZ to kill TMZ-resistant GBM. By growing U87 cells for 3 weeks in media that contained 100 μM TMZ, we selected for a TMZ-resistant variant of U87 (designated U87R) that expressed significantly higher levels of MGMT [26]. We compared the ability of free TMZ and scL-TMZ to kill U87 and U87R cells by an XTT assay, and **Figure 5B** shows the viability curves for U87 (left graph) and U87R (right graph). We determined that

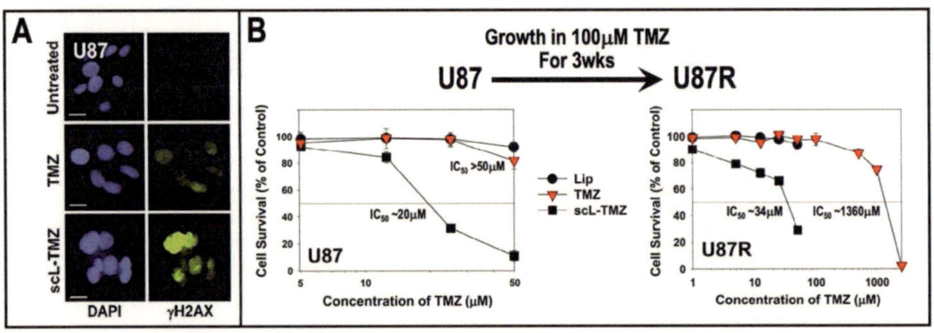

Figure 5.
The nanocomplex formulation scL-TMZ is more effective than free TMZ in U87 GBM cells and in TMZ-resistant variant of U87 (termed U87R). (A) U87 GBM cells were exposed to 100 μM TMZ or the TMZ-equivalent amount of scL-TMZ for 3 h. At 48 h after exposures to the two formulations, the cells were stained with antibody that detects γH2AX, a marker of double-strand DNA breaks (green) and DAPI counterstain for nuclei (blue). The extent of DNA damage is clearly higher in the U87 cells treated with scL-TMZ than in cells treated with free TMZ. (B) TMZ-resistant variant of U87 GBM was produced by growing U87 cells for 3 weeks in medium containing 100 μM TMZ as previously described [26, 32]. This TMZ-resistant cell line (termed U87R) expressed higher levels of MGMT accounting for its TMZ-resistance [26]. Cell survival was assessed using an XTT assay for cell viability and apparent IC_{50} values are provided from bead-to-head comparisons of free TMZ and scL-TMZ for their ability to kill U87 cells (left graph) or U87R cells (right graph). As a control, DOTAP/DOPE liposome (Lip) vehicle without payload was also assessed for ability to kill cells based on the toxicity of the lipids. The scL-TMZ was more effective in killing both U87 and U87R cells than was free TMZ, and the liposomes were non-toxic. In the case of U87R, it appears that scL-TMZ (IC_{50} of ~1360 μM) is approximately 40-times more effective than free TMZ (IC_{50} of ~34 μM).

the lipids (Lip) used to create scL-TMZ were not themselves cytotoxic at the levels employed. Both free TMZ and scL-TMZ were capable of killing the cultured TMZ-resistant tumor cells. However, whereas the IC_{50} for free TMZ in U87R is ~1360 μM, the IC_{50} for scL-TMZ is ~34 μM *i.e.*, the efficacy of scL-TMZ in killing TMZ-resistant U87R is approximately 40-fold higher than that seen with free TMZ. Using a second TMZ-resistant GBM line (T98G), we also observed an IC_{50} for scL-TMZ that was >35-fold lower than that for free TMZ (data not shown). The active pharmaceutical agent in scL-TMZ remains TMZ, and the fundamental mechanism of action of TMZ as a DNA alkylating agent is not changed by its encapsulation within the scL nanocomplex. The most straightforward explanation for the observed 40-fold shift in IC_{50} is that the level of TMZ achieved in the nucleus of the cells with scL-TMZ taken into cells *via* TfR-mediated endocytosis is at least 40-fold higher than that achieved by exposing the GBM cells to an equimolar dose of unencapsulated TMZ.

3.2 Comparing nano-encapsulated scL-TMZ with free TMZ against intracranial GBM tumors

Brain tumors are notoriously difficult to treat in part because a given chemotherapeutic drug that may be fully capable of killing brain tumor cells in a tissue culture dish does not effectively cross the BBB to reach the same tumor cells growing intracranially. The scientific literature is replete with promising drug candidates against brain cancers that have failed in clinical development [41]. Having demonstrated that GBM cells in culture are more sensitive to TMZ formulated as scL-TMZ than to free TMZ at an equimolar concentration, we sought to test the scL nanoformulation of TMZ against intracranial GBM tumors *in vivo*. For these experiments we utilized U87-luc2, a variant of U87 GBM cells engineered to constitutively expresses firefly luciferase. The luciferase expressed by these cells generates a luminescence signal that is proportional to the number of tumor cells. When U87-luc2 GBM cells are inoculated into the brains of nude mice, intracranial tumors form and as these tumors grow over time, tumor growth can be monitored using an IVIS® imaging system that can quantify the luciferase-generated luminescence that reflects tumor size (**Figure 3A**). This methodology allows one to monitor intracranial tumor growth over time in living mice. To compare scL-TMZ with free TMZ for their ability to prevent brain tumor growth, mice bearing intracranial U87-luc2 tumor received the two distinct forms of TMZ (i.e., scL-encapsulated and unencapsulated) on the treatment schedule shown at the top of **Figure 3B**. Note that chemotherapy was always administered systemically *via* the tail veins of the mice. Absent treatment, all tumor-bearing mice succumb to their brain tumors or had to be euthanized by Day 26 of the protocol. Both free TMZ and scL-TMZ were capable of impeding tumor growth in these mice, but the sizes of intracranial tumors were significantly smaller in those mice receiving scL-TMZ compared to the mice receiving free TMZ (**Figure 3C**). Survival analysis demonstrated a significant improvement in life-span extension for mice getting the scL-TMZ treatments (**Figure 3D**). Compared to Lip-treated mice that all succumbed to disease by day 26 (or were euthanized), treatment with free TMZ increased survival by 18 days. However, all of these mice also had succumbed to their brain tumors by day 58. In contrast, 37.5% of mice receiving scL-TMZ survived until day 77 (45 days after the end of treatment) when this experiment was terminated. Mean survival times of mice treated with scL-TMZ were 2.4-fold longer than mice treated with Lip and 1.4-fold longer than mice treated with free TMZ, respectively. A log-rank statistical analysis showed statistical significance ($p < 0.001$). More details on the uses of scL-TMZ to treat mice with intracranial GBM are provided in a previous publication [26]. There, we demonstrated using FACS analyses that the percentage of apoptotic cells present was significantly higher in tumors from the mice receiving scL-TMZ than in tumors from mice getting free TMZ. We had analyzed cells on the basis of expression of CD133 (Prominin-1), a marker for cancer stem cells (CSCs) in pediatric and adult brain tumors [42, 43] with CD133- cells representing the bulk of tumor cells and CD133+ cells representing the CSCs that are implicated in resistance to chemotherapy and radiotherapy [44, 45]. It has been suggested that a way to improve outcomes of TMZ therapy in GBM patients would be to design a TMZ formulation that is more effective in the killing of CD133+ stem cells of the tumors [39]. The fact that scL-TMZ can reach and affect the CSCs *in vivo* suggests that this nanomedicine formulation may be useful in overcoming the chemoresistance and recurrence often seen in GBM patients.

3.3 Comparing nano-encapsulated scL-TMZ with free TMZ against non-GBM tumor cells

Although TMZ is currently approved only for astrocytoma and GBM, its mechanism of action would suggest that this drug might also be useful against neoplasms beyond its formal indications [46, 47]. Given our results showing superiority of scL-TMZ over free TMZ in killing GBM cells *in vitro* and *in vivo*, we sought to do head-to-head comparisons using cells derived from tumors other than GBM. In these experiments, we used the XTT assay for cell viability and exposed various tumor cell lines to increasing doses of free TMZ or scL-TMZ that would allow for the estimation of IC_{50} values as had been done for U87 cells and U87R cells (**Figure 5B**). Comparisons of IC_{50} values for free TMZ and scL-TMZ in cells from breast, lung, colon, melanoma, pancreas, and prostate cancers are provided in **Figure 6**.

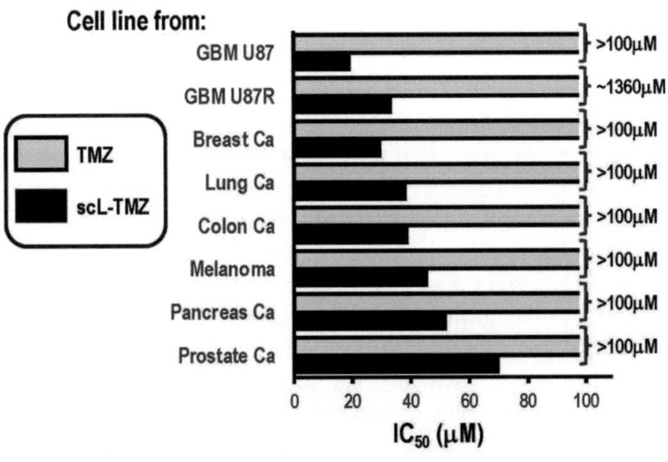

Figure 6.
Sensitivity of GBM and non-GBM tumor cells to TMZ and scL-TMZ. Assessment of cell viability via *XTT assays were conducted using cell lines derived from breast (MDA-MB-231), lung (A549), colon (HT-29), melanoma (MDA-MB-435), pancreas (PANC-1), and prostate (DU145) cancers [26]. The IC_{50} values for TMZ (lighter bars) and for scL-TMZ (darker bars) were estimated by interpolation using the viability curves for each cell line. Note that the IC_{50} value for scL-TMZ in the TMZ-resistant GBM cell line (U87R) is only modestly higher than that seen in the parental U87 cells despite a much larger difference in their sensitivity to free TMZ.*

In all cell lines examined, the IC_{50} for scL-TMZ was markedly lower than that seen for free TMZ in the same cancer cell line. The IC_{50} values observed in the breast, lung, and colon cancer lines assessed were all between 1x and 2x of the IC_{50} seen in U87 GBM (~20 μM). The IC_{50} values for scL-TMZ against the other cancer cell lines assessed were only modestly higher. Our interpretation of these results is that scL-TMZ treatment of the various tumor lines is resulting in higher levels of the DNA-alkylating agent in the nucleus of the cells than is achieved with an equimolar dose of free TMZ. These results suggest that scL-TMZ might have usefulness beyond treating malignancies of the central nervous system. In considering possible use of scL-TMZ for an expanded constellation of tumors, it is noteworthy that TMZ has been associated with severe hematologic adverse events (HAE) that can include fatalities [48]. To assess toxicity, we have administered free TMZ or scL-TMZ at 75 mg/m^2 to mice without tumors on each of five consecutive days and examined hematological parameters 3 days later. We found that leukocytes, lymphocytes and thrombocytes were all reduced in numbers by >25% in mice receiving free TMZ, but not in mice treated with scL-TMZ [26]. If these results are extrapolatable to human patients, scL-TMZ may have less HAE that might allow their chemotherapy to proceed without HAE-related interruption or discontinuation and thereby increase the probability of a better outcome of the chemotherapy. Results from our toxicology study in mice also indicated treatment with free TMZ resulted elevated alanine transaminase (ALT) and aspartate transaminase (AST), which can reflect liver damage, elevated blood urea nitrogen (BUN), which can reflect renal damage, and elevated creatine phosphokinase (CPK) that can indicate muscle or brain tissue damage. With scL-TMZ, these elevated values for these markers of possible toxicity were absent Neither free TMZ nor scL TMZ resulted in abnormalities in creatine, total protein, sodium or potasium in the blood of the mice [26]. No additional indications of overt toxicity were observed in mice given scL-TMZ.

3.4 Comparing nano-encapsulated imatinib with free imatinib against prostate cancer cells

Imatinib (a.k.a. Glivec®, Gleevec®, or STI571) is a protein kinase inhibitor of 494 Da that was first approved by the U.S. FDA in 2001 for chronic myelogenous leukemia (CML) and subsequently for gastrointestinal stromal tumor (GIST). Imatinib was the first kinase inhibitor approved and is considered the paradigm of rationally designed, molecularly targeted cancer therapeutics [49]. Imatinib kills tumor cells by inducing mitochondria-mediated apoptosis of gastric cancer cells involving reactive oxygen species and endoplasmic reticulum stress [50, 51]. We have formulated imatinib as an scL nanocomplex and performed head-to-head comparisons with unencapsulated imatinib. Using the XTT assay for cell viability and cultured DU145 prostate cancer cells, we observed an IC_{50} for free imatinib of >100 μM whereas the IC_{50} for scL-Imatinib was just ~35 μM representing an improvement in apparent efficacy of >3-fold for the scL nanomedicine formulation (**Figure 7**).

3.5 Comparing nano-encapsulated scL-Sunitinib with free sunitinib against prostate cancer cells

Sunitinib (*a.k.a.* Sutent® or SU11248) is a protein kinase inhibitor of 398 Da that the U.S. FDA approved for renal cell carcinoma and imatinib-resistant GIST in 2006 [52]. Sunitinib became available as a generic in 2021. A number of trials aimed at expanding

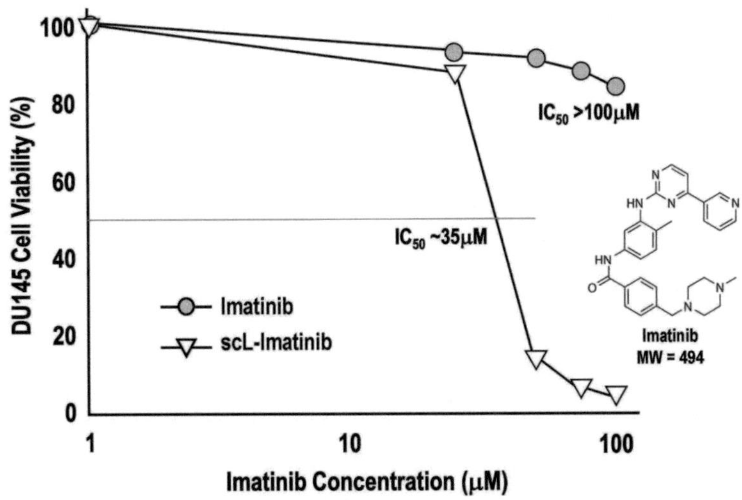

Figure 7.
Sensitivity of prostate cancer cells (DU145) to free imatinib and scL-Imatinib. Cell survival was assessed using an XTT assay and apparent IC_{50} values are provided. Based on the respective IC_{50} values, it appears that scL-Imatinib (IC_{50} of ~35 μM) is at least 3-times more effective in killing prostate cancer cells than free imatanib (IC_{50} of >100 μM).

sunitinib's usage to other solid tumor indications have been conducted over the years since its original approval. These trials included one that aimed to assess sunitinib against brain tumors [53] wherein its ability to cross the BBB would be relevant. We have formulated sunitinib as an scL nanocomplex and assessed its ability to kill cancer cells with unencapsulated sunitinib in head-to-head comparisons. Using the XTT assay for cell viability and DU145 prostate cancer cells, we observed an IC_{50} for free sunitinib of ~13 μM whereas the IC_{50} for scL-Sunitinib was only ~5.3 μM representing an improvement in apparent efficacy of ~2.5-fold for the scL nanomedicine formulation of sunitinib (**Figure 8**).

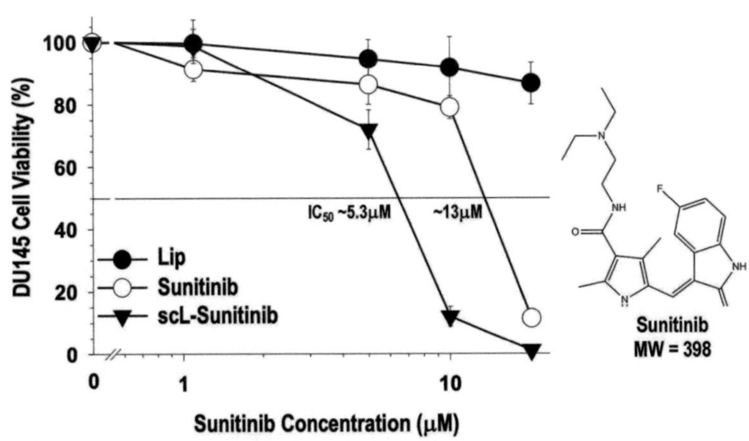

Figure 8.
Sensitivity of prostate cancer cells (DU145) to free sunitinib and scL-Sunitinib. Cell survival was assessed using an XTT assay for cell viability and apparent IC_{50} values are provided. As a control, liposomes without payload (Lip) were also assessed for ability to kill DU145 cells. Based on the respective IC_{50} values, it appears that scL-Sunitinib (IC_{50} of ~5.3 μM) is approximately 2.5-times more effective in killing prostate cancer cells than free sunitinib (IC_{50} of ~13 μM).

3.6 Comparing nano-encapsulated scL-Erlotinib with free erlotinib against prostate & pancreas cancer cells

Erlotinib (*a.k.a.* Tarceva®) is a 393 Da tyrosine kinase inhibitor of the epidermal growth factor receptor (EGFR). EGFR has been implicated in cancer-related cellular signal transduction pathways including cellular proliferation, adhesion, migration, angiogenesis and apoptosis inhibition [54, 55]. Erlotinib followed gefitinib, which was the first approved drug in this class. Erlotinib was approved by the U.S. FDA in 2005 for treatment of non-small cell lung cancer and in combination with gemcitabine (Gemzar®) for treatment of locally advanced, unresectable, or metastatic pancreatic cancer. We have formulated erlotinib as an scL nanocomplex and assessed its ability to kill cancer cells with unencapsulated erlotinib in head-to-head comparisons. Using the XTT assay for cell viability and prostate cancer cells (DU145), we observed an IC_{50} for free erlotinib of >30 μM, whereas the IC_{50} for scL-erlotinib was only ~11 μM representing an improvement in apparent efficacy of ~3-fold (**Figure 9A**). The observed IC_{50} in pancreas cancer cells (PANC-1) for free erlotinib of >30 μM whereas the IC_{50} for scL-Erlotinib was only ~3.5 μM representing an improvement in apparent efficacy of ~10-fold for the scL nanomedicine formulation of erlotinib against pancreas cancer cells (**Figure 9B**).

3.7 Comparing nano-encapsulated scL-Irinotecan with free irinotecan against lung cancer cells and lung cancer xenografts

Irinotecan (*a.k.a.* Onivyde®, Camptosar®, or CPT-11) is a 587 Da chemotherapeutic agent related to the natural product camptothecin. It was first approved for clinical use in Japan in 1994 and then in the U.S. in 1996 [56]. Irinotecan is in the class of topoisomerase I inhibitors that results in DNA breaks, which can push cells into apoptotic death if not repaired [57, 58]. In causing DNA damage leading to

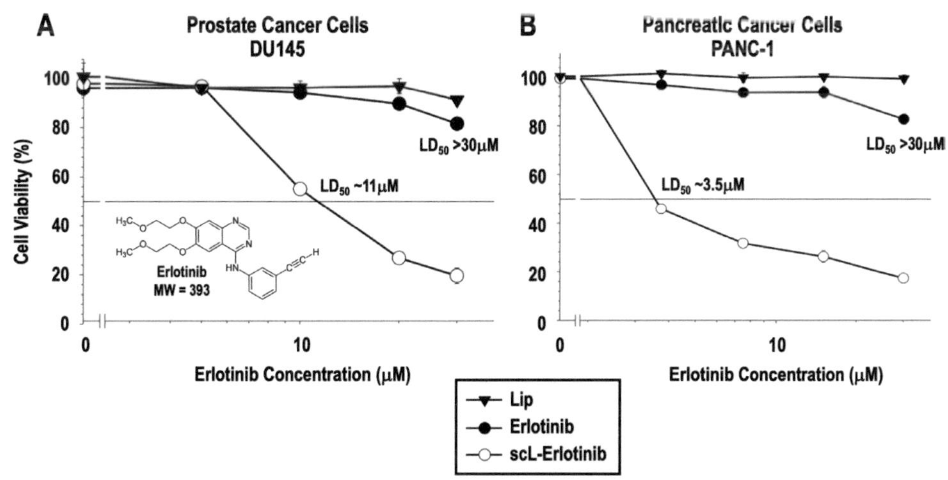

Figure 9.
Sensitivity of prostate cancer cells (DU145) and pancreas cancer cells (PANC-1) to free erlotinib and scL-Erlotinib. Cell survival was assessed using an XTT assay for cell viability and apparent IC_{50} values are provided. (A) Based on the respective IC_{50} values, it appears that against prostate cancer cells, scL-Erlotinib (IC_{50} of >30 μM) is at least 3-times more effective than free erlotinib (IC_{50} of ~11 μM). (B) Against pancreas cancer cells, scL-Erlotinib (IC_{50} of >30 μM) is at least 10-times more effective than free erlotinib (IC_{50} of ~3.5 μM).

apoptosis, irinotecan resembles TMZ although irinotecan's mechanism of introducing DNA damage is distinct. Major uses of irinotecan are as a component of the chemotherapeutic combination known as FOLFIRI (comprising 5-fluorouracil, leucovorin and irinotecan) for use in patients with metastatic or recurrent colon cancer and FOLFIRINOX (a version of FOLFIRI plus oxaliplatin) for advanced pancreatic cancers. Irinotecan has also been approved as a liposomal formulation (irinotecan hydrochloride liposome) for advanced pancreatic cancer in conjunction with fluorouracil and leucovorin. Irinotecan, and irinotecan hydrochloride liposome are also being studied in other types of cancer including GBM [59, 60].

We have formulated irinotecan as an scL nanocomplex and assessed its ability to kill cancer cells with unencapsulated irinotecan and untargeted Lip-Irinotecan in head-to-head comparisons. Because lung cancer remains the most common and lethal of cancers and novel therapeutic approaches are urgently needed, we assessed a nanoformulation of irinotecan against lung cancer both *in vitro* and *in vivo* using subcutaneous xenograft tumors in mice. Using the XTT assay for cell viability in A549 lung cancer cells *in vitro*, we observed an IC_{50} for free irinotecan of >10 μM, whereas the IC_{50} for scL-Irinotecan was ~5.5 μM representing an improvement in apparent efficacy of >2-fold for the scL nanomedicine formulation of irinotecan (**Figure 10A**). We have also assessed scL-Irinotecan *in vivo* using mice bearing subcutaneous A549 lung cancer xenografts. Treatments involved twice per week tail vein injections of 200 μg of either irinotecan or an equivalent amount of nanoformulated irinotecan as either untargeted Lip-Irinotecan or TfR-targeting scL-Irinotecan. As shown in **Figure 10B**, only scL-Irinotecan treatments resulted in any appreciable reduction in the size of tumors confirming that its antitumor activity requires the TfRscFv targeting.

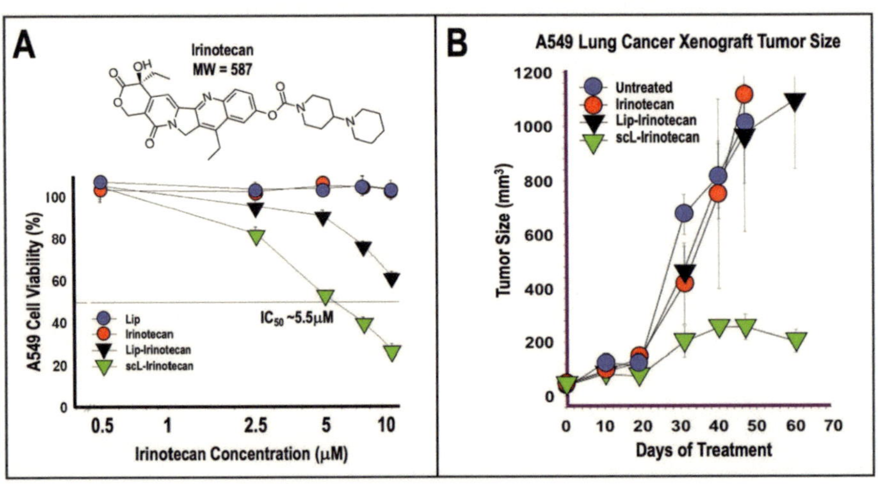

Figure 10.
Sensitivity of A549 lung cancer to free irinotecan and scL-Irinotecan. (A) Survival of A549 cells was assessed in vitro *using an XTT assay for cell viability and apparent IC_{50} values are provided. Based on the respective IC_{50} values, it appears that against A549 lung cancer cells, scL-Irinotecan (IC_{50} of ~5.5 μM) is at least 2-times more effective than free irinotecan (IC_{50} of >10 μM). (B) Mice bearing A549 subcutaneous xenografts were intravenously administered the indicated treatment with twice weekly injections (15 total injections). The sizes of tumors assessed on the indicated days. Tumor sizes in mice treated with free irinotecan or untargeted Lip-Irinotecan were not significantly different from those in untreated mice, whereas tumors in mice receiving scL-Irinotecan were significantly smaller. Since Lip-Irinotecan is relatively ineffective in impeding tumor growth, these data confirm that the* in vivo *antitumor activity of scL-Irinotecan requires the TfRscFv targeting moiety on the nanocomplex. Data points represent mean tumor sizes and error bars reflect their standard deviations.*

4. Discussion

We are developing scL nanocomplexes (depicted schematically in **Figures 1A**) as a delivery vehicle capable carrying diverse therapeutic molecules. The size of the scL nanoparticles (<300 nm) allows them to participate in the enhanced permeability component of the EPR effect, with their retention and uptake into cells mediated by the elevated TfR expression, which appears to be a universal biomarker for tumors [18]. We have previously shown that the scL nanocomplexes are capable of encapsulating a variety of payloads including plasmid DNAs for gene therapy [22] as well as antisense oligonucleotides or siRNAs to modulate gene expression [23–25]. Two products that utilize the scL platform technology for gene therapy (SGT-53 and SGT-94) are now in human clinical trials. SGT-53 for p53 gene therapy has completed phase Ia and Ib clinical trials [29, 30] and is currently in Phase II for metastatic pancreatic cancer in combination with gemcitabine/nab-paclitaxel (ClinicalTrials.gov Identifier: NCT02340117). Another investigational new drug application (IND) involving SGT-53 for children with advanced tumors of the central nervous system has been approved (ClinicalTrials.gov Identifier: NCT03554707). Two children have already been treated with SGT-53 under an extended access IND with no serious safety issues observed, and evidence of tumor responses was apparent *via* CT scans (unpublished data). A second investigational agent (SGT-94) that is based on the gene encoding a truncated form of the RB1 tumor suppressor (RB94) has also completed a Phase I clinical trial (ClinicalTrials.gov Identifier: NCT01517464) with an acceptable safety profile [28]. SGT-53 and SGT-94 are among a few TfR-targeting nanomedicines now undergoing clinical evaluation [61]. The safety profiles in trials for both SGT-53 and SGT-94 suggest that some "regulatory risk" of products utilizing the scL delivery system has been effectively reduced by these trials of products using this drug delivery system.

This article focuses exclusively on chemotherapeutic drugs as scL cargoes. It is not intended to be an in-depth study of any particular chemotherapeutic agent but rather to highlight the potential of nanotechnology to improve the efficacy of cancer drugs. Because the BBB effectively blocks ~98% of small molecule drugs from entering the brain [11], various strategies have been employed to get chemotherapeutics for cancer (and for other neurological conditions) into the brain with some approaches using various receptor-mediated pathways [12, 62]. Strategies for drug delivery to the brain have also included intranasal administration aimed at direct nose-to-brain drug delivery to bypass the BBB. The numerous attempts to deliver drugs to the brain *via* the direct nose-to-brain pathway have been reviewed, but there remains no evidence of any clinical benefits to patients coming from these efforts [12, 63]. There have also been attempts to disrupt temporarily the BBB to allow drugs to enter the brain from the bloodstream. In reviewing these efforts, Pardridge has concluded that BBB disruption by any means is not likely to yield a favorable therapeutic index and that BBB disruption would likely cause neurotoxicity as plasma proteins and other agents in the blood enter the brain without the protection normally afforded by the BBB [12]. Because cancer patients are likely to be given multiple administrations of chemotherapy in the course of their treatment, repeating highly invasive procedures including those aimed at disrupting the BBB would clearly be suboptimal. The administration route for the chemotherapeutic agents used in all of our mouse studies has been tail vein injections that rely on the targeting moiety of the scL nanocomplex facilitating brain entry *via* the physiological pathway of TfR-mediated transcytosis (depicted schematically in **Figure 1**). Our liposomal nanocomplexes fall into the category of drug delivery strategies referred to as "Trojan Horse Liposomes" [12] and might allow patients to be treated systemically using the intravenous administration commonly used in chemotherapy.

The current standard of care for GBM patients involves TMZ chemotherapy, but as currently used, TMZ improves median survival by only ~2.5 months, and even this modest effect is seen in only about 30% of patients [36–38]. When brain tumors recur after treatment, these tumors are likely to be TMZ-resistant. Although TMZ is routinely used in treatment of brain tumors, its use is limited by dose-related side effects, and it has been recognized that there is a need for TMZ reformulation, using carriers or functionalization to reduce toxicity and improve BBB crossing [64]. We have produced a novel TfR-targeted nanocomplex formulation of TMZ designed to actively crosses the BBB by receptor-mediated transcytosis of the endothelial cells and then actively targets cancer cells in the brain [26]. This nanocomplex formulation (scL-TMZ) has been shown to be markedly more active than free TMZ in killing GBM cells including U87R and T98G, both of which are TMZ-resistant. The superiority of scL-TMZ over free TMZ is also seen in mice with intracranial human GBM tumors. Our previous data indicated that scL nanocomplexes deliver their payloads to both bulk tumor and to the CSCs implicated in treatment resistance and tumor recurrence [22, 26, 65]. Encapsulation of TMZ in the nanocomplex also enhances the agent's activity against other types of tumor cell lines (lung, prostate, pancreas, breast, melanoma, and colorectal). Based on these findings, there is every reason to expect that scL-TMZ could prove to be effective against a range of cancer types beyond brain tumors.

Here, we summarize the use of the scL delivery technology for encapsulation of several smaller cancer chemotherapeutic agents. Our data involve scL formulations of five different chemotherapeutic drugs (TMZ, imatinib, sunitinib, erlotinib, and irinotecan) that have molecular weights between 194 Da to 587 Da. For each of these chemotherapeutics, we find that their scL nanomedicine formulations are markedly more effective than their unencapsulated counterparts in killing cancer cells (i.e. the scL nanocomplexes display reduced IC_{50} values). The nanomedicine scL-TMZ was assessed for killing cell lines coming from seven distinct types of cancer (GBM, melanoma, breast, colon, lung, pancreas, and prostate). It is also noteworthy that scL-TMZ was ~40-times more effective than free TMZ against a TMZ-resistant GBM cell line (U87R) and displayed improved efficacy in preventing tumor growth and extending lifespan in mice bearing intracranial GBM tumors. The scL formulation of irinotecan likewise displayed both enhanced potency against cultured lung cancer cells and improved efficacy in reducing tumor size *in vivo*. Given the ability to encapsulate the various agents used here and to improve the apparent efficacy of each agent examined, we would speculate that it should be possible to create scL formulations of other chemotherapeutics to improve their effectiveness against tumors in like manner. The scL formulations may also decrease toxic side effects associated with chemotherapy, as we have observed with scL-TMZ in mice toxicology studies [26].

Enhancing the efficacy of anticancer drugs and decreasing their undesirable side effects have long been aspirational goals, and numerous approaches have been employed to pursue one or both objectives. Among these efforts have been a substantial number of attempts to encapsulate drugs within nanoparticles of one kind or another [4–6]. Particularly attractive have been attempts to deliver chemotherapeutics to tumors *via* some form of selective targeting of the cancer cells [8, 9]. Our scL nanocomplexes are certainly not conceptually unique, but they do serve as a paradigm for how tumor-targeting nanoparticles can actually work to enhance cancer cell killing and to impede *in vivo* tumor growth. We have previously shown that when administered intravenously to mice with widely disseminated metastatic pancreatic cancer, scL nanocomplexes carrying a plasmid encoding the gene for β-galactosidase home to the metastatic cancer cells throughout the body with a very high degree of selectivity for expression of the reporter gene without expression in adjacent normal tissues [21]. The scL delivery system also has the advantage of having already been manufactured as two clinical-grade investigational agents for cancer gene therapy with three Phase I clinical trials completed with excellent safety profiles for the scL-based products [28–30].

The focus in this article is on anticancer drugs, but because scL nanocomplexes can ferry diverse payloads across the BBB, their utility in producing brain-penetrant pharmaceutical formulations is certainly not restricted to oncology. The BBB has long been recognized as a 'bottleneck for brain drug development" for both brain tumors and for neurological diseases and conditions in general [11]. In this regard, we have shown that scL nanocomplexes carrying an siRNA targeting TNFα reduces neuroinflammation triggered by administration to mice of bacterial endotoxin [24]. We have recently demonstrated that the scL formulation of a 137 Da oxime capable of reactivating brain acetylcholinesterase after exposure to an organophosphate toxin is superior to its unencapsulated counterpart as an organophosphate countermeasure [66, 67]. The original patents on the cancer drugs discussed in this article have all expired. However, new formulations of older drugs have their own potential for coverage as intellectual property. In this regard, a patent was recently allowed to cover certain aspects of TMZ delivered *via* an scL formulation. Based the paradigm of this newly allowed patent, it may be possible to breathe new life into the intellectual property coverage of drugs that are off-patent by converting these agents into novel nanomedicines. For all five chemotherapeutic drugs examined here, encapsulation within a scL nanocomplex that has a targeting moiety that binds the TfR rendered each of the drugs more potent in killing cells from a variety of human tumors. In the case of TMZ, the nano-encapsulated formulation (scL-TMZ) was also shown to be more effective in treating intracranial GBM as judged by reduction in tumor size and extension of the lifespans of GBM-bearing mice. The nanomedicine scL-TMZ was markedly more active against a TMZ-resistant variant of GBM than was free TMZ. Within intracranial GBM tumors, nano-encapsulated TMZ triggered apoptosis in both bulk tumor cells in the CSCs that are thought to contribute to therapeutic resistance and cancer recurrence. Nano-encapsulated irinotecan was also shown to be more effective *in vivo* using mice bearing human lung cancer xenografts. It is likely that the improved chemotherapeutic potency observed with all five drugs examined in this article could be extended to other chemotherapeutic agents not yet tested. By creating nanomedicine formulations capable of selectively targeting tumor cells, chemotherapeutic drugs could be rendered both more potent against tumor cells and less toxic to normal cells. Beyond brain tumors, the ability of the scL drug delivery system to cross the BBB may be useful in improving therapeutics for other neurological diseases and conditions.

5. Conclusions

For the five chemotherapeutic drugs examined, encapsulation within a scL nanocomplex that has a targeting moiety that binds TfRs rendered each of the drugs more potent in killing cells from a variety of human tumors. In the case of TMZ, the nano-encapsulated formulation (scL-TMZ) has also been shown to be more effective in treating intracranial GBM as judged by reduction in tumor size and extension of the lifespans of GBM-bearing mice. The nanomedicine scL-TMZ was markedly more active against a TMZ-resistant variant of GBM than was free TMZ. Within intracranial GBM tumors, nano-encapsulated TMZ triggered apoptosis in both bulk tumor cells in the CSCs that are thought to contribute to therapeutic resistance and cancer recurrence. Nano-encapsulated irinotecan was also shown to be more effective *in vivo* using mice bearing human lung cancer xenografts. It is likely that the improved chemotherapeutic potency observed with all five drugs examined in this article could be extended to other chemotherapeutic agents not yet tested. By creating nanomedicine formulations capable of selectively targeting tumor cells, chemotherapeutic drugs could at once be rendered both more potent against tumor cells and less toxic to normal cells. Beyond use against brain tumors, the ability of the scL drug delivery system to cross the BBB may prove useful in improving therapeutics for other neurological diseases and conditions.

Acknowledgements

The authors thank former members of the Chang laboratory at Georgetown, Sung Hee Hwang and Venkata M. Yenugonda, for their technical assistance in testing early versions of encapsulated chemotherapeutics. The authors also thank Karen Creswell for her technical assistance with flow cytometry.

Author contributions

Conceptualization: Joe B. Harford, Sang-Soo Kim, Kathleen F. Pirollo and Esther H. Chang; Laboratory Experiments: Sang-Soo Kim, Kathleen F. Pirollo and Antonina S. Rait; Supervision: Esther H. Chang; Writing – original draft: Joe B. Harford; Writing – review & editing: Joe B. Harford, Sang-Soo Kim, Kathleen F. Pirollo and Esther H. Chang; Figure Preparation: Joe B. Harford. All authors have read and approved the submission.

Funding

Studies described here were supported in part by the NCI (5R01CA132012–02 to E.H.C.), NCI SBIR contract (HHSN261201400038C to SynerGene Therapeutics, Inc.), the National Foundation for Cancer Research (HU0001 to E.H.C.), and a research grant from SynerGene Therapeutics Inc. (to K.F.P.). This study was conducted in part using the Flow Cytometry & Cell Sorting Shared Resource, Preclinical Imaging Research Laboratory, Microscopy & Imaging Shared Resource, Tissue Culture & Biorepository for Cell Lines and Biofluids Shared Resource, and Animal Core Facilities supported by NCI Cancer Center Support grant (2P30CA51008) and U.S. Public Health Service grant (1S10RR15768–01). This investigation was performed in part in a facility constructed with support from Research Facilities Improvement grant from the National Center for Research Resources, NIH (C06RR14567).

DOI: http://dx.doi.org/10.5772/intechopen.1007332

Conflict of interest

S.S.K., K.F.P. A.S.R and E.H.C. are inventors on patent applications related to the of the described scL technology. These patents are owned by Georgetown University and have been licensed to SynerGene Therapeutics, Inc. for commercial development. K.F.P. serves as Principal Investigator for research at Georgetown University that is supported by SynerGene Therapeutics, Inc. E.H.C. owns an equity interest in SynerGene Therapeutics, Inc. E.H.C., K.F.P. and A.S.R. serve as paid scientific consultants to SynerGene Therapeutics, Inc. S.S.K. is salaried employee of SynerGene Therapeutics, Inc. J.B.H. serves as salaried President & CEO of SynerGene Therapeutics, Inc. and owns stock in same. The authors report no other conflicts of interest in this work.

Data availability

The datasets generated during and/or analyzed during the current study are available from the corresponding author on reasonable request.

Ethics approval

All animal experiments were approved by the Georgetown University Institutional Animal Care and Use Committee. All animal experiments were performed in the AAALAC-accredited, USDA-registered animal facility of Georgetown University adhering to the *Guide for the Care and Use of Laboratory Animals* as required by the Office of Laboratory Animal Welfare (OLAW).

Author details

Joe B. Harford[1]*, Sang-Soo Kim[1,2], Kathleen F. Pirollo[2], Antonina S. Rait[1] and Esther H. Chang[2]

1 SynerGene Therapeutics, Inc., Potomac, MD, United States

2 Department of Oncology, Lombardi Comprehensive Cancer Center, Georgetown University Medical Center, Washington, DC, United States

*Address all correspondence to: harfordj@synergeneus.com

References

[1] Sung H, Ferlay J, Siegel RL, Laversanne M, Soerjomataram I, Jemal A, et al. Global cancer statistics 2020: GLOBOCAN estimates of incidence and mortality worldwide for 36 cancers in 185 countries. CA: a Cancer Journal for Clinicians. 2021;**71**(3):209-249

[2] Wilson BE, Jacob S, Yap ML, Ferlay J, Bray F, Barton MB. Estimates of global chemotherapy demands and corresponding physician workforce requirements for 2018 and 2040: A population-based study. The Lancet Oncology. 2019;**20**(6):769-780

[3] DeVita VT Jr, Rosenberg SA. Two hundred years of cancer research. The New England Journal of Medicine. 2012;**366**(23):2207-2214

[4] Ajith S, Almomani F, Elhissi A, Husseini GA. Nanoparticle-based materials in anticancer drug delivery: Current and future prospects. Heliyon. 2023;**9**(11):e21227

[5] Kandula S, Singh PK, Kaur GA, Tiwari A. Trends in smart drug delivery systems for targeting cancer cells. Materials Science and Engineering B. 2023;**297**:116816

[6] Sell M, Lopes AR, Escudeiro M, Esteves B, Monteiro AR, Trindade T, et al. Application of nanoparticles in cancer treatment: A concise review. Nanomaterials (Basel). 2023;**13**(21):2887

[7] Maeda H. Toward a full understanding of the EPR effect in primary and metastatic tumors as well as issues related to its heterogeneity. Advanced Drug Delivery Reviews. 2015;**91**:3-6

[8] Bazak R, Houri M, El Achy S, Kamel S, Refaat T. Cancer active targeting by nanoparticles: A comprehensive review of literature. Journal of Cancer Research and Clinical Oncology. 2015;**141**(5):769-784

[9] Rasool M, Malik A, Waquar S, Arooj M, Zahid S, Asif M, et al. New challenges in the use of nanomedicine in cancer therapy. Bioengineered. 2022;**13**(1):759-773

[10] Abbott NJ. Blood-brain barrier structure and function and the challenges for CNS drug delivery. Journal of Inherited Metabolic Disease. 2013;**36**(3):437-449

[11] Pardridge WM. The blood-brain barrier: Bottleneck in brain drug development. NeuroRx. 2005;**2**(1):3-14

[12] Pardridge WM. A historical review of brain drug delivery. Pharmaceutics. 2022;**14**(6):1283

[13] Liu HJ, Xu P. Strategies to overcome/penetrate the BBB for systemic nanoparticle delivery to the brain/brain tumor. Advanced Drug Delivery Reviews. 2022;**191**:114619

[14] Lundy DJ, Nguyen H, Hsieh PCH. Emerging Nano-carrier strategies for brain tumor drug delivery and considerations for clinical translation. Pharmaceutics. 2021;**13**(8):1193

[15] Johnsen KB, Burkhart A, Thomsen LB, Andresen TL, Moos T. Targeting the transferrin receptor for brain drug delivery. Progress in Neurobiology. 2019;**181**:101665

[16] Vega-Vasquez P, Mosier NS, Irudayaraj J. Nanoscale drug delivery

systems: From medicine to agriculture. Frontiers in Bioengineering and Biotechnology. 2020;**8**:79

[17] Daniels TR, Delgado T, Rodriguez JA, Helguera G, Penichet ML. The transferrin receptor part I: Biology and targeting with cytotoxic antibodies for the treatment of cancer. Clinical Immunology. 2006;**121**(2):144-158

[18] Essaghir A, Demoulin JB. A minimal connected network of transcription factors regulated in human tumors and its application to the quest for universal cancer biomarkers. PLoS One. 2012;**7**(6):e39666

[19] Daniels TR, Bernabeu E, Rodriguez JA, Patel S, Kozman M, Chiappetta DA, et al. The transferrin receptor and the targeted delivery of therapeutic agents against cancer. Biochimica et Biophysica Acta. 2012;**1820**(3):291-317

[20] Tortorella S, Karagiannis TC. Transferrin receptor-mediated endocytosis: A useful target for cancer therapy. The Journal of Membrane Biology. 2014;**247**(4):291-307

[21] Pirollo KF, Dagata J, Wang P, Freedman M, Vladar A, Fricke S, et al. A tumor-targeted nanodelivery system to improve early MRI detection of cancer. Molecular Imaging. 2006;**5**(1):41-52

[22] Kim SS, Rait A, Kim E, Pirollo KF, Nishida M, Farkas N, et al. A nanoparticle carrying the p53 gene targets tumors including cancer stem cells, sensitizes glioblastoma to chemotherapy and improves survival. ACS Nano. 2014;**8**(6):5494-5514

[23] Pirollo KF, Rait A, Zhou Q, Hwang SH, Dagata JA, Zon G, et al. Materializing the potential of small interfering RNA via a tumor-targeting nanodelivery system. Cancer Research. 2007;**67**(7):2938-2943

[24] Kim SS, Rait A, Garrido-Sanabria ER, Pirollo KF, Harford JB, Chang EH. Nanotherapeutics for gene modulation that prevents apoptosis in the brain and fatal Neuroinflammation. Molecular Therapy. 2018;**26**(1):84-94

[25] Kim SS, Harford JB, Moghe M, Rait A, Pirollo KF, Chang EH. Targeted nanocomplex carrying siRNA against MALAT1 sensitizes glioblastoma to temozolomide. Nucleic Acids Research. 2018;**46**(3):1424-1440

[26] Kim SS, Rait A, Kim E, DeMarco J, Pirollo KF, Chang EH. Encapsulation of temozolomide in a tumor-targeting nanocomplex enhances anti-cancer efficacy and reduces toxicity in a mouse model of glioblastoma. Cancer Letters. 2015;**369**(1):250-258

[27] Hwang SH, Rait A, Pirollo KF, Zhou Q, Yenugonda VM, Chinigo GM, et al. Tumor-targeting nanodelivery enhances the anticancer activity of a novel quinazolinone analogue. Molecular Cancer Therapeutics. 2008;**7**(3):559-568

[28] Siefker-Radtke A, Zhang XQ, Guo CC, Shen Y, Pirollo KF, Sabir S, et al. A phase I study of a tumor-targeted systemic Nanodelivery system, SGT-94, in genitourinary cancers. Molecular Therapy. 2016;**24**(8):1484-1491

[29] Senzer N, Nemunaitis J, Nemunaitis D, Bedell C, Edelman G, Barve M, et al. Phase I study of a systemically delivered p53 nanoparticle in advanced solid tumors. Molecular Therapy. 2013;**21**(5):1096-1103

[30] Pirollo KF, Nemunaitis J, Leung PK, Nunan R, Adams J, Chang EH. Safety and efficacy in advanced solid Tumors of a targeted Nanocomplex carrying the p53

gene used in combination with docetaxel: A phase 1b study. Molecular Therapy. 2016;**24**(9):1697-1706

[31] Leung CP, Barve MA, Wu M-S, Pirollo KF, Strauss JF, Liao W-C, et al. A phase II trial combining tumor-targeting TP53 gene therapy with gemcitabine/nab-paclitaxel as a second-line treatment for metastatic pancreatic cancer. Journal of Clinical Oncology. 2021;**39**(suppl. 15):4139-4139

[32] Kohsaka S, Takahashi K, Wang L, Tanino M, Kimura T, Nishihara H, et al. Inhibition of GSH synthesis potentiates temozolomide-induced bystander effect in glioblastoma. Cancer Letters. 2013;**331**(1):68-75

[33] Xu L, Huang CC, Huang W, Tang WH, Rait A, Yin YZ, et al. Systemic tumor-targeted gene delivery by anti-transferrin receptor scFv-immunoliposomes. Molecular Cancer Therapeutics. 2002;**1**(5):337-346

[34] Yu W, Pirollo KF, Yu B, Rait A, Xiang L, Huang W, et al. Enhanced transfection efficiency of a systemically delivered tumor-targeting immunolipoplex by inclusion of a pH-sensitive histidylated oligolysine peptide. Nucleic Acids Research. 2004;**32**(5):e48

[35] Miller KD, Ostrom QT, Kruchko C, Patil N, Tihan T, Cioffi G, et al. Brain and other central nervous system tumor statistics, 2021. CA: a Cancer Journal for Clinicians. 2021;**71**(5):381-406

[36] Stupp R, Mason WP, van den Bent MJ, Weller M, Fisher B, Taphoorn MJ, et al. European organisation for, R.; treatment of cancer brain, T.; radiotherapy, G.; National Cancer Institute of Canada clinical trials, G., radiotherapy plus concomitant and adjuvant temozolomide for glioblastoma. The New England Journal of Medicine. 2005;**352**(10):987-996

[37] Villano JL, Seery TE, Bressler LR. Temozolomide in malignant gliomas: Current use and future targets. Cancer Chemotherapy and Pharmacology. 2009;**64**(4):647-655

[38] Zhang J, Stevens MF, Bradshaw TD. Temozolomide: Mechanisms of action, repair and resistance. Current Molecular Pharmacology. 2012;**5**(1):102-114

[39] Iturrioz-Rodriguez N, Sampron N, Matheu A. Current advances in temozolomide encapsulation for the enhancement of glioblastoma treatment. Theranostics. 2023;**13**(9):2734-2756

[40] Mah LJ, El-Osta A, Karagiannis TC. gammaH2AX: A sensitive molecular marker of DNA damage and repair. Leukemia. 2010;**24**(4):679-686

[41] Sokolov AV, Dostdar SA, Attwood MM, Krasilnikova AA, Ilina AA, Nabieva AS, et al. Brain cancer drug discovery: Clinical trials, drug classes, targets, and combinatorial therapies. Pharmacological Reviews. 2021;**73**(4):1-32

[42] Hemmati HD, Nakano I, Lazareff JA, Masterman-Smith M, Geschwind DH, Bronner-Fraser M, et al. Cancerous stem cells can arise from pediatric brain tumors. Proceedings of the National Academy of Sciences of the United States of America. 2003;**100**(25):15178-15183

[43] Singh SK, Hawkins C, Clarke ID, Squire JA, Bayani J, Hide T, et al. Identification of human brain tumour initiating cells. Nature. 2004;**432**(7015):396-401

[44] Bao S, Wu Q, McLendon RE, Hao Y, Shi Q, Hjelmeland AB, et al. Glioma stem cells promote radioresistance

by preferential activation of the DNA damage response. Nature. 2006;**444**(7120):756-760

[45] Liu Q, Nguyen DH, Dong Q, Shitaku P, Chung K, Liu OY, et al. Molecular properties of CD133+ glioblastoma stem cells derived from treatment-refractory recurrent brain tumors. Journal of Neuro-Oncology. 2009;**94**(1):1-19

[46] Tatar Z, Thivat E, Planchat E, Gimbergues P, Gadea E, Abrial C, et al. Temozolomide and unusual indications: Review of literature. Cancer Treatment Reviews. 2013;**39**(2):125-135

[47] Li RH, Hou XY, Yang CS, Liu WL, Tang JQ, Liu YQ, et al. Temozolomide for treating malignant melanoma. Journal of the College of Physicians and Surgeons–Pakistan. 2015;**25**(9):680-688

[48] Villano JL, Letarte N, Yu JM, Abdur S, Bressler LR. Hematologic adverse events associated with temozolomide. Cancer Chemotherapy and Pharmacology. 2012;**69**(1):107-113

[49] Cohen P, Cross D, Janne PA. Kinase drug discovery 20 years after imatinib. Nature Reviews. Drug Discovery. 2022. DOI: 10.1038/s41573-022-00418-2

[50] Chang SP, Shen SC, Lee WR, Yang LL, Chen YC. Imatinib mesylate induction of ROS-dependent apoptosis in melanoma B16F0 cells. Journal of Dermatological Science. 2011;**62**(3):183-191

[51] Kim JL, Lee DH, Jeong S, Kim BR, Na YJ, Park SH, et al. Imatinib-induced apoptosis of gastric cancer cells is mediated by endoplasmic reticulum stress. Oncology Reports. 2019;**41**(3):1616-1626

[52] Gan HK, Seruga B, Knox JJ. Sunitinib in solid tumors. Expert Opinion on Investigational Drugs. 2009;**18**(6):821-834

[53] Chaskis C, Sadones J, Michotte A, Dujardin M, Everaert H, Neyns B. A phase II trial of sunitinib in patients with recurrent high-grade glioma. Journal of Clinical Oncology. 2008;**26**(suppl. 15):13001-13001

[54] Tang PA, Tsao MS, Moore MJ. A review of erlotinib and its clinical use. Expert Opinion on Pharmacotherapy. 2006;7(2):177-193

[55] Steins M, Thomas M, Geissler M. Erlotinib. Recent Results in Cancer Research. 2018;**211**:1-17

[56] Bailly C. Irinotecan: 25 years of cancer treatment. Pharmacological Research. 2019;**148**:104398

[57] Weekes J, Lam AK, Sebesan S, Ho YH. Irinotecan therapy and molecular targets in colorectal cancer: A systemic review. World Journal of Gastroenterology. 2009;**15**(29):3597-3602

[58] Thomas A, Pommier Y. Targeting topoisomerase I in the era of precision medicine. Clinical Cancer Research. 2019;**25**(22):6581-6589

[59] Louis N, Liu S, He X, Drummond DC, Noble CO, Goldman S, et al. New therapeutic approaches for brainstem tumors: A comparison of delivery routes using nanoliposomal irinotecan in an animal model. Journal of Neuro-Oncology. 2018;**136**(3):475-484

[60] Lu G, Rao M, Zhu P, Liang B, El-Nazer RT, Fonkem E, et al. Triple-drug therapy with bevacizumab, Irinotecan, and Temozolomide plus tumor treating fields for recurrent

glioblastoma: A retrospective study. Frontiers in Neurology. 2019;**10**:42

[61] van der Meel R, Vehmeijer LJ, Kok RJ, Storm G, van Gaal EV. Ligand-targeted particulate nanomedicines undergoing clinical evaluation: Current status. Advanced Drug Delivery Reviews. 2013;**65**(10):1284-1298

[62] Jones AR, Shusta EV. Blood-brain barrier transport of therapeutics via receptor-mediation. Pharmaceutical Research. 2007;**24**(9):1759-1771

[63] Dhuyvetter D, Tekle F, Nazarov M, Vreeken RJ, Borghys H, Rombouts F, et al. Direct nose to brain delivery of small molecules: Critical analysis of data from a standardized in vivo screening model in rats. Drug Delivery. 2020;**27**(1):1597-1607

[64] Krajcer A, Grzywna E, Lewandowska-Łańcucka J. Strategies increasing the effectiveness of temozolomide at various levels of anti-GBL therapy. Biomedicine & Pharmacotherapy. 2023;**165**:115174

[65] Kim SS, Rait A, Rubab F, Rao AK, Kiritsy MC, Pirollo KF, et al. The clinical potential of targeted nanomedicine: Delivering to cancer stem-like cells. Molecular Therapy. 2014;**22**(2):278-291

[66] Pirollo KF, Moghe M, Guan M, Rait AS, Wang A, Kim SS, et al. A Pralidoxime Nanocomplex formulation targeting transferrin receptors for reactivation of brain acetylcholinesterase after exposure of mice to an anticholinesterase organophosphate. International Journal of Nanomedicine. 2024;**19**:307-326

[67] Moghe M, Kim S-S, Guan M, Rait A, Pirollo KF, Harford JB, et al. scL-2PAM: A novel countermeasure that ameliorates Neuroinflammation and neuronal losses in mice exposed to an anticholinesterase organophosphate. International Journal of Molecular Sciences. 2024;**25**:7539

Chapter 13

Perspective Chapter: Targeting the Myeloid Compartment – Innovative Immunotherapy Strategies for Malignant Brain Tumors

Jenny Christine Kienzler

Abstract

This chapter explores the complex immune landscape of malignant brain tumors and the potential of immunotherapy in their treatment. It focuses on the predominant role of tumor-associated macrophages in the tumor microenvironment, including monocyte-derived macrophages, microglia, and border-associated macrophages. We discuss the results of various immunotherapy trials, including immune checkpoint blockade. While some approaches have shown promise, particularly in brain metastases, many have faced challenges in improving patient outcomes, especially in glioblastoma. The section highlights the importance of understanding the diverse functions of myeloid cells in the tumor microenvironment and proposes strategies for targeting these cells. Finally, we emphasize the need for more comprehensive research on the macrophage niche to develop effective immunotherapies for malignant brain tumors, potentially revolutionizing treatment approaches in this challenging field.

Keywords: malignant brain tumors, glioblastoma, brain metastases, immune microenvironment, immunotherapy, myeloid cells, tumor-associated macrophages, monocyte-derived macrophages, microglia, border-associated macrophages

1. Introduction

Central nervous system (CNS) tumors comprise a diverse range of both benign and malignant entities. In the adult population, meningioma, glioma, and brain metastases are the most prevalent. Malignant brain tumors, in particular, are associated with a poor prognosis [1]. Recent advancements in the single-cell analysis have shed light on the immune landscape of these tumors, revealing a predominance of tissue-resident and monocyte-derived macrophages (MoMacs), which are thought to contribute to an environment that promotes tumorigenesis [2, 3]. The identification of PDL1 expression in brain tumor cells led to clinical trials that explored the use of immune checkpoint inhibitors [4]. However, these treatments have demonstrated limited efficacy in brain metastases and have been largely unsuccessful in glioma [5]. The causes of treatment failure are believed to be linked to the immune microenvironment, characterized by a low mutational burden, poor infiltration of cytotoxic T cells, a lack of neoantigens, and the "corruption" of macrophages toward an immunosuppressive milieu [6, 7]. Several immunotherapeutic approaches are being examined, including CAR-T cells, oncolytic viral therapy, dendritic cell (DC) vaccination, and cytokine antibody fusions. These strategies aim to enhance the local immune cell infiltrate and foster a proinflammatory milieu.

This chapter will discuss the current understanding of the immune landscape in malignant brain tumors and give an overview of the results of completed immunotherapy trials. We will focus on the role of the myeloid compartment in the tumor microenvironment and explore various strategies to target these cells for immunotherapy. Additionally, we will discuss the challenges and future directions in developing effective immunotherapies for malignant brain tumors.

2. Immune infiltrate in malignant brain tumors

The tumor microenvironment of brain cancers is delineated by a predominant presence of tumor-associated macrophages (TAMs) that exhibit an immunosuppressive phenotype, which has been shown to support tumor growth and progression [2, 3, 8–10]. These TAMs can have two distinct origins within the CNS: They can arise from resident microglia or from blood-derived monocytes that infiltrate the tumor microenvironment [2, 7]. Previous research has demonstrated that as tumors progress, they trigger the recruitment of monocytes from the bloodstream. Once these monocytes enter the tumor microenvironment, they differentiate into monocyte-derived macrophages (MoMacs) [11–13]. The presence of these immunosuppressive TAMs, whether derived from resident microglia or infiltrating monocytes, plays a crucial role in forming the immune landscape of brain tumors and adds to the challenges faced in developing effective immunotherapies for these malignancies.

Recently, two back-to-back papers investigated the leukocyte landscape in brain cancer, focusing on the constitution of immune cells within the tumor microenvironment [2, 3]. Their findings revealed striking differences between glioblastoma and brain metastases (BrM). The glioblastoma microenvironment was found to be primarily dominated by TAMs, while the microenvironment of brain metastases contained a higher proportion of tumor-infiltrating lymphocytes [2, 3]. Upon further analysis of the myeloid compartment, the researchers discovered that the tumor type significantly influences the differentiation and phenotype of MoMacs [2, 14]. In glioblastoma, the tumor microenvironment predominantly consisted of TAMs, originating from resident microglia. In contrast, brain metastases exhibited a high abundance of MoMacs [2, 14] Interestingly, the studies also found that IDH mutant glioblastomas mainly comprised TAMs derived from microglia, whereas the more aggressive IDH wildtype glioblastomas had a higher proportion of MoMacs [2, 3].

T cells on the other hand are often not efficiently primed, are terminally exhausted, or inactivated by immune checkpoints [6, 14]. Brain metastases typically exhibit higher T cell infiltration compared to glioblastoma, making them potentially more responsive to immunotherapy approaches that aim to reinvigorate T cells. However, in brain metastases, these T cells are often concentrated in the tumor stroma rather than within the tumor tissue itself [14]. The distinct immune profiles of glioblastoma and brain metastases revealed by these studies could inform the development of more effective, targeted immunotherapies for these brain cancers.

3. Results of immunotherapy trials

3.1 Immune checkpoint blockade

The immune system has evolved regulatory mechanisms known as immune checkpoints to ensure a balanced immune response. These checkpoints are crucial in maintaining self-tolerance and preventing autoimmune reactions by mitigating excessive immune activation [15]. The concept of immune checkpoints encompasses several inhibitory pathways that help control T cell responses. The PD-1 (programmed cell death protein-1) pathway is one of the most well-known and clinically significant immune checkpoints. PD-1 is expressed on the surface of activated T cells, and its interaction with ligands PD-L1 and PD-L2 induces decreased T cell effector functions, inhibited cytotoxic activity, and reduced cytokine production. Another key immune checkpoint is cytotoxic T-lymphocyte-associated protein 4 (CTLA-4), which inactivates T cells by competing with the co-stimulatory molecule CD28 for binding to B7 ligands [15]. Cancer cells often exploit these regulatory pathways to evade immune detection and resist destruction [16]. Immune checkpoint inhibitors (ICIs) have transformed cancer immunotherapy, unleashing the immune system's natural capacity to detect and destroy malignant cells. This groundbreaking approach has significantly altered the landscape of cancer treatment [17]. By blocking inhibitory immune checkpoint pathways, the immune system's brakes are lifted, thereby enhancing the antitumor response [18]. Monoclonal antibodies targeting PD-1 and/or CTLA-4, such as pembrolizumab, nivolumab, and ipilimumab, have demonstrated excellent clinical outcomes and effectiveness in various cancers, including melanoma, non-small cell lung cancer, and renal carcinoma. Immunotherapy approaches for malignant brain tumors have shown mixed results in clinical trials, particularly phase 3 trials. For glioblastoma (GBM), immune checkpoint blockade (ICB) has had limited success. While some small studies showed promise in recurrent, hypermutated high-grade gliomas [4, 19], larger randomized phase 3 trials, such as CheckMate 143, compared anti-PD-1 treatment with bevacizumab (anti-VEGF) in recurrent GBM and found no significant survival benefit [5]. Two phase 3 trials investigated anti-PD-1 ICB treatment in newly diagnosed glioblastoma. CheckMate 498 compared anti-PD-1 combined with radiotherapy against standard treatment [20]. CheckMate 548 evaluated anti-PD-1 added to standard of care versus placebo plus standard of care [21]. Unfortunately, ICB failed to improve overall survival in newly diagnosed GBM compared to standard of care. Various other immune checkpoint blockade (ICB) therapies are under investigation for glioblastoma treatment. These include combination approaches using anti-CTLA-4 and anti-PD-1 agents together. Additionally, studies are exploring other ICB targets, such as TIM-3, LAG-3, TIGIT, and 4-1BB. Factors, such as the immunosuppressive tumor microenvironment, lack of T cell infiltrate, tumor heterogeneity, and poor blood–brain barrier penetration, may contribute to ICB's ineffectiveness in glioblastoma.

3.2 Vaccines: tumor-associated antigens and dendritic cell vaccines

Vaccination strategies have also been explored for glioblastoma treatment. Phase 3 trials have evaluated vaccines targeting epidermal growth factor receptor (EGFR) and the active mutant form EGFRvIII. These vaccines used either peptide-based formulations or antibody-drug conjugates [22, 23]. Unfortunately, these trials did not meet their primary endpoints and failed to demonstrate improved survival outcomes for patients.

Other vaccine trials have focused on targeting specific tumor mutations, showing promising results. For instance, a phase 1 trial evaluated an IDH1-specific peptide vaccine in 33 patients with gliomas harboring IDH1 mutations [24]. The encouraging outcomes from this study suggest that mutation-specific vaccines merit further investigation in larger trials.

Dendritic cell vaccines represent an alternative vaccination strategy. This approach involves exposing dendritic cells (specialized antigen-presenting cells) to tumor antigens before administering them as a vaccine. The pre-exposure to tumor antigens aims to enhance the dendritic cells' ability to stimulate a targeted immune response against the cancer. A recent phase 3 trial evaluated DCVax-L, a dendritic cell vaccine loaded with autologous tumor lysate, in addition to standard of care [25]. The study reported improved survival outcomes for both newly diagnosed and recurrent glioblastoma patients treated with this vaccine [25]. Despite these promising results, the trial's design attracted criticism from some researchers, raising questions about the interpretation of its findings [26].

3.3 Oncolytic viruses

Oncolytic viral therapies utilize replication-competent viruses to stimulate an immune response against tumors [27, 28]. Various viral types have been explored for this purpose, including polioviruses, adenoviruses, herpes simplex viruses, retroviruses, and measles viruses. Large-scale trials have not demonstrated significant survival benefits. The largest completed trial of an oncolytic viral therapy for glioblastoma evaluated a replicating retrovirus targeting tumor cells, known as Toca 511, used in combination with Toca flucytosine [29]. The virus was injected into the cavity wall during surgery to resect recurrent glioblastoma or anaplastic astrocytoma tumors. This procedure was performed for either the first or second instance of tumor recurrence, followed by a six-week course of oral Toca flucytosine. This study compared outcomes between 201 patients receiving the viral therapy combination and 202 patients undergoing standard treatment [29]. The trial results revealed no statistically significant difference in median overall survival between the groups [29]. Various phase 2 trials examining the impact of oncolytic viral therapy in high-grade gliomas have yielded inconsistent outcomes, without demonstrating a definitive survival advantage [30–32].

3.4 Engineered chimeric antigen receptor (CAR)-T cell therapy

Engineered chimeric antigen receptor (CAR)-T cell therapy is currently under investigation in clinical trials for the treatment of high-grade gliomas. CAR-T cells are autologous T cells that have been genetically modified *ex vivo* to express a specific T cell receptor targeting a predefined tumor antigen. Upon reinfusion into the patient, these engineered cells can recognize and eliminate cancer cells expressing the target antigen. While this approach has shown remarkable efficacy in hematological malignancies, its application to solid tumors, including brain tumors, has proven challenging. A pioneering study tested CAR-T cell therapy targeting EGFR variant

III in 10 individuals with recurring glioblastoma. The trial successfully showed that it is possible to safely produce and deliver personalized CAR-T cells for this condition. The study found no cases of cytokine release syndrome or unintended toxic effects. Notably, one participant exhibited stable disease throughout an 18-month observation period [33]. Recent phase 1 trials reported promising interim results. In one study, the authors report six patients with recurrent glioblastoma administered with intrathecal bivalent chimeric antigen receptor (CAR) T cells targeting EGFR and interleukin-13 receptor alpha 2 [34]. Although neurotoxicity was observed and needed treatment, the study demonstrated the preliminary safety and bioactivity of this CAR-T cell therapy, with an encouraging early efficacy signal that requires further investigation [34]. The second study examined three patients with recurrent glioblastoma. These patients were treated using CAR-T cells engineered to target both the EGFR variant III and wildtype EGFR through a T cell-engaging antibody molecule [35]. The treatment showed promising initial results, with rapid and significant tumor regression observed radiographically in all patients. Importantly, no adverse events above grade 3 were reported. However, the therapeutic response proved to be short-lived in two of the three patients [35]. Ongoing research is exploring CAR-T cells targeting various tumor antigens, including HER2, IL-13 Ra2, GD2, and B7-H3 [36]. Despite showing promise in early-phase clinical trials for glioblastoma, CAR-T cell therapy has generally elicited limited responses, and some instances of toxicity have been observed. Additional research is required to refine this therapeutic strategy for solid tumors, especially those affecting the central nervous system. This refinement process encompasses the enhancement of CAR-T cell efficacy, including innovative approaches such as in vivo CAR-T cell induction [37].

3.5 Immunotherapy approaches in brain metastases

Recent research has demonstrated that ICB therapy shows promise in treating brain metastases [14]. Several ongoing phase 3 clinical trials are appraising the potential of anti-CTLA-4 and anti-PD-1 antibodies in managing brain metastases originating from melanoma and non-small cell lung cancer (NSCLC). These studies assess the effectiveness of ICB therapy as a standalone treatment and in combination with radiotherapy and chemotherapy.

A phase 2 trial with asymptomatic, untreated melanoma brain metastasis demonstrated that anti-PD-1 therapy resulted in a median overall survival of 17 months [38]. The CheckMate 204 phase 2 study investigated the combined use of anti-PD-1 and anti-CTLA-4 in patients with one or more melanoma brain metastases [39]. For patients in the asymptomatic cohort, 36-month overall survival was 71.9%, while for patients with stable neurological symptoms and corticosteroid use, it was 36.6% [39]. In NSCLC patients, a phase 2 trial of anti-PD-1 treatment in 42 patients resulted in a 29.7% response rate [40]. Another phase 2 trial treated 26 patients with unirradiated brain metastases from NSCLC or renal cell carcinoma using anti-PD-1 and stereotactic radiosurgery within 14 days after the first dose of immune checkpoint blockade (ICB) [41]. The median overall survival for these patients was 21.4 months [41].

Currently, numerous studies are exploring additional treatment options for brain metastases. These include trials investigating dendritic cell vaccination and the combination of ICB treatment with stereotactic radiation for brain metastases originating from melanoma, lung, and breast cancers. Several additional immunotherapy trials are ongoing, with results expected in the coming years.

4. Role of myeloid cells in the tumor microenvironment

The malignant brain tumor microenvironment is populated by various macrophage subsets. However, emerging evidence suggests that these cells play diverse and multifaceted roles in tumor progression and immune regulation. These subsets can be broadly categorized into three main groups: monocyte-derived macrophages (MoMacs), microglia, and border-associated macrophages (BAMs).

4.1 Microglia

Microglia, the resident immune cells of the brain parenchyma originate from embryonic cells and possess the ability to self-renew [42]. The exact functions of microglia within the glioma microenvironment remain incompletely understood. Microglia in healthy brain tissue typically express specific homeostatic markers, including SALL1, TMEM119, and P2RY12 [2]. However, in the presence of brain tumors, the expression of these markers may be reduced [2]. Analysis of human brain cancer samples reveals that microglia exhibit a reactive state characterized by increased expression of CD14 and CD64. These microglia also express HMOX1, which may contribute to the exhaustion of CD8 T cells [2, 43]. However, depletion of HMOX1 in microglia resulted in reactivated effector T cells in *in vivo* experiments [43]. TREM2 is a marker found in high levels expressed on both microglia and MoMacs in the context of gliomas and brain metastases. Its presence has been correlated with poor survival outcomes in glioma patients, suggesting a potential role in tumor progression [44]. Inhibition of TREM2 in preclinical models yielded promising results, inhibiting tumor growth and inducing a proinflammatory polarization in the tumor microenvironment [45].

Intriguingly, analysis of both human and mouse samples revealed a distinct spatial distribution pattern of immune cells within brain metastases. The spatial distribution of immune cells showed a distinct pattern. MoMacs were primarily located in the center of the tumor, whereas microglia were more commonly found in the surrounding brain tissue [46].

4.2 Border-associated macrophages

Border-associated macrophages (BAMs) are a group of immune cells found at the interfaces of the CNS. This category includes three distinct populations: Perivascular macrophages, meningeal macrophages, and choroid plexus macrophages [47]. Research on BAMs and their developmental origins has been more extensively conducted in mouse brains. A recent comprehensive single-cell analysis of mouse brain macrophages revealed six distinct major subsets of BAMs [48]. BAMs are characterized by the expression of several key markers, including CD163, CD206, Lyve1, Folr2, NRP1, P2RX7, CLEC12A, CD63, and MHCII [48].

4.2.1 Perivascular macrophages

In various tumor types, perivascular macrophages (PVMs) within the tumor microenvironment have been linked to several pro-tumor functions. These include facilitating the intravasation of cancer cells, promoting tumor angiogenesis, and contributing to the establishment of distant metastases [49]. Preclinical studies using intravital imaging techniques have revealed that PVMs play two key roles in breast cancer progression: They facilitate the escape of tumor cells from the primary site and influence the permeability of blood vessels in the local tumor environment [50]. A recent analysis of human samples treated with ICB uncovered distinct patterns of PVM distribution in different brain tumors. In recurrent glioblastoma, PVMs were found to accumulate in the perivascular space. In contrast, PVMs infiltrated the tumor tissue in brain metastases [14].

4.2.2 Meningeal macrophages

The dural layer enveloping the brain contains both meningeal macrophages and T cells in close proximity. Studies using encephalomyelitis models have shown that meningeal macrophages play a role in presenting antigens and activating T cells [51]. Moreover, the microvascular network in the dura mater lacks a blood–brain barrier, and it also contains lymphatics, which enables immune cells to access the central nervous system. These insights may pave the way for novel immunotherapy strategies.

4.2.3 Choroid plexus macrophages

The choroid plexus is a unique region within the brain's ventricles, characterized by a diverse cellular composition. Its primary function is cerebrospinal fluid production and choroid plexus epithelial cells form the blood-cerebrospinal fluid barrier [52]. The choroid plexus stroma contains choroid plexus macrophages and features a dense network of microvessels lacking a blood–brain barrier [52]. This structure facilitates the recruitment and infiltration of peripheral immune cells into the brain. Manipulating choroid plexus macrophages could potentially be used to modulate the infiltration of proinflammatory cell subsets specifically.

4.3 MoMacs

The composition of microglia and MoMacs varies across different brain tumor types. Myeloid cells in the tumor microenvironment seem to contribute significantly to immunotherapy treatment failure in glioblastoma [6]. Interestingly, the appearance of MoMacs increases progressively from melanoma to breast and lung brain metastases, while the opposite trend is observed for microglia, highlighting the dynamic nature of myeloid cell populations across different brain tumor types [3]. Current evidence indicates that MoMacs in brain tumors are influenced by the specific tumor type and tend to adopt immunosuppressive properties [2]. These MoMacs are characterized by the expression of various markers, including CD206, CD209, CD204, LILRB2, CD163, CD169, and PD-L1, which collectively contribute to their immunomodulatory functions in the tumor microenvironment [2, 3, 6]. CSF1-receptor (CSF1R) is expressed on both macrophages and microglia in the brain tumor microenvironment. This receptor is crucial for the proliferation, differentiation, and survival of these myeloid cells, contributing to their recruitment and maintenance in tumors. CSF1R inhibition has shown promise as an immunotherapy approach in preclinical glioblastoma models, demonstrating survival benefits [53]. This preclinical research uncovered a competitive relationship between microglia and MoMacs, where impeding monocyte influx triggered compensatory mechanisms that maintained overall tumor-associated macrophage numbers by increasing microglia in the tumor [54]. Despite these promising preclinical results, clinical trials using CSF1R inhibition in glioblastoma patients have not yet demonstrated effectiveness, highlighting the challenges of translating these findings to human therapies [55].

The distinct classification of MoMacs in the M1 and M2 categories has been found to be overly simplistic and not reflective of their true nature. Instead, current research reveals that MoMacs exist with overlapping phenotypes that can shift based on environmental cues [56]. This more nuanced understanding highlights the plasticity of macrophage populations and the need to characterize and target these cells in the context of brain tumors [57].

5. Future immunotherapy targets

The aforementioned studies have shed light on the specific markers expressed by myeloid cells within the tumor microenvironment (**Figure 1**). However, despite these valuable insights, targeted therapies specifically designed for these cells have yet to be developed. The future of immunotherapy for malignant brain tumors holds promise, particularly in targeting the understudied innate immune compartment. While previous efforts have largely focused on T cell-based approaches, the abundant myeloid cell population in brain cancers presents an untapped opportunity for therapeutic intervention. As the predominant immune cell population in malignant brain tumors, myeloid cells present a promising target for novel therapeutic approaches. Antibody-cytokine fusions, for instance, could be effectively delivered by targeting these cells. However, a more nuanced understanding of the various myeloid

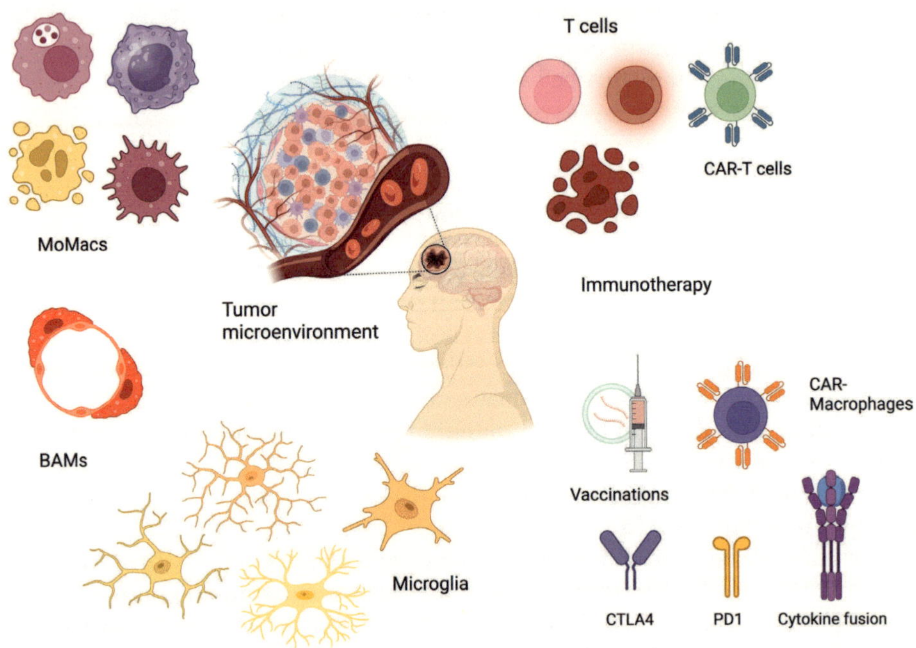

Figure 1
The tumor microenvironment in malignant brain tumors is dominated by monocyte-derived macrophages (MoMacs) and microglia. While their exact function remains unclear, current research suggests they exhibit an immunosuppressive phenotype. Border-associated macrophages (BAMs) are less prevalent but may play a crucial role in regulating the blood–brain barrier and immune cell infiltration, potentially influencing immunotherapy responses. T cells within the tumor often remain inactive due to insufficient exposure to tumor antigens or become terminally exhausted, losing their ability to eliminate cancer cells. Researchers are currently exploring various immunotherapy approaches for malignant brain tumors, including dendritic cell and mRNA vaccines, as well as combinations of immune checkpoint blockade (ICB) and antibody-cytokine fusion therapies.

subgroups and their functions within the tumor microenvironment is crucial. Within the MoMacs population, identifying and distinguishing between pro-tumoral and antitumoral subsets could enable more precise targeting and reeducation of the immune environment. MoMacs in the tumor microenvironment frequently display an anti-inflammatory or pro-tumorigenic phenotype. Therapeutic strategies aimed at reprogramming these cells toward a more proinflammatory state could shift the balance of the immune response in favor of antitumor activity. Monocytes and macrophages possess a natural ability to home in on brain tumors, making them ideal candidates for targeted drug delivery in cancer therapy. These cells can be loaded with anticancer drugs, effectively turning them into living delivery vehicles that bring therapeutic agents directly to the tumor site, potentially increasing local drug concentrations while minimizing systemic side effects. Additionally, monocytes and macrophages can be engineered to express therapeutic genes, enabling sustained, localized production of anticancer proteins or immunomodulatory factors directly within the tumor microenvironment, thus enhancing the antitumor response.
By expressing CAR on macrophages, one could potentially enhance the targeting specificity of these cells while leveraging their natural ability to infiltrate tumors. This approach combines the precision of CAR technology with the innate tumor-targeting capabilities of macrophages, offering a novel and potentially powerful method of immunotherapy for brain cancers. To fully leverage these opportunities, more comprehensive research on the myeloid compartment is essential. This deeper understanding will be critical in designing novel, more effective strategies for the treatment of brain cancers, potentially revolutionizing immunotherapy approaches in this challenging field.

6. Conclusions

The complex immune landscape of malignant brain tumors presents both challenges and opportunities for immunotherapy. While T cell-based approaches have shown limited success, the abundant myeloid cell population offers a promising avenue for future interventions. The diverse roles of monocyte-derived macrophages, microglia, and border-associated macrophages highlight the need for novel targeting strategies. Emerging approaches, such as reprogramming myeloid cells, utilizing macrophages as drug delivery vehicles, and developing CAR-macrophage therapies, show potential for enhancing antitumor responses. However, translating preclinical successes into effective clinical treatments remains challenging. A deeper understanding of the myeloid compartment's complexity is crucial for developing better immunotherapies. By leveraging the unique properties of myeloid cells and their interactions within the tumor microenvironment, we may overcome current limitations of immunotherapy in malignant brain tumors, potentially revolutionizing treatment strategies and improving patient outcomes.

Acknowledgements

Funding information: Dr. Kienzler received funding from the "Filling the Gap" Grant from the University of Zurich, UZH, Switzerland.

The figure has been created using Biorender.com.

Conflict of interest

The author declares no conflict of interest.

Author details

Jenny Christine Kienzler[1,2]

1 Institute of Experimental Immunology, University of Zurich, Zurich, Switzerland

2 Department of Neurosurgery, University Hospital of Lausanne, Lausanne, Switzerland

*Address all correspondence to: kienzler@immunology.uzh.ch

References

[1] Vaz-Salgado MA, Villamayor M, Albarrán V, Alía V, Sotoca P, Chamorro J, et al. Recurrent glioblastoma: A review of the treatment options. Cancers. 2023;**15**:1-22, 4279. DOI: 10.3390/cancers15174279

[2] Friebel E, Kapolou K, Unger S, Nunez NG, Utz S, Rushing EJ, et al. Single-cell mapping of human brain cancer reveals tumor-specific instruction of tissue-invading leukocytes. Cell. 2020;**181**(7):1626-42e20

[3] Klemm F, Maas RR, Bowman RL, Kornete M, Soukup K, Nassiri S, et al. Interrogation of the microenvironmental landscape in brain Tumors reveals disease-specific alterations of immune cells. Cell. 2020;**181**(7):1643-60e17

[4] Cloughesy TF, Mochizuki AY, Orpilla JR, Hugo W, Lee AH, Davidson TB, et al. Neoadjuvant anti-PD-1 immunotherapy promotes a survival benefit with intratumoral and systemic immune responses in recurrent glioblastoma. Nature Medicine. 2019;**25**(3):477-486

[5] Reardon DA, Brandes AA, Omuro A, Mulholland P, Lim M, Wick A, et al. Effect of Nivolumab vs bevacizumab in patients with recurrent glioblastoma: The CheckMate 143 phase 3 randomized clinical trial. JAMA Oncology. 2020;**6**(7):1003-1010

[6] Lee AH, Sun L, Mochizuki AY, Reynoso JG, Orpilla J, Chow F, et al. Neoadjuvant PD-1 blockade induces T cell and cDC1 activation but fails to overcome the immunosuppressive tumor associated macrophages in recurrent glioblastoma. Nature Communications. 2021;**12**(1):6938

[7] Kienzler JC, Becher B. Immunity in malignant brain tumors: Tumor entities, role of immunotherapy, and specific contribution of myeloid cells to the brain tumor microenvironment. European Journal of Immunology. 2024;**54**(2):e2250257

[8] Fischer GM, Jalali A, Kircher DA, Lee WC, McQuade JL, Haydu LE, et al. Molecular profiling reveals unique immune and metabolic features of melanoma brain metastases. Cancer Discovery. 2019;**9**(5):628-645

[9] Pinton L, Masetto E, Vettore M, Solito S, Magri S, D'Andolfi M, et al. The immune suppressive microenvironment of human gliomas depends on the accumulation of bone marrow-derived macrophages in the center of the lesion. Journal for Immunotherapy of Cancer. 2019;**7**(1):58

[10] Yeo AT, Rawal S, Delcuze B, Christofides A, Atayde A, Strauss L, et al. Single-cell RNA sequencing reveals evolution of immune landscape during glioblastoma progression. Nature Immunology. 2022;**23**(6):971-984

[11] Bowman RL, Klemm F, Akkari L, Pyonteck SM, Sevenich L, Quail DF, et al. Macrophage ontogeny underlies differences in tumor-specific education in brain malignancies. Cell Reports. 2016;**17**(9):2445-2459

[12] Goldmann T, Wieghofer P, Jordao MJ, Prutek F, Hagemeyer N, Frenzel K, et al. Origin, fate and dynamics of macrophages at central nervous system interfaces. Nature Immunology. 2016;**17**(7):797-805

[13] Mrdjen D, Pavlovic A, Hartmann FJ, Schreiner B, Utz SG, Leung BP, et al. High-dimensional single-cell mapping of central nervous system immune

cells reveals distinct myeloid subsets in health, aging, and disease. Immunity. 2018;**48**(2):380-395 e6

[14] Sun L, Kienzler JC, Reynoso JG, Lee A, Shiuan E, Li S, et al. Immune checkpoint blockade induces distinct alterations in the microenvironments of primary and metastatic brain tumors. The Journal of Clinical Investigation. 2023;**133**(17)

[15] Sharma P, Allison JP. The future of immune checkpoint therapy. Science. 2015;**348**(6230):56-61

[16] Topalian SL, Drake CG, Pardoll DM. Immune checkpoint blockade: A common denominator approach to cancer therapy. Cancer Cell. 2015;**27**(4):450-461

[17] Pardoll D, Drake C. Immunotherapy earns its spot in the ranks of cancer therapy. The Journal of Experimental Medicine. 2012;**209**(2):201-209

[18] Ribas A, Wolchok JD. Cancer immunotherapy using checkpoint blockade. Science. 2018;**359**(6382):1350-1355

[19] Zhao J, Chen AX, Gartrell RD, Silverman AM, Aparicio L, Chu T, et al. Immune and genomic correlates of response to anti-PD-1 immunotherapy in glioblastoma. Nature Medicine. 2019;**25**(3):462-469

[20] Omuro A, Brandes AA, Carpentier AF, Idbaih A, Reardon DA, Cloughesy T, et al. Radiotherapy combined with nivolumab or temozolomide for newly diagnosed glioblastoma with unmethylated MGMT promoter: An international randomized phase III trial. Neuro-Oncology. 2023;**25**(1):123-134

[21] Lim M, Weller M, Idbaih A, Steinbach J, Finocchiaro G, Raval RR, et al. Phase III trial of chemoradiotherapy with temozolomide plus nivolumab or placebo for newly diagnosed glioblastoma with methylated MGMT promoter. Neuro-Oncology. 2022;**24**(11):1935-1949

[22] Weller M, Butowski N, Tran DD, Recht LD, Lim M, Hirte H, et al. Rindopepimut with temozolomide for patients with newly diagnosed, EGFRvIII-expressing glioblastoma (ACT IV): A randomised, double-blind, international phase 3 trial. The Lancet Oncology. 2017;**18**(10):1373-1385

[23] Lassman AB, Pugh SL, Wang TJC, Aldape K, Gan HK, Preusser M, et al. Depatuxizumab mafodotin in EGFR-amplified newly diagnosed glioblastoma: A phase III randomized clinical trial. Neuro-Oncology. 2022;**25**(2):339-350

[24] Platten M, Bunse L, Wick A, Bunse T, Le Cornet L, Harting I, et al. A vaccine targeting mutant IDH1 in newly diagnosed glioma. Nature. 2021;**592**(7854):463-468

[25] Liau LM, Ashkan K, Brem S, Campian JL, Trusheim JE, Iwamoto FM, et al. Association of Autologous Tumor Lysate-Loaded Dendritic Cell Vaccination with Extension of survival among patients with newly diagnosed and recurrent glioblastoma: A phase 3 prospective externally controlled cohort trial. JAMA Oncology. 2023;**9**(1):112-121

[26] Mandel JJ, de Groot JF. External control arms and data analysis methods in nonrandomized trial of patients with glioblastoma. JAMA Oncology. 2023;**9**(7):1006

[27] Foreman PM, Friedman GK, Cassady KA, Markert JM. Oncolytic Virotherapy for the treatment of malignant glioma. Neurotherapeutics. 2017;**14**(2):333-344

[28] Lawler SE. Shifting the balance of power? The combination of oncolytic virotherapy and immune checkpoint blockade for glioblastoma treatment. Neuro-Oncology. 2017;**19**(4):463-465

[29] Cloughesy TF, Petrecca K, Walbert T, Butowski N, Salacz M, Perry J, et al. Effect of Vocimagene Amiretrorepvec in combination with Flucytosine vs standard of care on survival following tumor resection in patients with recurrent high-grade glioma: A randomized clinical trial. JAMA Oncology. 2020;**6**(12):1939-1946

[30] Nassiri F, Patil V, Yefet LS, Singh O, Liu J, Dang RMA, et al. Oncolytic DNX-2401 virotherapy plus pembrolizumab in recurrent glioblastoma: A phase 1/2 trial. Nature Medicine. 2023;**29**(6):1370-1378

[31] Ji N, Weng D, Liu C, Gu Z, Chen S, Guo Y, et al. Adenovirus-mediated delivery of herpes simplex virus thymidine kinase administration improves outcome of recurrent high grade glioma. Oncotarget. 2016;7(4):4369-4378

[32] Wheeler LA, Manzanera AG, Bell SD, Cavaliere R, McGregor JM, Grecula JC, et al. Phase II multicenter study of gene-mediated cytotoxic immunotherapy as adjuvant to surgical resection for newly diagnosed malignant glioma. Neuro-Oncology. 2016;**18**(8):1137-1145

[33] O'Rourke DM, Nasrallah MP, Desai A, Melenhorst JJ, Mansfield K, Morrissette JJD, et al. A single dose of peripherally infused EGFRvIII-directed CAR T cells mediates antigen loss and induces adaptive resistance in patients with recurrent glioblastoma. Science Translational Medicine. 2017;**9**(399):eaaa0984

[34] Bagley SJ, Logun M, Fraietta JA, Wang X, Desai AS, Bagley LJ, et al. Intrathecal bivalent CAR T cells targeting EGFR and IL13Rα2 in recurrent glioblastoma: Phase 1 trial interim results. Nature Medicine. 2024;**30**(5):1320-1329

[35] Choi BD, Gerstner ER, Frigault MJ, Leick MB, Mount CW, Balaj L, et al. Intraventricular CARv3-TEAM-E T cells in recurrent glioblastoma. The New England Journal of Medicine. 2024;**390**(14):1290-1298

[36] Karschnia P, Teske N, Thon N, Subklewe M, Tonn J-C, Dietrich J, et al. Chimeric antigen receptor T cells for glioblastoma. Neurology. 2021;**97**(5):218-230

[37] Short L, Holt RA, Cullis PR, Evgin L. Direct *in vivo* CAR T cell engineering. Trends in Pharmacological Sciences. 2024;**45**(5):406-418

[38] Kluger HM, Chiang V, Mahajan A, Zito CR, Sznol M, Tran T, et al. Long term survival of patients with melanoma with active brain metastases treated with Pembrolizumab on a phase II trial. Journal of Clinical Oncology. 2019;**37**(1):52-60

[39] Tawbi HA, Forsyth PA, Hodi FS, Algazi AP, Hamid O, Lao CD, et al. Long-term outcomes of patients with active melanoma brain metastases treated with combination nivolumab plus ipilimumab (CheckMate 204): Final results of an open-label, multicentre, phase 2 study. The Lancet Oncology. 2021;**22**(12):1692-1704

[40] Goldberg SB, Schalper KA, Gettinger SN, Mahajan A, Herbst RS, Chiang AC, et al. Pembrolizumab for management of patients with NSCLC and brain metastases: Long-term results and biomarker analysis from a non-randomised, open-label,

phase 2 trial. The Lancet Oncology. 2020;**21**(5):655-663

[41] Wong P, Masucci L, Florescu M, Plourde ME, Panet-Raymond V, Pavic M, et al. Phase II multicenter trial combining nivolumab and radiosurgery for NSCLC and RCC brain metastases. Neuro-Oncology Advances. 2023;**5**(1):vdad018

[42] Crotti A, Ransohoff RM. Microglial physiology and pathophysiology: Insights from genome-wide transcriptional profiling. Immunity. 2016;**44**(3):505-515

[43] Ravi VM, Neidert N, Will P, Joseph K, Maier JP, Kuckelhaus J, et al. T-cell dysfunction in the glioblastoma microenvironment is mediated by myeloid cells releasing interleukin-10. Nature Communications. 2022;**13**(1):925

[44] Yu M, Chang Y, Zhai Y, Pang B, Wang P, Li G, et al. TREM2 is associated with tumor immunity and implies poor prognosis in glioma. Frontiers in Immunology. 2022;**13**:1089266

[45] Sun R, Han R, McCornack C, Khan S, Tabor GT, Chen Y, et al. TREM2 inhibition triggers antitumor cell activity of myeloid cells in glioblastoma. Science Advances. 2023;**9**(19):eade3559

[46] Schulz M, Michels B, Niesel K, Stein S, Farin H, Rodel F, et al. Cellular and molecular changes of brain metastases-associated myeloid cells during disease progression and therapeutic response. iScience. 2020;**23**(6):101178

[47] Li Q, Barres BA. Microglia and macrophages in brain homeostasis and disease. Nature Reviews. Immunology. 2018;**18**(4):225-242

[48] Van Hove H, Martens L, Scheyltjens I, De Vlaminck K, Pombo Antunes AR, De Prijck S, et al. A single-cell atlas of mouse brain macrophages reveals unique transcriptional identities shaped by ontogeny and tissue environment. Nature Neuroscience. 2019;**22**(6):1021-1035

[49] Lewis CE, Harney AS, Pollard JW. The multifaceted role of perivascular macrophages in Tumors. Cancer Cell. 2016;**30**(1):18-25

[50] Harney AS, Arwert EN, Entenberg D, Wang Y, Guo P, Qian BZ, et al. Real-time imaging reveals local, transient vascular permeability, and tumor cell Intravasation stimulated by TIE2hi macrophage-derived VEGFA. Cancer Discovery. 2015;**5**(9):932-943

[51] Montilla A, Zabala A, Er-Lukowiak M, Rissiek B, Magnus T, Rodriguez-Iglesias N, et al. Microglia and meningeal macrophages depletion delays the onset of experimental autoimmune encephalomyelitis. Cell Death & Disease. 2023;**14**(1):16

[52] Engelhardt B, Vajkoczy P, Weller RO. The movers and shapers in immune privilege of the CNS. Nature Immunology. 2017;**18**(2):123-131

[53] Pyonteck SM, Akkari L, Schuhmacher AJ, Bowman RL, Sevenich L, Quail DF, et al. CSF-1R inhibition alters macrophage polarization and blocks glioma progression. Nature Medicine. 2013;**19**(10):1264-1272

[54] Pombo Antunes AR, Scheyltjens I, Lodi F, Messiaen J, Antoranz A, Duerinck J, et al. Single-cell profiling of myeloid cells in glioblastoma across species and disease stage reveals macrophage competition and specialization. Nature Neuroscience. 2021;**24**(4):595-610

[55] Butowski N, Colman H, De Groot JF, Omuro AM, Nayak L, Wen PY, et al.

Orally administered colony stimulating factor 1 receptor inhibitor PLX3397 in recurrent glioblastoma: An ivy foundation early phase clinical trials consortium phase II study. Neuro-Oncology. 2016;**18**(4):557-564

[56] Mulder K, Patel AA, Kong WT, Piot C, Halitzki E, Dunsmore G, et al. Cross-tissue single-cell landscape of human monocytes and macrophages in health and disease. Immunity. 2021;**54**(8):1883-900e5

[57] Silvin A, Uderhardt S, Piot C, Da Mesquita S, Yang K, Geirsdottir L, et al. Dual ontogeny of disease-associated microglia and disease inflammatory macrophages in aging and neurodegeneration. Immunity. 2022;**55**(8):1448-65e6

Chapter 14

The Role of Stem Cells in Targeted Glioblastoma Treatment

Elvira M. Carbonell-Martínez, Julia L. Gutiérrez-Arroyo, Pia Gallego-Porcar, Luis G. González-Bonet, Conrado Martínez-Cadenas and Maria Angeles Marqués-Torrejón

Abstract

Gliomas represent a fascinating contemporary challenge in the field of neuroscience. These tumours account for almost a quarter of all primary central nervous system (CNS) tumours; they are particularly intriguing because of their high-grade variant, glioblastoma, which has a particularly poor prognosis due to its aggressiveness and the adverse effects of radiotherapy and chemotherapy on the brain. This makes them valuable for reducing the side effects of radiotherapy and chemotherapy and for targeted drug delivery to tumours. Stem cell therapy is a promising treatment for several diseases, and it offers multiple treatment options, since stem cells can be genetically engineered to produce substances that inhibit tumour growth or they can be used as carriers for oncolytic viral vectors. Combining stem cells with prodrugs that are activated when they reach the tumour is also a possible approach. While much research into the efficacy of stem cell therapy is based on animal studies, many clinical trials are underway to investigate its efficacy in humans.

Keywords: glioblastoma, brain tumour, neural stem cells, cancer relapse, cancer treatment

1. Introduction

The 2021 World Health Organisation (WHO) classification of gliomas represents a major change, advancing the role of molecular diagnostics in stratifying central nervous system (CNS) tumours, while still incorporating established approaches such as histology and immunohistochemistry. Gliomas, which are primary brain tumours that originate from glial cells, are classified into four grades (1–4). Each grade reflects the degree of malignancy, which is determined by histopathological criteria. Grade 1 gliomas are low-proliferation lesions that can often be cured by surgery, whereas grade 2–4 gliomas are considered malignant and invasive. Glioblastoma (GB) is classified as grade 4. In addition, according to the WHO CNS classification, the term

GB is no longer used for children and adolescents; instead, the term paediatric-type diffuse high-grade glioma is now used to describe the more aggressive paediatric brain tumours [1].

GB in adults should be diagnosed as an isocitrate dehydrogenase wild-type (IDHwt) diffuse astrocytic glioma and/or at least one of the following three criteria: concomitant gain of chromosome 7 and loss of chromosome 10 (+7/−10), telomerase reverse transcriptase (TERT) promoter mutations, and epidermal growth factor receptor (EGFR) amplification, even in the absence of microvascular proliferation or necrosis (**Figure 1**) [1, 2].

The incidence of primary malignant brain tumours is approximately 7 per 100,000 people. Approximately 49% of primary malignant brain tumours are GBs, which are the most common, complex, and aggressive. In children, paediatric-type diffuse high-grade glioma is extremely rare, affecting approximately 0.87 per 100,000 children; however, it accounts for more than 40% of all childhood brain tumour deaths [3].

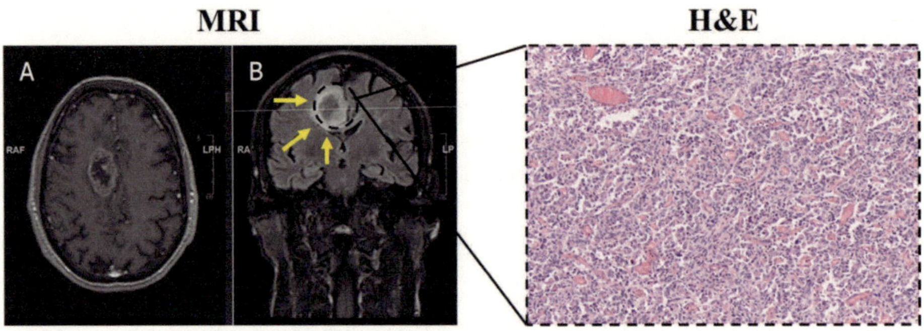

Figure 1.
Left, MRI image axial (A) and coronal (B) of GB patient. Yellow arrows indicate the tumour mass. Right, histological haematoxylin and eosin section of GB resection. Increased cellularity and the presence of significant cellular pleomorphism, palisade necrosis and microvascular proliferation.

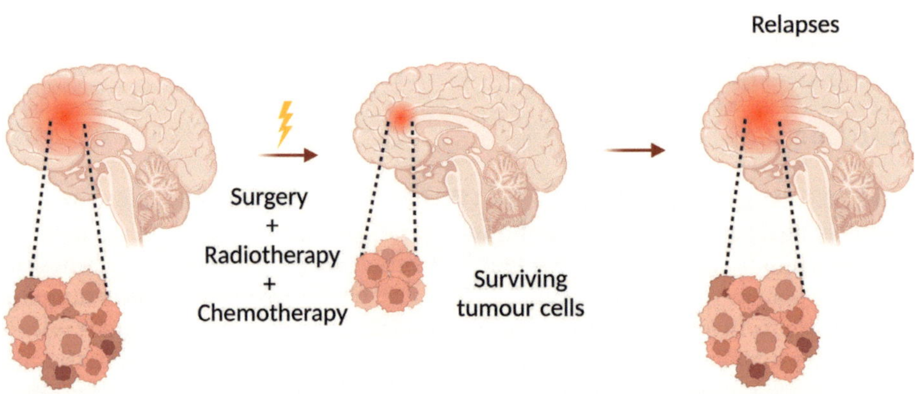

Figure 2.
Progression of GB following standard treatment. On the left, the brain is shown before treatment, with a significant tumour mass. In the centre, after therapeutic intervention (surgery, radiotherapy, and chemotherapy), a significant reduction in tumour size is observed. On the right, the tumour re-grows, representing the characteristic recurrence of GB despite treatment. This highlights the challenges of GB management and the need for new therapeutic strategies. The recurrence is in part due to the presence of glioma stem cells. Image created with BioRender.com.

The incidence of GB is 1.6 times more common in males than females, and it is also more frequent in Caucasians relative to other ethnicities [3, 4].

The treatment for GB has remained largely unchanged since the landmark study by Stupp et al. [5]. The standard therapy includes maximal safe surgical resection, followed by radiation therapy (RT) and chemotherapy (CT) [5, 6]. Patients typically receive radiation five times per week for 6 weeks post-surgery, along with daily oral temozolomide (TMZ), an alkylating agent that has shown antitumour activity as a single agent in recurrent GB treatment. The standard Stupp regimen includes concurrent temozolomide at a dose of 75 mg/m^2 daily during radiotherapy, followed by adjuvant temozolomide at a dose of 150–200 mg/m^2 for 5 days every 28-day cycle [7]. Despite this treatment regimen, GB remains incurable, with a median survival of 15 months and inevitable relapses (**Figure 2**) [8]. The lack of significant improvements in survival highlights the need for ongoing research to develop more effective treatments and provide better options for patients.

2. Neural stem cells (NSCs) in the subventricular zone (SVZ)

The tumour microenvironment (TME) refers to the complex and dynamic environment surrounding a tumour, which plays a crucial role in its development, progression, and resistance to treatments. In GB, the TME includes a variety of cellular and non-cellular components. Additionally, glioma stem cells (GSCs) with stem-like characteristics (**Figure 3**) also exist within this niche [9]. These cells have the capacity to self-renew, differentiate into various cell types, exhibit significant resistance to both cytotoxic and radiotherapies, and possess a high potential for tumour formation [4, 9, 10].

The concept of the cellular origin of GB refers to the normal cells that are prone to oncogenic mutations and can transform into cancerous cells, leading to tumour formation. This is distinct from GSCs, which are a specific cellular subtype within the tumour that serves as a reservoir for tumour regeneration. While the cell of origin

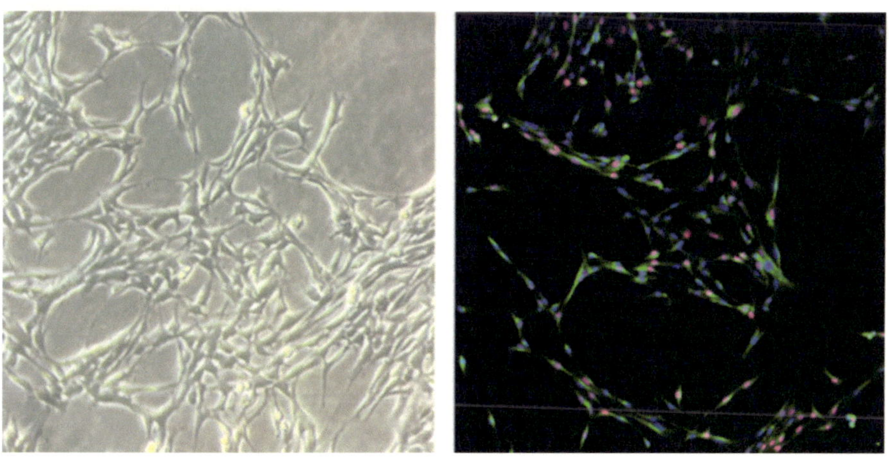

Figure 3.
GSCs growing in vitro. *Left: phase contrast image of GSCs. Right: immunocytochemistry shows that GSCs express the neural stem cell marker and intermediate filament protein, Nestin (green). GSCs proliferate, so they incorporate the thymidine analogue, EdU (red). Nuclear counterstaining with DAPI (blue).*

is the initial cell type that starts the glioma, GSCs are responsible for sustaining and propagating the tumour within the TME [4, 10].

GSCs are mainly found in the tumour mass, though they have also been detected in the subventricular zone (SVZ), a region that contains neural stem cells (NSCs) [10]. The SVZ is composed of different cell types organised in a specific pattern. Although neurogenesis in this area persists throughout life, its capacity gradually decreases with age [10].

The term "neural stem cell" is used loosely to describe cells that (i) can generate neural tissue or are derived from the nervous system, (ii) have some capacity for self-renewal, and (iii) can give rise to differentiated neural cells as astrocytes, neurons, and oligodendrocytes (multipotency capacity) [11]. These cells could first acquire the driver mutations of human GB [10]. In addition, human SVZ NSCs are more susceptible to malignant transformation, as they generate mainly oligodendrocyte precursor cells (OPCs) which are a group of undifferentiated cells that remain undifferentiated during adulthood. In addition to NSCs and OPCs, astrocytes, although they are differentiated cells, maintain some capacity for proliferation, especially after brain injury. Because of their regenerative potential, both NSCs, OPCs, and astrocytes could act as sources of glioma-initiating cells [4].

SVZ is chemo-attractive for glioma cells, and microglia act as supporting cells for neurogenesis. SVZ NSCs line the lateral ventricles and are in contact with cerebrospinal fluid (CSF), which is rich in factors that could promote and maintain the tumour [4, 10].

Many genes or molecules such as tumour oncogenes and transcription factors involved in biological functions may affect the development of GB. It is now known that SVZ NSCs that have acquired mutations in the *TP53* or *IDH1* genes can lead to uncontrolled proliferation and tumourigenesis. In addition, p53 deficiency can induce the accumulation of oncogenic alterations. This indicates that mutations in *p53* or *IDH1* in SVZ NSCs are key in gliomagenesis, as they alter the characteristics and phenotypes of these cells [12].

Recent preclinical and clinical studies have confirmed that SVZ NSCs are closely linked to the origin and progression of gliomas through gene mutations and factor delivery (**Figure 4**). Although gliomas are typically located far from the SVZ, they

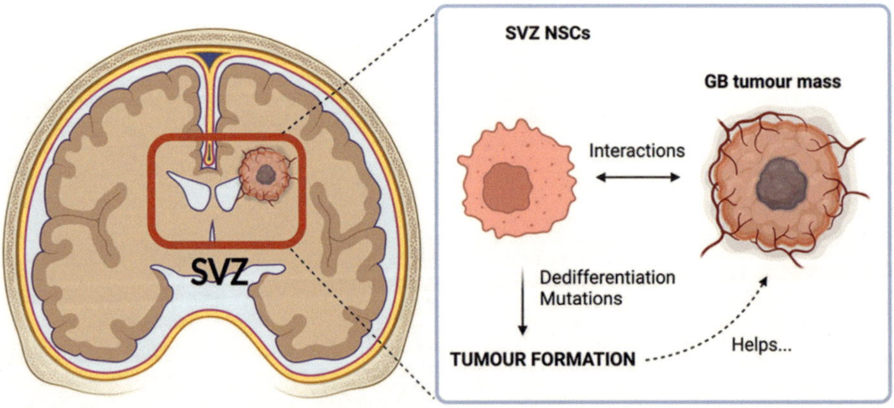

Figure 4.
Relationship between the SVZ, NSCs, and GB development. The left panel shows a cross-section of the brain, highlighting the SVZ as a source of NSCs and its proximity to a GB tumour. The inset on the right illustrates a potential progression from NSCs to tumour cells, suggesting that NSCs from the SVZ may play a role in GB formation and recurrence. This figure emphasises the SVZ as a critical niche in the origin and progression of GB. Image created with BioRender.com.

can interact *via* paracrine signalling pathways, including secreted cytokines and extracellular vesicles (EVs) [12].

3. Tropism, migration, and tumour-homing properties of neural stem cells

NSCs are a type of cell predominantly located in the SVZ and hippocampus, specifically in the dentate gyrus of the human brain [13]. These cells possess distinctive tropic properties, which have been instrumental in the development of innovative therapies that employ NSCs as vectors for the localisation and tracking of invasive tumour cells, as well as for targeted drug delivery to tumours [14]. Consequently, NSCs have been the subject of intense research for their use in the delivery of oncolytic drugs and viruses in brain neoplasms, with particular emphasis on medulloblastomas and gliomas [15, 16]. NSCs demonstrate a remarkable ability to migrate to cancerous masses derived from glial precursors, as well as to tumours of non-glial origin, such as medulloblastoma [17, 18]. In addition, these cells show the ability to migrate towards metastatic cancers, including melanoma and mammary neoplasms [19, 20].

In vivo studies in mice have shown that migration of NSCs begins approximately 50 minutes after transplantation, with a marked increase in the number of NSCs in the tumour region during the first 5 days after transplantation, followed by a further expansion over the next 15 days [21]. Migration of NSCs into the tumour mass is influenced by both number of cells administered [22] and the components of the tumour microenvironment [23]. In addition, the cytotoxic capacity of NSCs depends on the proximity between the site of administration and the tumour. NSC migration is mediated by chemotactic factors, although the exact mechanistic pathways that guide NSCs into gliomas are not yet fully understood [24]. Tumour masses have been documented to continuously secrete chemoattractants that recruit NSCs to the tumour site [25]. These chemoattractants include cytokines such as monocyte chemotactic protein-1 (MCP-1) [26], stem cell stimulating factor (SCF) [27], and hepatocyte growth factor (HGF) [28], as well as proangiogenic growth factors such as vascular endothelial growth factor (VEGF) [29], hypoxia-inducible factors [30], extracellular matrix components [31] and other inflammatory mediators [32]. In response to these tumour-derived factors, NSCs express specific surface receptors, such as CCL2 [26], c-Kit [27], c-Met [28], VEGF receptors [29], and hypoxia-sensitive receptors [30], which trigger their migration towards the tumour mass.

It has been observed *in vivo* (in mice) that hypoxia can also activate tumour properties through the secretion of hypoxia-induced transcription factor 1 (HIF-1) [33]. This factor upregulates the production of chemoattractants. Furthermore, since conventional cancer therapies, such as radiotherapy and chemotherapy, are associated with increased hypoxia-induced chemokine expression in cancer cells, combining these therapies with the administration of NSCs may amplify chemotactic pathways and signals, thereby enhancing NSC migration and, consequently, overall therapeutic efficacy [34].

4. Neuroprotective and neurotropic functions of neural stem cell therapy

NSCs located in the SVZ, which is the main neurogenic niche in the mammalian brain, possess the ability to self-renew and generate neural progenitor cells (NPCs) [35].

These cells have the ability to migrate to areas affected by neuronal injury, such as those caused by stroke or other CNS pathologies, and can differentiate into mature cells involved in damage repair [36, 37]. Research on the therapeutic use of NSCs is promising due to their potential to improve recovery after CNS injury and mitigate the effects of neurodegenerative diseases [38, 39].

The multipotent and self-renewing properties of NSCs are essential for CNS tissue repair [40]. These cells are capable of continuously generating both glial cells and neurons, which play a crucial role in the repair of damaged areas of the CNS through mechanisms of cell migration and replacement. In addition, NSCs can enhance the effects of nutritional supplements and trophic factors by secreting paracrine signals [41–43]. These therapies also have the potential to promote angiogenesis, thereby improving intracranial blood perfusion by increasing the expression of angiogenic factors in the brain [44].

NSCs of both human and animal origin express multiple chemokine receptors that facilitate their migration to areas of the CNS where proinflammatory chemokines are produced [45]. Several *in vivo* studies in mice models have shown that stromal cell-derived factor 1 alpha (SDF-1α/CXCL12) interacts with CXCR4 receptors present on NSCs, constituting a crucial mechanism for the migration of these cells to sites of injury [46–48]. Furthermore, it has been observed that intravenously administered NSCs are able to cross the blood-brain barrier (BBB) and exert their functions without inducing brain toxicity [49, 50]. This ability to cross the BBB has been associated with the expression of cell surface adhesion molecules, such as CD44 and VLA-4, as well as with the inflammatory state of the CNS [50, 51].

Numerous preclinical trials have demonstrated positive results in neurogenesis following transplantation of NSCs in rodent models of stroke (*in vivo*). Treatment using human embryonic stem cells (hESCs) and NSCs derived from foetal tissues have promoted cell proliferation and migration in the subventricular zone, dentate gyrus and striatum [52]. In addition, these cells have produced regenerative trophic factors that promote angiogenesis, reduce inflammation and support tissue regeneration after stroke [53]. NSC transplantation has also been shown to stimulate endogenous neurogenesis, as evidenced by the expression of markers such as DCX, a marker of neuroblasts, and Fox3, a marker of mature neurons [44, 54].

NSC therapy has also shown promising results in the treatment of Huntington's disease (HD) [55], motor coordination disorders caused by degeneration of Purkinje neurons [56], amyotrophic lateral sclerosis [57], Alzheimer's disease [58, 59], and multiple sclerosis [60], among other pathologies.

5. Immunomodulation and immunotherapy

Immunomodulators are molecules that modulate the activity of the immune system, either by stimulating or suppressing it, and can help the body fight cancer, infections, or other diseases. These substances play a key role in the regulation of stem cells, both at different stages of embryonic development and in adult life. Immune and inflammatory responses, including cytokine action and Toll-like receptor (TLR)-mediated signalling, have been shown to influence the differentiation capacity of NSCs and tissue-specific mesenchymal stem cells (MSCs) [61].

Genetic modification of NSCs has been shown to induce the production of antineoplastic compounds in the tumour microenvironment, including various immunomodulators (**Figure 5**). In several experimental studies, NSCs have been programmed

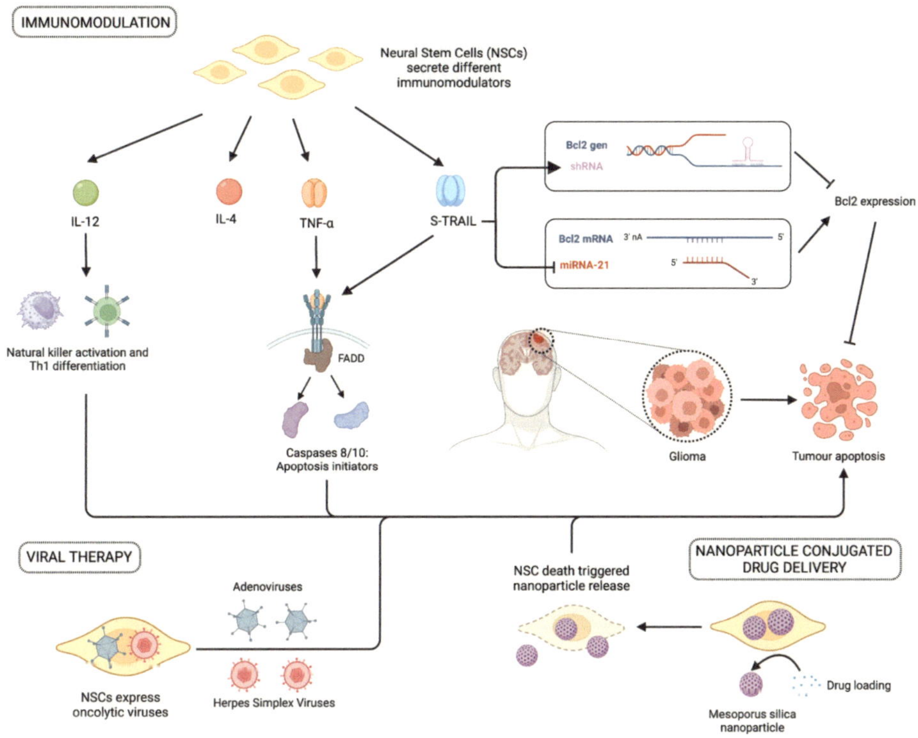

Figure 5.
Novel strategies for GB. Scheme showing different new strategies using NSCs to tackle GB: immunomodulation, viral vectors and nanotherapy. Image created with BioRender.com.

to express interleukins such as IL-4 and IL-12, reducing tumour burden and improving survival in *in vivo* murine models [62, 63]. In addition, other immunomodulators, including interleukins such as IL-23 and IL-24, as well as interferon-β, have been used with promising results [63–67]. Another molecule of interest is the tumour necrosis factor-related apoptosis-inducing ligand (TRAIL), which interacts with death receptors (DR) 4 and 5 to trigger apoptosis in malignant cells [68]. This binding activates the recruitment of FAS-associated protein with death domain (FADD), which in turn activates caspases 8 and 10, essential in the apoptotic cascade [69, 70].

The use of a secreted form of TRAIL (called S-TRAIL), in combination with complementary antitumour agents, can significantly enhance its ability to fight tumours. One approach is to employ short hairpin RNA (shRNA) to silence the expression of the Bcl2 gene, which encodes a protein well-known for its anti-apoptotic function [71]. Alternatively, inhibition of microRNA-21, which promotes Bcl2 expression, can also enhance the proapoptotic effect of TRAIL [72]. Both methods amplify the ability of S-TRAIL to induce apoptosis, thereby increasing its therapeutic efficacy.

Another strategy is to sensitise tumour cells to S-TRAIL to maximise its apoptotic effects. Combining TRAIL with proteasome inhibitors has been shown to increase the expression of DR5, the key TRAIL receptor. Proteasome inhibitors generate reactive oxygen species (ROS), which activates the binding of p53 to the regulatory introns of the DR5 gene, increasing its expression [73]. In addition, reduced levels of nuclear factor kappa-beta (NF-κB) inhibitors are observed, which, like p53, promote the binding of NF-κB to DR5 introns, contributing to its overexpression. The increased expression of DR5 enhances the proapoptotic effect of S-TRAIL, improving its therapeutic potential.

Recently, Liu et al. [74] developed a novel combined immunotherapeutic compound using induced neural stem cells (iNSCs) derived from peripheral blood mononuclear cells (PBMCs) genetically modified to express herpes simplex virus type 1 thymidine kinase (HSV-TK) and second-generation CAR-NK cells (Chimeric Antigen Receptors-Natural Killer cells that are T cells genetically modified to express chimeric natural killer lymphocyte antigen receptors), directed against GB. These PBMC-derived iNSCsTKs were found to show tumour tropism and significant antitumour activity in the presence of ganciclovir. Furthermore, when combined with GD2-CAR-NK92 cells (GD2-specific CAR-NK92 cells generated from NK92 cell lines) [75], the therapeutic efficacy of iNSCsTKs improved median survival in animal *in vivo* models with tumours [74].

6. Other therapies

A variety of innovative therapies for GB are under investigation, each offering unique mechanisms for targeting tumour cells. Recent advancements include the use of viral vectors, nanotechnology-based delivery systems, and stem cell engineering, which are increasingly recognised for their potential in overcoming challenges posed by conventional therapies [76].

6.1 Viral vectors

Viral vectors, particularly oncolytic viruses, have gained interest for their ability to selectively infect and lyse tumour cells (**Figure 5**). This approach leverages stem cells (SCs) as delivery vehicles for viral agents, using their inherent tumour-homing properties to enhance delivery precision, especially in challenging tumour microenvironments. Studies with mesenchymal stem cells (MSCs) demonstrate that these cells can carry a significantly higher viral load than direct injections, leading to improved survival rates in glioma models [77]. Additionally, research by ***Ahmed et al. [78] suggests that neural stem cells (NSCs) might outperform MSCs due to their superior tumour-targeting capabilities [79].

Oncolytic herpes simplex virus (HSV) mutants, such as G207—having reached Phase I and Phase II in paediatric and adult glioblastoma patients, demonstrating safety and preliminary efficacy—and G47Δ—currently undergoing Phase III trials in Japan for malignant glioma, marking significant progress in the clinical development of viral vector therapies—represent another promising vector. Modifications in these strains, including deletion of pathogenic genes, enhance both safety and efficacy, with G47Δ also stimulating immune cell recruitment, further strengthening its therapeutic impact [80]. In tandem with viral vectors, some approaches engineer NSCs to express therapeutic enzymes, such as carboxylesterase (CE), which convert prodrugs into active.

6.2 Nanotherapy

Innovative nanotherapy approaches complement viral vector strategies (**Figure 5**). Loading NSCs with mesoporous nanoparticles containing the chemotherapeutic drug doxorubicin targets malignant glial cell proliferation. The death of NSCs releases these nanoparticles into gliomas [81, 82]. NSC-loaded gold nanorods have also shown promising results. Pseudomonas exotoxin (PE) arrests cellular protein synthesis and exhibits antitumour properties against various cancers. Engineered NSCs secreting PE-cytotoxins can inhibit GB growth and recurrence. Preclinical research on NSC-engineered therapies has laid the groundwork for Phase I trials, aiming to evaluate safety and feasibility in glioblastoma patients [83, 84].

NSCs have garnered significant attention as potential delivery vehicles for anti-cancer agents due to their inherent tumour-tropic properties [85]. Mesoporous silica nanoparticles (MSNs) have emerged as versatile drug delivery systems due to their high surface area, tuneable pore size, and ease of functionalisation. When loaded with chemotherapeutic drugs like doxorubicin and delivered *via* NSCs, these nanoparticles can effectively target proliferating glioma cells [86].

The integration of nanotherapies with viral vector strategies offers a multifaceted approach to GB treatment. Oncolytic viruses delivered by NSCs have shown synergistic effects when combined with conventional chemotherapy and radiation [86, 87].

As research in this field progresses, the combination of NSC-based therapies with nanotechnology and viral vectors holds great promise for improving GB treatment outcomes.

7. Conclusions

The treatment of GB has remained largely unchanged for over two decades. GB is a very aggressive tumour, which spreads in the brain very easily. This is a major problem for the neurosurgeon when it comes to resection, as there are limitations in accessing and completely clearing the tumour.

It has been known for years that GBs contain stem cells with neural stem cell characteristics that can be in a continuum of cellular states: proliferation, quiescence, and differentiation. These quiescent cells are known to survive conventional therapies and eventually regenerate the tumour. There is also a high genetic heterogeneity in GB tumours which complicates their study and therefore their successful treatment. Conversely, genetic, viral vectors, nanotherapy, and cellular immunotherapeutic strategies founded upon stem and immune cells are emerging as promising treatments for GB.

In recent years, immunotherapy strategies have transformed the treatment of numerous types of cancer, inspiring optimism regarding their potential for GB. However, the efficacy of immunotherapy in GB remains low, primarily due to the presence of multiple immunosuppressive factors within the microenvironment, the incomplete understanding of the neuroimmune system, and the presence of the blood-brain barrier. Recently, new strategies for the treatment of GB have employed immunotherapy combinations, with encouraging results observed in both preclinical and clinical studies.

To design effective immunotherapy trials in GB, multidisciplinary teams are needed to find out why current therapies are not working and to improve the prognosis of this devastating disease.

Acknowledgements

We thank K. Ferguson for the corrections in editing. E.C thanks the Spanish Association against Cancer (AECC) fellowship. J.L.G-A. thanks to an "Epriex" contract from *Plan Nacional de Recuperación, Transformación y Resiliencia*, and Industrial fellowship Research co-financed by the Generalitat and the European Social Fund within the framework of the collaboration agreement between the

Generalitat Valenciana, through the Department of Education, Culture, Universities and Employment, and the Universitat Jaume I for the promotion of doctorates in collaboration with companies. M.A.M.-T was supported by a 'Maria Zambrano' research contract (number MAZ/2021/03 UP2021-021) funded by the European Union-Next generation EU, UJI grant (23I469 UJI-2023-2029) and Ramon y Cajal Research Fellow RYC2022-038481-by MCIN/AEI/10.13039/501100011033.

Conflict of interest

The authors declare no conflict of interest.

Abbreviations

BBB	blood-brain barrier
CAR-NK	chimeric antigen receptors-natural killer
CNS	central nervous system
CSF	cerebrospinal fluid
CT	chemotherapy
DR	death receptors
EGFR	epidermal growth factor receptor
EVs	extracellular vesicles
FADD	FAS-associated protein with death domain
GB	glioblastoma
GSCs	glioma stem cells
hESCs	human embryonic stem cells
HD	Huntington's disease
HGF	hepatocyte growth factor
HIF-1	hypoxia-induced factor 1
HSV-TK	herpes simplex virus type I thymidine kinase
IDHwt	isocitrate dehydrogenase wild-type
iNSCs	induced neural stem cells
MCP-1	monocyte chemotactic protein-1
MSCs	mesenchymal stem cells
NF-κβ	nuclear factor kappa-beta
NPCs	neural progenitor cells
NSCs	neural stem cells
OPCs	oligodendrocyte precursor cells
PBMCs	peripheral blood mononuclear cells
pHGG	paediatric high-grade glioma
ROS	reactive oxygen species
RT	radiation therapy
SCF	cell stimulating factor
SDF-1α	stromal cell-derived factor 1 alpha
shRNA	short hairpin RNA
SVZ	subventricular zone
TERT	telomerase reverse transcriptase
TLR	Toll-like receptor
TMZ	temozolomide

TME	tumour microenvironment
TRAIL	tumour necrosis factor-related apoptosis-inducing ligand
VEGF	vascular endothelial growth factor
WHO	World Health Organization

Author details

Elvira M. Carbonell-Martínez[1†], Julia L. Gutiérrez-Arroyo[1†],
Pia Gallego-Porcar[1†], Luis G. González-Bonet[2], Conrado Martínez-Cadenas[1]
and Maria Angeles Marqués-Torrejón[1*]

1 Department of Medicine, Jaume I University of Castellon, Castellon, Spain

2 Department of Neurosurgery, Castellon General University Hospital, Castellon, Spain

*Address all correspondence to: torrejom@uji.es

† These authors contributed equally.

References

[1] Louis DN, Perry A, Wesseling P, Brat DJ, Cree IA, Figarella-Branger D, et al. The 2021 WHO classification of tumors of the central nervous system: A summary. Neuro-Oncology. 2021;**23**(8):1231-1251

[2] Berger TR, Wen PY, Lang-Orsini M, Chukwueke UN. World Health Organization 2021 classification of central nervous system tumors and implications for therapy for adult-type gliomas: A review. JAMA Oncology. 2022;**8**(10):1493-1501

[3] Ostrom QT, Price M, Neff C, Cioffi G, Waite KA, Kruchko C, et al. CBTRUS statistical report: Primary brain and other central nervous system tumors diagnosed in the United States in 2015-2019. Neuro-Oncology. 2022;**24**(Suppl. 5):v1-v95

[4] Loras A, Gonzalez-Bonet LG, Gutierrez-Arroyo JL, Martinez-Cadenas C, Marques-Torrejon MA. Neural stem cells as potential glioblastoma cells of origin. Life. 2023;**13**(4):905

[5] Stupp R, Mason WP, Bent MJ v d, Weller M, Fisher B, Taphoorn MJB, et al. Radiotherapy plus concomitant and adjuvant temozolomide for glioblastoma. The New England Journal of Medicine. 2005;**352**(10):987-996

[6] Colopi A, Fuda S, Santi S, Onorato A, Cesarini V, Salvati M, et al. Impact of age and gender on glioblastoma onset, progression, and management. Mechanisms of Ageing and Development. 2023;**211**:111801

[7] Wong S, Rosenthal MA, Dowling A, Jennens R, Woods AM, Ashley D, et al. Phase II study of two-weekly temozolomide in patients with high-grade gliomas. Journal of Clinical Neuroscience is the official journal of the Neurosurgical Society of Australasia. 2006;**13**(1):18-22

[8] Alifieris C, Trafalis DT. Glioblastoma multiforme: Pathogenesis and treatment. Pharmacology & Therapeutics. 2015;**152**:63-82

[9] Sharma P, Aaroe A, Liang J, Puduvalli VK. Tumor microenvironment in glioblastoma: Current and emerging concepts. Neuro-Oncology Advances. 2023;**5**(1):vdad009

[10] Li S, Dong L, Pan Z, Yang G. Targeting the neural stem cells in subventricular zone for the treatment of glioblastoma: an update from preclinical evidence to clinical interventions. Stem Cell Research & Therapy. 2023;**14**(1):125

[11] Gage FH. Mammalian neural stem cells. Science. 2000;**287**(5457):1433-1438

[12] Zhang GL, Wang CF, Qian C, Ji YX, Wang YZ. Role and mechanism of neural stem cells of the subventricular zone in glioblastoma. World Journal of Stem Cells. 2021;**13**(7):877-893

[13] Urbán N, Blomfield IM, Guillemot F. Quiescence of adult mammalian neural stem cells: A highly regulated rest. Neuron. 2019;**104**(5):834-848

[14] Ahmed AU, Alexiades NG, Lesniak MS. The use of neural stem cells in cancer gene therapy: Predicting the path to the clinic. Current Opinion in Molecular Therapeutics. 2010;**12**(5):546-552

[15] Fares J, Ahmed AU, Ulasov IV, Sonabend AM, Miska J, Lee-Chang C,

et al. Neural stem cell delivery of an oncolytic adenovirus in newly diagnosed malignant glioma: A first-in-human, phase 1, dose-escalation trial. The Lancet Oncology. 2021;**22**(8):1103-1114

[16] Parker Kerrigan BC, Hossain A, Yamashita S, Lang FF. Stem cell therapy of gliomas. Progress in Neurological Surgery. 2018;**32**:124-151

[17] Kim SK, Kim SU, Park IH, Bang JH, Aboody KS, Wang KC, et al. Human neural stem cells target experimental intracranial medulloblastoma and deliver a therapeutic gene leading to tumor regression. Clinical cancer research : an official journal of the American Association for Cancer Research. 2006;**12**(18):5550-5556

[18] Swartling FJ, Čančer M, Frantz A, Weishaupt H, Persson AI. Deregulated proliferation and differentiation in brain tumors. Cell and Tissue Research. 2015;**359**(1):225-254

[19] Aboody KS, Bush RA, Garcia E, Metz MZ, Najbauer J, Justus KA, et al. Development of a tumor-selective approach to treat metastatic cancer. PLoS One. 2006;**1**(1):e23

[20] Joo KM, Park IH, Shin JY, Jin J, Kang BG, Kim MH, et al. Human neural stem cells can target and deliver therapeutic genes to breast cancer brain metastases. Molecular Therapy: The Journal of the American Society of Gene Therapy. 2009;**17**(3):570-575

[21] Kim JH, Lee JE, Kim SU, Cho KG. Stereological analysis on migration of human neural stem cells in the brain of rats bearing glioma. Neurosurgery. 2010;**66**(2):333

[22] Barish ME, Herrmann K, Tang Y, Argalian Herculian S, Metz M, Aramburo S, et al. Human neural stem cell biodistribution and predicted tumor coverage by a diffusible therapeutic in a mouse glioma model. Stem Cells Translational Medicine. 2017;**6**(6):1522-1532

[23] Stabenfeldt SE, Munglani G, García AJ, LaPlaca MC. Biomimetic microenvironment modulates neural stem cell survival, migration, and differentiation. Tissue Engineering. Part A. 2010;**16**(12):3747-3758

[24] Mooney R, Hammad M, Batalla-Covello J, Abdul Majid A, Aboody KS. Concise review: Neural stem cell-mediated targeted cancer therapies. Stem Cells Translational Medicine. 2018;**7**(10):740-747

[25] Kendall SE, Najbauer J, Johnston HF, Metz MZ, Li S, Bowers M, et al. Neural stem cell targeting of glioma is dependent on phosphoinositide 3-kinase signaling. Stem Cells. 2008;**26**(6):1575-1586

[26] Magge SN, Malik SZ, Royo NC, Chen HI, Yu L, Snyder EY, et al. Role of monocyte chemoattractant protein-1 (MCP-1/CCL2) in migration of neural progenitor cells toward glial tumors. Journal of Neuroscience Research. 2009;**87**(7):1547-1555

[27] Sun L, Lee J, Fine HA. Neuronally expressed stem cell factor induces neural stem cell migration to areas of brain injury. Journal of Clinical Investigation. 2004;**113**(9):1364-1374

[28] Heese O, Disko A, Zirkel D, Westphal M, Lamszus K. Neural stem cell migration toward gliomas in vitro. Neuro-Oncology. 2005;7(4):476-484

[29] Schmidt NO, Przylecki W, Yang W, Ziu M, Teng YD, Kim SU, et al. Brain tumor tropism of transplanted human neural stem cells is induced by vascular endothelial growth factor. Neoplasia. 2005;7(6):623-630

[30] Zhao D, Najbauer J, Garcia E, Metz MZ, Gutova M, Glackin CA, et al. Neural stem cell tropism to glioma: Critical role of tumor hypoxia. Molecular Cancer Research. 2008;**6**(12):1819-1829

[31] Ziu M, Schmidt NO, Cargioli TG, Aboody KS, Black PM, Carroll RS. Glioma-produced extracellular matrix influences brain tumor tropism of human neural stem cells. Journal of Neuro-Oncology. 2006;**79**(2):125-133

[32] Zhao D, Najbauer J, Annala AJ, Garcia E, Metz MZ, Gutova M, et al. Human neural stem cell tropism to metastatic breast cancer. Stem Cells. 2012;**30**(2):314-325

[33] In Park K, Hack MA, Ourednik J, Yandava B, Flax JD, Stieg PE, et al. Acute injury directs the migration, proliferation, and differentiation of solid organ stem cells: Evidence from the effect of hypoxia–ischemia in the CNS on clonal "reporter" neural stem cells. Experimental Neurology. 2006;**199**(1):156-178

[34] Kim SM, Oh JH, Park SA, Ryu CH, Lim JY, Kim DS, et al. Irradiation enhances the tumor tropism and therapeutic potential of tumor necrosis factor-related apoptosis-inducing ligand-secreting human umbilical cord blood-derived mesenchymal stem cells in glioma therapy. Stem Cells. 2010;**28**(12):2217-2228

[35] Zarco N, Norton E, Quiñones-Hinojosa A, Guerrero-Cázares H. Overlapping migratory mechanisms between neural progenitor cells and brain tumor stem cells. Cellular and Molecular Life Sciences. 2019;**76**(18):3553-3570

[36] Pieczonka K, Nakashima H, Nagoshi N, Yokota K, Hong J, Badner A, et al. Human spinal oligodendrogenic neural progenitor cells enhance pathophysiological outcomes and functional recovery in a clinically relevant cervical spinal cord injury rat model. Stem Cells Translational Medicine. 2023;**12**(9):603-616

[37] Yin D, Wang C, Qi Y, Wang YC, Hagemann N, Mohamud Yusuf A, et al. Neural precursor cell delivery induces acute post-ischemic cerebroprotection, but fails to promote long-term stroke recovery in hyperlipidemic mice due to mechanisms that include pro-inflammatory responses associated with brain hemorrhages. Journal of Neuroinflammation. 2023;**20**(1):210

[38] Clifford T, Finkel Z, Rodriguez B, Joseph A, Cai L. Current advancements in spinal cord injury research—Glial scar formation and neural regeneration. Cells. 2023;**12**(6):853

[39] Boese AC, Hamblin MH, Lee JP. Neural stem cell therapy for neurovascular injury in Alzheimer's disease. Experimental Neurology. 2020;**324**:113112

[40] Gasperoni J, Dworkin S. Neural stem/progenitor cell (NSPC) extraction and culture. Methods in Molecular Biology (Clifton, N.J.). 2024;**2746**:109-120

[41] Hosseini SM, Borys B, Karimi-Abdolrezaee S. Neural stem cell therapies for spinal cord injury repair: An update on recent preclinical and clinical advances. Brain. 2024;**147**(3):766-793

[42] Zhang ZG, Buller B, Chopp M. Exosomes — Beyond stem cells for restorative therapy in stroke and neurological injury. Nature Reviews. Neurology. 2019;**15**(4):193-203

[43] Baker EW, Kinder HA, West FD. Neural stem cell therapy for stroke: A multimechanistic approach to restoring

neurological function. Brain and Behavior: A Cognitive Neuroscience Perspective. 2019;**9**(3):e01214

[44] Ryu S, Lee SH, Kim SU, Yoon BW. Human neural stem cells promote proliferation of endogenous neural stem cells and enhance angiogenesis in ischemic rat brain. Neural Regeneration Research. 2016;**11**(2):298

[45] Tran PB, Banisadr G, Ren D, Chenn A, Miller RJ. Chemokine receptor expression by neural progenitor cells in neurogenic regions of mouse brain. Journal of Comparative Neurology. 2007;**500**(6):1007-1034

[46] Carbajal KS, Schaumburg C, Strieter R, Kane J, Lane TE. Migration of engrafted neural stem cells is mediated by CXCL12 signaling through CXCR4 in a viral model of multiple sclerosis. Proceedings of the National Academy of Sciences. 2010;**107**(24):11068-11073

[47] Imitola J, Raddassi K, Park KI, Mueller FJ, Nieto M, Teng YD, et al. Directed migration of neural stem cells to sites of CNS injury by the stromal cell-derived factor 1α/CXC chemokine receptor 4 pathway. Proceedings of the National Academy of Sciences. 2004;**101**(52):18117-18122

[48] Itoh T, Satou T, Ishida H, Nishida S, Tsubaki M, Hashimoto S, et al. The relationship between SDF-1α/CXCR4 and neural stem cells appearing in damaged area after traumatic brain injury in rats. Neurological Research. 2009;**31**(1):90-102

[49] Aboody KS, Najbauer J, Metz MZ, D'Apuzzo M, Gutova M, Annala AJ, et al. Neural stem cell–mediated enzyme/prodrug therapy for glioma: Preclinical studies. Science Translational Medicine. 2013;**5**(184):184ra59-184ra59

[50] Boese AC, Le QSE, Pham D, Hamblin MH, Lee JP. Neural stem cell therapy for subacute and chronic ischemic stroke. Stem Cell Research & Therapy. 2018;**9**(1):154

[51] Deak D, Gorcea-Andronic N, Sas V, Teodorescu P, Constantinescu C, Iluta S, et al. A narrative review of central nervous system involvement in acute leukemias. Annals of Translational Medicine. 2021;**9**(1):68-68

[52] Grochowski C, Radzikowska E, Maciejewski R. Neural stem cell therapy—Brief review. Clinical Neurology and Neurosurgery. 2018;**173**:8-14

[53] Watanabe T, Nagai A, Sheikh AM, Mitaki S, Wakabayashi K, Kim SU, et al. A human neural stem cell line provides neuroprotection and improves neurological performance by early intervention of neuroinflammatory system. Brain Research. 2016;**1631**:194-203

[54] Mine Y, Tatarishvili J, Oki K, Monni E, Kokaia Z, Lindvall O. Grafted human neural stem cells enhance several steps of endogenous neurogenesis and improve behavioral recovery after middle cerebral artery occlusion in rats. Neurobiology of Disease. 2013;**52**:191-203

[55] Liszewska E, Jaworski J. Neural stem cell dysfunction in human brain disorders. Results and Problems in Cell Differentiation. 2018;**66**:283-305

[56] Higuera GA, Iaffaldano G, Bedar M, Shpak G, Broersen R, Munshi ST, et al. An expandable embryonic stem cell-derived Purkinje neuron progenitor population that exhibits in vivo maturation in the adult mouse cerebellum. Scientific Reports. 2017;7(1):8863

[57] Wang L, Yi F, Fu L, Yang J, Wang S, Wang Z, et al. CRISPR/Cas9-mediated targeted gene correction in amyotrophic lateral sclerosis patient iPSCs. Protein & Cell. 2017;**8**(5):365-378

[58] Xuan AG, Luo M, Ji WD, Long DH. Effects of engrafted neural stem cells in Alzheimer's disease rats. Neuroscience Letters. 2009;**450**(2):167-171

[59] Eckert A, Huang L, Gonzalez R, Kim HS, Hamblin MH, Lee JP. Bystander effect fuels human induced pluripotent stem cell-derived neural stem cells to quickly attenuate early stage neurological deficits after stroke. Stem Cells Translational Medicine. 2015;**4**(7):841-851

[60] Karussis D, Karageorgiou C, Vaknin-Dembinsky A, Gowda-Kurkalli B, Gomori JM, Kassis I, et al. Safety and immunological effects of mesenchymal stem cell transplantation in patients with multiple sclerosis and amyotrophic lateral sclerosis. Archives of Neurology. 2010;**67**(10):1187-1194

[61] Ulrich H, do Nascimento IC, Bocsi J, Tárnok A. Immunomodulation in stem cell differentiation into neurons and brain repair. Stem Cell Reviews and Reports. 2015;**11**(3):474-486

[62] Benedetti S, Pirola B, Pollo B, Magrassi L, Bruzzone MG, Rigamonti D, et al. Gene therapy of experimental brain tumors using neural progenitor cells. Nature Medicine. 2000;**6**(4):447-450

[63] Ehtesham M, Kabos P, Kabosova A, Neuman T, Black KL, Yu JS. The use of interleukin 12-secreting neural stem cells for the treatment of intracranial glioma. Cancer Research. 2002;**62**(20):5657-5663

[64] Dickson PV, Hamner JB, Burger RA, Garcia E, Ouma AA, Kim SU, et al. Intravascular administration of tumor tropic neural progenitor cells permits targeted delivery of interferon-beta and restricts tumor growth in a murine model of disseminated neuroblastoma. Journal of Pediatric Surgery. 2007;**42**(1):48-53

[65] Yuan X, Hu J, Belladonna ML, Black KL, Yu JS. Interleukin-23–expressing bone marrow–derived neural stem-like cells exhibit antitumor activity against intracranial glioma. Cancer Research. 2006;**66**(5):2630-2638

[66] Hingtgen S, Kasmieh R, Elbayly E, Nesterenko I, Figueiredo JL, Dash R, et al. A first-generation multi-functional cytokine for simultaneous optical tracking and tumor therapy. PLoS ONE. 2012;**7**(7):e40234

[67] Dent P, Yacoub A, Hamed HA, Park MA, Dash R, Bhutia SK, et al. MDA-7/IL-24 as a cancer therapeutic: from bench to bedside. Anti-Cancer Drugs. 2010;**21**(8):725

[68] Pitti RM, Marsters SA, Ruppert S, Donahue CJ, Moore A, Ashkenazi A. Induction of apoptosis by Apo-2 ligand, a new member of the tumor necrosis factor cytokine family. The Journal of Biological Chemistry. 1996;**271**(22):12687-12690

[69] Oberst A, Pop C, Tremblay AG, Blais V, Denault JB, Salvesen GS, et al. Inducible dimerization and inducible cleavage reveal a requirement for both processes in Caspase-8 activation. The Journal of Biological Chemistry. 2010;**285**(22):16632-16642

[70] Wang J, Chun HJ, Wong W, Spencer DM, Lenardo MJ. Caspase-10 is an initiator caspase in death receptor signaling. Proceedings of the National Academy of Sciences. 2001;**98**(24):13884-13888

[71] Balyasnikova IV, Ferguson SD, Han Y, Liu F, Lesniak MS. Therapeutic

effect of neural stem cells expressing TRAIL and bortezomib in mice with glioma xenografts. Cancer Letters. 2011;**310**(2):148-159

[72] Chen JJ, Chou CW, Chang YF, Chen CC. Proteasome inhibitors enhance TRAIL-induced apoptosis through the intronic regulation of DR5: Involvement of NF-κB and reactive oxygen species-mediated p53 activation. Journal of Immunology. 2008;**180**(12):8030-8039

[73] Kohlhaas SL, Craxton A, Sun XM, Pinkoski MJ, Cohen GM. Receptor-mediated endocytosis is not required for tumor necrosis factor-related apoptosis-inducing ligand (TRAIL)-induced apoptosis. The Journal of Biological Chemistry. 2007;**282**(17):12831-12841

[74] Liu W, Zhao Y, Liu Z, Zhang G, Wu H, Zheng X, et al. Therapeutic effects against high-grade glioblastoma mediated by engineered induced neural stem cells combined with GD2-specific CAR-NK. Cellular Oncology. 2023;**46**(6):1747-1762

[75] Woo SR, Oh YT, An JY, Kang BG, Nam DH, Joo KM. Glioblastoma specific antigens, GD2 and CD90, are not involved in cancer stemness. Anatomy & Cell Biology. 2015;**48**(1):44

[76] Obrador E, Moreno-Murciano P, Oriol-Caballo M, López-Blanch R, Pineda B, Gutiérrez-Arroyo JL, et al. Glioblastoma therapy: Past, present and future. International Journal of Molecular Sciences. 2024;**25**(5):2529

[77] Yong RL, Shinojima N, Fueyo J, Gumin J, Vecil GG, Marini FC, et al. Human bone marrow-derived mesenchymal stem cells for intravascular delivery of oncolytic adenovirus Delta24-RGD to human gliomas. Cancer Research. 2009;**69**(23):8932-8940

[78] Ahmed AU, Thaci B, Alexiades NG, Han Y, Qian S, Liu F, et al. Neural stem cell-based cell carriers enhance therapeutic efficacy of an oncolytic adenovirus in an orthotopic mouse model of human glioblastoma. Molecular Therapy. 2011;**19**(9):1714-1726

[79] Sonabend AM, Ulasov IV, Tyler MA, Rivera AA, Mathis JM, Lesniak MS. Mesenchymal stem cells effectively deliver an oncolytic adenovirus to intracranial glioma. Stem Cells. 2008;**26**(3):831-841

[80] Mineta T, Rabkin SD, Yazaki T, Hunter WD, Martuza RL. Attenuated multi-mutated herpes simplex virus-1 for the treatment of malignant gliomas. Nature Medicine. 1995;**1**(9):938-943

[81] Kranzler J, Tyler MA, Sonabend AM, Ulasov IV, Lesniak MS. Stem cells as delivery vehicles for oncolytic adenoviral virotherapy. Current Gene Therapy. 2009;**9**(5):389

[82] Racles C, Zaltariov MF, Peptanariu D, Vasiliu T, Cazacu M. Functionalized mesoporous silica as doxorubicin carriers and cytotoxicity boosters. Nanomaterials (Basel, Switzerland). 2022;**12**(11):1823

[83] Fang J, Zhang S, Xue X, Zhu X, Song S, Wang B, et al. Quercetin and doxorubicin co-delivery using mesoporous silica nanoparticles enhance the efficacy of gastric carcinoma chemotherapy. International Journal of Nanomedicine. 2018;**13**:5113-5126

[84] Shen J, He Q, Gao Y, Shi J, Li Y. Mesoporous silica nanoparticles loading doxorubicin reverse multidrug resistance: performance and mechanism. Nanoscale. 2011;**3**(10):4314-4322

[85] Mooney R, Roma L, Zhao D, Van Haute D, Garcia E, Kim SU, et al. Neural stem cell-mediated intratumoral

delivery of gold nanorods improves photothermal therapy. ACS Nano. 2014;**8**(12):12450-12460

[86] Yu J, Chlebanowski L, Hammer J, Thapa P, Shrestha T, Wang H, et al. Assembly of mesoporous silica nanoparticle drug conjugates for enhanced delivery. Supramolecular Nanotechnology: Advanced Design of Self-Assembled Functional Materials. 2023;**2**:765-794

[87] Tobias AL, Thaci B, Auffinger B, Rincón E, Balyasnikova IV, Kim CK, et al. The timing of neural stem cell-based virotherapy is critical for optimal therapeutic efficacy when applied with radiation and chemotherapy for the treatment of glioblastoma. Stem Cells Translational Medicine. 2013;**2**(9):655-666

Chapter 15

Modern Strategies in Treatment of the Most Common Central Nervous System Tumors in Pediatric Patients

Miroslav Vukić and Ivan Pašalić

Abstract

Primary tumors of the central nervous system (CNS) represent 20% of all solid pediatric tumors. In this chapter, we want to present the latest approaches in the treatment of the most common CNS tumors that occur in the pediatric population. Those are pilocytic astrocytomas, medulloblastomas, ependymomas, and craniopharyngiomas. CNS tumors can be benign or malignant. Their clinical manifestations, in the form of a focal neurological deficit, an epileptic seizure, or simply symptoms of increased intracranial pressure, are the reason for establishing a working diagnosis and indications for active treatment. While in the case of benign CNS tumors, complete surgical resection generally leads to a cure, in the case of malignant tumors, surgery is frequently only one of the stages in the treatment process. In addition to the open surgical approach, radiosurgery (RS) as well as oncological treatment that includes radiotherapy (RT) and chemotherapy (CT) are often part of the treatment scheme for the abovementioned CNS tumors. Also, it is important to highlight that in the treatment of craniopharyngiomas, due to damage to the pituitary stalk, hormonal therapy (HT) is often necessary. Therefore, the treatment of CNS tumors is often complex and with a questionable outcome.

Keywords: CNS tumors, pediatric population, open surgery (OS), radiosurgery (RS), radiotherapy (RT), chemotherapy (CT), hormonal therapy (HT)

1. Introduction

Tumors of the central nervous system (CNS) often occur in the pediatric population. Moreover, some of the tumors occur most frequently in the pediatric population and are significantly rarer in adults. In this chapter, we will look at the CNS tumors that are most frequent in the pediatric population. These tumors include pilocytic astrocytomas (PCA), medulloblastomas, ependymomas, and craniopharyngiomas (CP). Although all the mentioned tumors appear in the intracranial space, some can also be found in the intraspinal canal in the form of spinal cord tumors. This chapter aims to present a detailed etiology, epidemiology, clinical picture, diagnostic methods used in establishing the working diagnosis, differential diagnosis, therapeutic approach, and prognosis for pediatric patients suffering from the mentioned tumors.

With the progress of every profession, including medicine, the systematization of knowledge occurs over time. This is what happened with oncological diseases of the central nervous system (CNS). The first official version of the classification of CNS tumors was issued by the World Health Organization (WHO) back in 1979 (known as the WHO Blue book) [1]. Since then, WHO has periodically issued revised versions of CNS tumor classification in 1993, 2000, 2007, 2016, and, most recently, 2021 [1, 2]. Therefore, WHO CNS5, the last current 2021 revision of the classification of CNS tumors, is generally accepted and as such used worldwide. The WHO CNS5 classification classifies tumors based on molecular biomarkers in combination with the clinicopathological characteristics of individual tumors [3]. This development of knowledge enables constant progress in the understanding and treatment of oncological diseases of the CNS both in adults and in pediatric patients.

2. Pilocytic astrocytomas

2.1 Definition, WHO classification, and grading

Pilocytic astrocytoma (PCA) is a benign tumor that can occur in any location within the CNS but is most commonly found in the posterior cranial fossa region of the cerebellum [4]. According to the latest available official WHO CNS5 classification of CNS tumors from 2021, PCA belongs to the group of gliomas, glioneuronal tumors, and neuronal tumors and to the subgroup of circumscribed astrocytic gliomas [3]. The aforementioned subgroup also includes astroblastoma, MN1-altered, chordoid glioma, high-grade astrocytoma with piloid features, pleomorphic xanthoastrocytoma, and subependymal giant cell astrocytoma (SEGA) [3]. Of all the mentioned tumors, only PCA and SEGA are WHO grade 1 tumors [4]. All the others either have a higher grade or are without an officially assigned grade [3].

2.2 Etiology

The main causes of PCA are still to be clarified [4]. However, it is known that PCA is caused by an overgrowth of astrocyte cells, which is related to BRAF gene mutations and changes in the mitogen-activated kinase (MAPK) pathway [4, 5]. The vast majority of PCA occur sporadically; however, it is also known that in patients with neurofibromatosis type 1 (NF1), PCA occurs in as many as 20% of patients [4, 5].

2.3 Epidemiology

PCA is the most common primary brain tumor that occurs in children [6]. It appears equally in both genders and most often occurs in the second half of the first decade of life [7].

2.4 Pathology

Macroscopically, PCAs are sharply demarcated, grayish tumors with a soft consistency [6, 8]. An important feature of PCA is the existence of a solid and cystic tumor component [6, 8]. Microscopically, PCAs are tumors of small to medium cellularity [6, 8]. They consist of bipolar cells with Rosenthal fibers and multipolar cells with microcysts [6, 8]. When it comes to immunohistochemistry, PCA tumors are GFAP- and OLIG2-positive and p53-negative [4, 6]. From the genetic point of view, BRAF mutations are present in over 70% of PCA cases [6].

2.5 Clinical presentation

PCAs can occur in any part of the central nervous system [4], and the clinical presentation depends on the location of the tumor. PCAs by far most often appear in the cerebellum, although they are also found in the optic nerve, the hypothalamus, and the spinal cord [4]. Thus, patients with PCA located in the area of the posterior cranial fossa most often present with symptoms of elevated intracranial pressure (ICP). In addition to headache, nausea, and vomiting, common symptoms are ataxia, drifting while walking, cranial nerve palsies and dysmetria, dysarthria, and nystagmus [4].

2.6 Diagnostics

The gold standard for establishing a working diagnosis of PCA is MRI of the brain [4]. In the T1 sequence, the solid component is iso- to hypointense compared to the adjacent brain, while the cystic component has a similar signal to CSF [4]. In the T2 sequence, the solid component is hyperintense compared to the adjacent brain, while the cystic component has a high signal [4]. Ultimately, the T1C sequence shows vivid contrast enhancement of the solid component; the cyst wall often also demonstrating contrast enhancement [4]. However, it should be emphasized that it often happens, especially in patients with acute presentation of symptoms, that a post-contrast MSCT of the brain is performed as the first line of diagnosis. The final diagnosis is made by histopathological, immunohistochemical, and genetic analysis of the tumor tissue.

2.7 Differential diagnosis

In the pediatric population, especially when it comes to tumors in the area of the posterior cranial fossa, medulloblastoma and ependymoma come into consideration in the differential diagnosis in addition to PCA [4, 5]. Other less common tumors include hemangioblastoma, atypical teratoid/rhabdoid tumor, and choroid plexus papilloma [4, 5].

2.8 Treatment

PCAs are benign tumors in which surgical resection of the tumor, if possible, leads to a complete cure [4]. If the PCA is located in the area of the brain stem or the optic nerve, surgical resection is limited to tumor reduction, and it is impossible to achieve the complete eradication of the tumor [4].

In case a residual tumor remains after the surgical treatment, clinical and radiological follow-up of the patient is recommended [9]. It should be considered that PCAs are slow-growing tumors, and if the clinical and radiological picture in patients with a residual tumor is favorable, it is advisable to adopt a conservative attitude in their treatment [9].

Obstructive hydrocephalus is the main cause of exacerbation of the clinical condition in patients with a tumor in the posterior cranial fossa. There are several methods for treating hydrocephalus. They include placement of external ventricular drainage (EVD), ventriculoperitoneal shunt (VPS), and endoscopic third ventriculostomy (ETV) [4]. EVD is actually an "open" system where the proximal end of the ventricular drain is placed in the frontal horn, usually of the right lateral ventricle, and the distal end is connected to an external tube and collection system. EVDs are typically temporary and are rarely used for longer than 14 days. VP is a surgical method in which a drainage system is passed through subcutaneous tunneling, the proximal end of which is placed in the ventricular system of the brain, and the distal end in the peritoneal port of the abdomen. ETV is an endoscopic method of resolving obstructive hydrocephalus in such a way that the endoscope first enters the area of the right lateral ventricle, then passes through the foramen of Monro and enters the third cerebral ventricle, in the bottom of which, premamillary, an opening is made to connect the ventricular system with the basal cisterns. There are ongoing debates in the literature as to whether it is necessary to treat obstructive hydrocephalus that is sampled by a tumor located in the posterior cranial fossa or whether it is necessary to treat the tumor immediately [10]. It is believed that by removing the tumor there is a great chance to resolve the hydrocephalus as well [10]. However, in about 30% of pediatric patients, the so-called postresection hydrocephalus remains [10]. The choice of treatment method for postresection hydrocephalus depends on the type of tumor [10]. Thus, although ETV is a surgical method with a significantly lower incidence of complications in patients with aggressive tumors that initially present with metastases, VP shunt is the preferred treatment [10].

The use of conventional RT is limited and most often not applied in the treatment of pediatric patients with PCA [4]. Nevertheless, some studies have shown good results in the treatment of recurrent tumors with stereotactic radiosurgery (SRS) [4]. The use of CT in the treatment of patients with PCA is very limited and can theoretically be used in advanced, inoperable tumors with the aim of delaying the use of RT in children [11].

2.9 Prognosis

If the postoperative follow-up MRI of the brain shows that gross total resection (GTR) of PCA has been successfully achieved, no further treatment is required, and the overall 10-year survival rate is over 90% [12].

2.10 Case presentation

The patient, a 10-year-old girl, clinically presented with torticollis, ataxia while walking, headaches, nausea, and vomiting. In the neurological status, there was instability in the Romberg position and an ataxic gait. As part of the diagnostic evaluation, the patient underwent MRI of the brain, which confirmed an expansive tumor process that invaded the fourth cerebral ventricle and consequently caused obstructive hydrocephalus (**Figures 1** and **2**). The patient underwent neurosurgery during which medial suboccipital osteoplastic craniotomy, a telovelar approach to the tumor, and a complete tumor resection were performed. Histopathological analysis confirmed that the tissue consisted of bipolar piloid astroglial cells (**Figure 3**). The tumor was slightly to moderately cellular, with no signs of mitosis. The blood vessel endothelium was swollen, in places proliferating and creating glomeruloid formations. Immunohistochemically, the tumor was GFAP-positive, OLIG2-positive, IDH1-negative, ATRX maintained, p53-negative, BRAF V600-negative, H3K27M-negative, and the

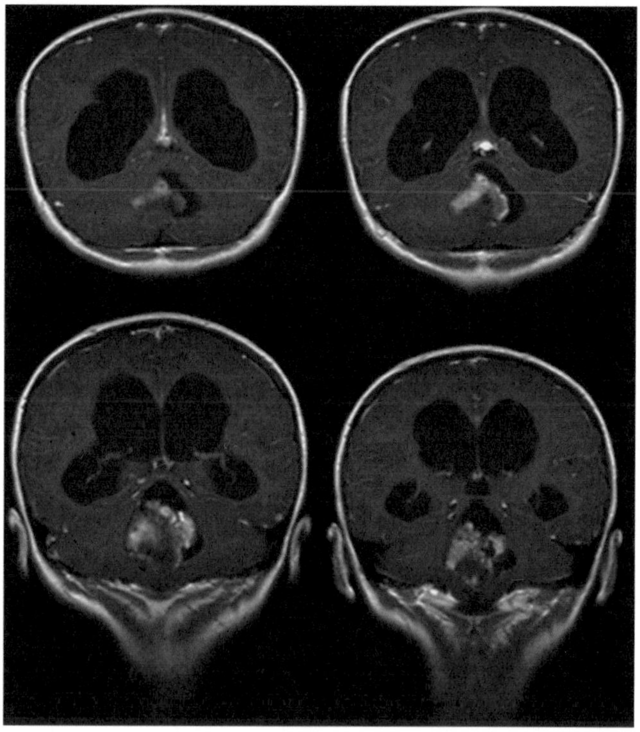

Figure 1.
Preoperative T1-weighted contrast-enhanced coronal MRI sequences showing a pilocytic astrocytoma in the posterior cranial fossa, filling the fourth ventricle and leading to hydrocephalus.

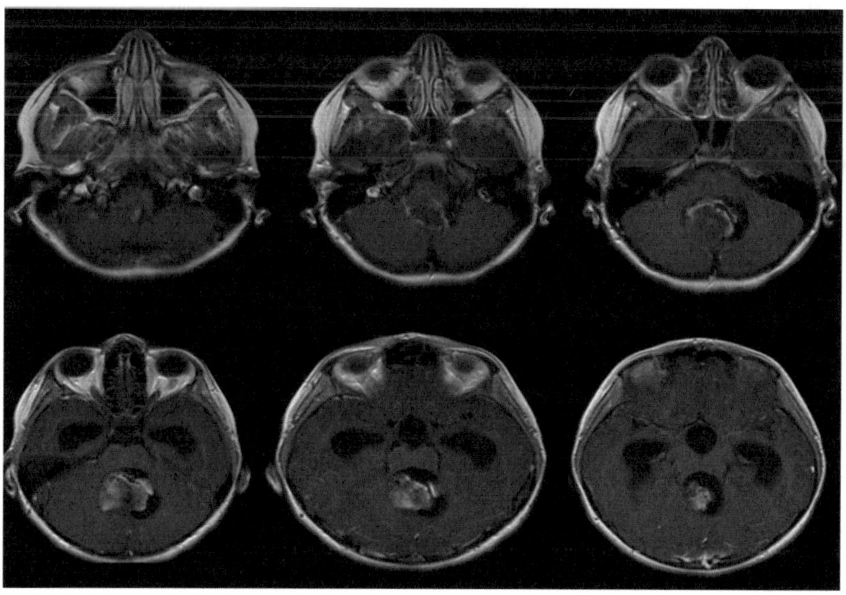

Figure 2.
Preoperative axial section of T1-weighted contrast-enhanced sequences of the brain MRI showing a pilocytic astrocytoma located in the fourth ventricle, with rounded temporal horns of both lateral ventricles and a ballooned third ventricle.

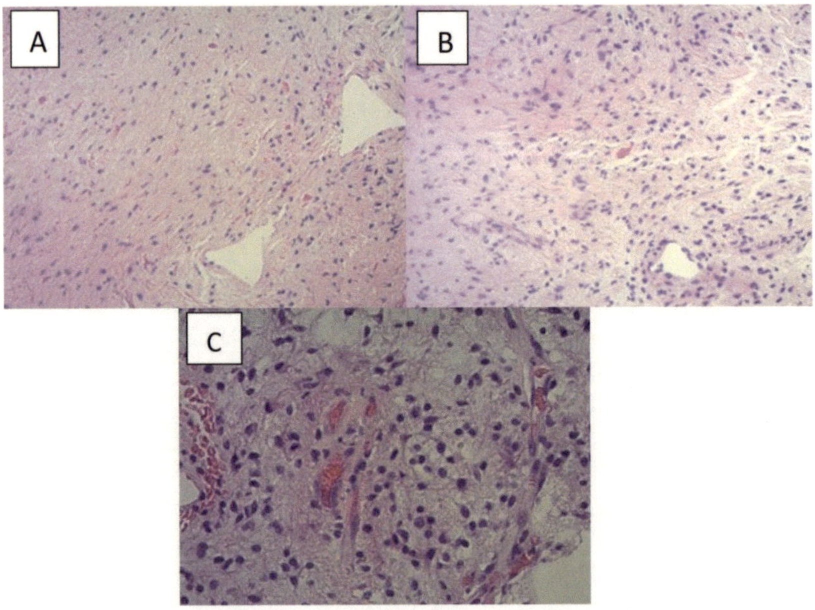

Figure 3.
A and B were stained with hematoxylin and eosin (HE) at 200× magnification; C was stained with HE at 400× magnification.

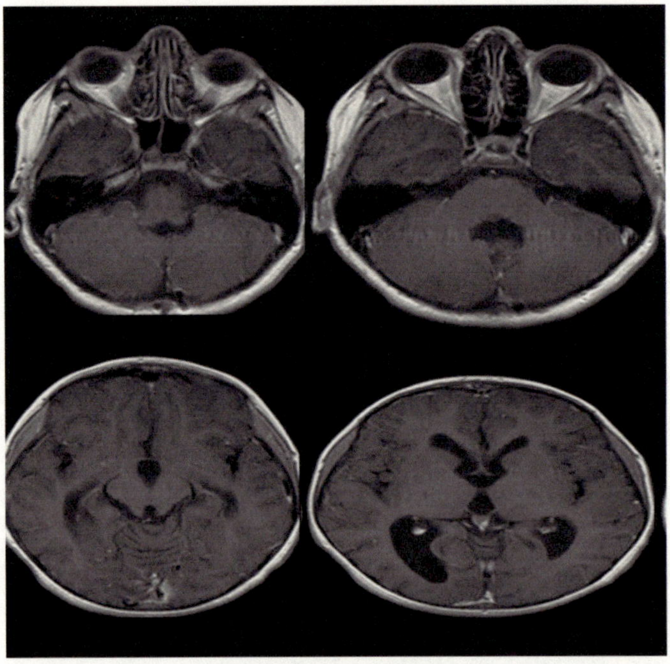

Figure 4.
Postoperative MRI of the brain, using the T1C sequence, shows the completely removed tumor (PA) and normal ventricular size in axial sections.

Ki67 proliferation index was 3.5%. Ultimately, the histopathology confirmed a pilocytic astrocytoma. Three months after the operation, a follow-up MRI of the brain was performed, which confirmed a complete resection of the tumor and a normal ventricular system (**Figure 4**).

3. Medulloblastomas

3.1 Definition, WHO classification, and grading

Medulloblastomas are malignant brain tumors that typically occur in children. They are the second most common tumors in the pediatric population. According to the latest WHO classification of CNS tumors from 2021, medulloblastomas are classified as embryonal tumors [2]. Accordingly, we distinguish several types of medulloblastoma entities that include medulloblastoma, histologically defined; medulloblastoma, WNT-activated; medulloblastoma, SHH-activated (TP53-wildtype/mutant); medulloblastoma non-WNT/non-SHH (group 3), and medulloblastoma non-WNT/non-SHH (group 4) [2, 13]. The last two are combined into the group of medulloblastoma, non-WNT/non-SHH [2, 13]. All medulloblastomas are graded as WHO grade 4 tumors [13].

3.2 Etiology

The exact cause of medulloblastoma is still unclear. However, it is known that the WNT group of medulloblastoma is associated with mutations in the CTNNB1 or APC genes [14]. On the other hand, the SHH group of medulloblastoma is associated with the activation of suppressor genes PTCH1 or SUFU [14]. The MBs of group 3 and group 4 are genetically significantly more heterogeneous and associated with SMARCA4, KDM6A, i(17q) and MYC amplifications are found in them [6, 15]. According to some research, the origin and occurrence of medulloblastoma is associated with viral infections or human cytomegalovirus (CMV) in childhood [16].

3.3 Epidemiology

Medulloblastomas are the second most frequent CNS tumors that occur in the pediatric population [5, 16]. They most often appear in the second half of the first decade of life and are 1.5 times more common in males [5, 16]. When it comes to subgroups of medulloblastoma, Group 4 MB occurs most often, in 35% of cases [17]. It is followed by SHH type MB with an incidence of 30% [17]. Group 3 MB occurs in 25% and WNT type MB in 10% of patients [17]. In 25% of patients with medulloblastoma, metastases occur through the cerebrospinal fluid (CSF) [14]. Group 3 and group 4 medulloblastomas metastasize most frequently [17].

3.4 Pathology

MBs are grayish tumors, usually of a soft consistency, with the possibility of necrosis [6]. MBs are highly cellular neoplasms with usually small- to medium-sized with hyperchromatic nuclei [6]. Homer-Wright rosettes are an important histological finding characteristic of MB [6].

Histologically, four types of MB are distinguished based on the WHO 2016 classification: classic medulloblastoma (CMB), desmoplastic/nodular medulloblastoma (DNMB), medulloblastoma with extensive nodularity (MBEN), and large cell/anaplastic medulloblastoma (LC/AMB) [6]. CMBs are so-called small blue cell tumors that are immunopositive for synaptophysin and NeuN [6]. The microscopic features of DNMB are characterized by the appearance of reticulin-free zones, which are surrounded by highly proliferative cells [6]. When it comes to immunophenotyping, this histological type of MB shows variable expression of synaptophysin and NeuN [6]. MBEN is a histological variant of medulloblastoma in which the main microscopic characteristics are unusually large reticulin-free zones containing small cells with round nuclei [6]. Immunophenotypic synaptophysin and NeuN play an important role [6]. Finally, LC/AMB is characterized by a high degree of mitosis and nuclear pleomorphism [6].

From the molecular and genetic point of view, according to the latest WHO 2021 classification, four entities of medulloblastoma can be distinguished: WNT-activated, SHH-activated and TP53 wildtype, SHH-activated and TP53 mutant, and non-WNT/non-SHH (previously groups 3 and 4) [14]. These molecular and genetic definitions do not recapitulate the prior histological subtypes.

3.5 Clinical presentation

Since medulloblastomas most often appear in the area of the posterior cranial fossa of the cerebellum, patients present clinically with symptoms of gait disturbances and clumsiness [14, 16]. Patients with medulloblastoma also often present with symptoms of obstructive hydrocephalus and elevated ICP, such as headache accompanied by nausea and vomiting, as well as drowsiness and impaired consciousness [14, 16]. Obstructive hydrocephalus occurs when the tumor growth spreads to the area of the fourth cerebral ventricle. It is important to note that medulloblastoma is a type of tumor that can metastasize through the CSF [14]. This can be seen in 20–25% of cases [14]. In this way, it can spread to the area of the spinal cord and present itself with symptoms such as pain syndromes, weakness of the extremities, and incontinence.

3.6 Diagnosis

In infants who present with symptoms of obstructive hydrocephalus, an increase in head circumference can be verified [16]. Additionally, determination of the fundus of the eye is used in the diagnosis of hydrocephalus [16]. When it comes to neuroradiological examinations in clinical practice, brain MSCT and MRI are usually performed [15]. On native MSCT of the brain, MB is most often presented as a hyperdense tumor mass of the vermis occupying the fourth cerebral ventricle [15]. In post-contrast MSCT sequences, enhancement of MB is present [15]. The gold standard in establishing a working diagnosis of MB is MRI of the brain, which is often supplemented with MRI spectroscopy. On both MSCT and MRI of the brain, MB is most commonly verified as a tumor formation of the vermis that fills the fourth cerebral ventricle and is hyperintense to gray matter in the T2 sequence [15]. In the T1 sequence, it is hypointense to gray matter, and in the T1C sequence, it shows heterogeneous enhancement, while in the DWI sequence, it is presented with a high signal, or diffusion restriction [15]. MRI spectroscopy in MB shows elevated choline and decreased NAA [15]. Since MB can spread through the CSF, lumbar puncture as well as MRI of the neuroaxis are essential in establishing the diagnosis, prognosis, as well as postoperative follow-up of patients [16].

3.7 Differential diagnosis

Differential diagnostic considerations include PA, ependymoma, choroid plexus papilloma, or carcinoma [2, 16].

3.8 Treatment

The treatment of MB consists of surgical resection and oncological treatment, which includes radiation and chemotherapy [5, 14–16]. The goal of surgical treatment involves tumor resection, resolution of obstructive hydrocephalus, and obtaining histopathology findings [16]. In 35% of patients, despite surgical resection of the tumor, additional treatment of obstructive hydrocephalus is required by placement of a VP shunt [15, 16]. Also, sometimes it is necessary to install an Ommaya reservoir to enable delivery of chemotherapy [16]. Complications of surgical treatment in the form of damage to the cerebellum and brainstem occur in 5–10% of patients and are presented as cerebellar mutism, ataxia, hemiparesis, and supranuclear cranial nerve palsies [14]. In pediatric MB patients older than 3 years, successful surgical treatment is followed by craniospinal radiation with a boost to the tumor site [14]. It is optimal to start radiation 4 weeks after successful surgical treatment [16]. Radiation is followed by chemotherapy in the treatment schedule [14]. Patients who are younger than 3 years do not undergo radiation but a special form of intensive chemotherapy [14].

One of the most significant historical forms of medulloblastoma grading is the one that resembles the TNM classification, known as Chang's criteria, which takes into account tumor volume and the presence of metastases [18]. Today, staging of patients with MB is based on three factors: the age of the patient, the presence of CSF metastases, and the volume of the residual tumor after surgical resection [14, 16]. Thus, patients who are at least 3 years old, have no detected CSF metastases, and whose residual tumor volume on the postoperative follow-up MRI of the brain is less than 1.5 cm^2 are classified as patients with an average risk [14, 16]. All others are considered as high-risk patients [14, 16]. The amount of prescribed craniospinal radiation is determined based on the above criteria [14]. Thus, patients with an average risk are administered 23.4 Gy, while high-risk patients are prescribed 36 Gy [14].

Patients with WNT subgroup MB generally have a fairly good prognosis [16]. Underlying the malignant transformation of these tumors is the insufficient breakdown of beta-carotene, and protein phosphatase inhibitors and cantharidin are used in their treatment [16]. Smoothened (SMO) inhibitors such as cyclopamine and vismodegib are essential in the treatment of patients suffering from the MB SHH subgroup, since they inhibit the key segment of the Smoothened (SMO) mediator signaling pathway [5, 16]. MYC inhibition and cell cycle checkpoint inhibitors could have promising results in the treatment of patients with MB of the non-SHH/WNT subgroup [16].

When it comes to immunotherapy, it has been shown that HER2 is overexpressed on the surface of MB, and preclinical studies of the effectiveness of anti-HER2 CAR-T cells for these tumors are underway [5].

3.9 Prognosis

Patients with WNT subgroup MB experience the best survival, with 5-year survival rates between 97% and 100% [16], followed by SHH subgroup MB patients with 5-year survival between 70% and 88% [16]. The worst prognosis is faced by those suffering from the non-SHH/WNT subgroups of MB [16]. Five-year survival of patients with group 4 MB is between 65% and 85%, while group 3 MB has survival rates between 40% and 65% [16]. It should be emphasized that average-risk patients have a 5-year survival rate of 85%, while the survival of high-risk patients is only 40% [16].

3.10 Case presentation

The patient, a 9-year-old boy, presented with symptoms of elevated ICP manifested by headache and vomiting. As part of the diagnostic workup, MRI of the brain was performed, which confirmed a tumor of the posterior cranial fossa that occupied the fourth cerebral ventricle with the presence of radiological signs of hydrocephalus (**Figure 5**). The patient presented with a normal neurological status. In view of the above, he underwent a neurosurgical procedure during which medial suboccipital osteoplastic craniotomy, laminectomy of the CI vertebra, and resection of the tumor were performed. The telovelar approach was used to access the tumor, whose margins were non-sharp compared to the surrounding cerebellar parenchyma, and which was very well vascularized. With the help of an aspirator and bipolar tweezers, the tumor was completely removed and sent for histopathological analysis. After the neurosurgical procedure, the patient was admitted to the pediatric intensive care unit, where he was extubated shortly and, hemodynamically and respiratorily stable, transferred to the Pediatric Department of the Clinic for Neurosurgery. Small, polymorphic cells with hyperchromatic nuclei were verified histologically in the analysis of the tumor tissue (**Figure 6A**). Numerous tumor cells were in division, and several necroses were

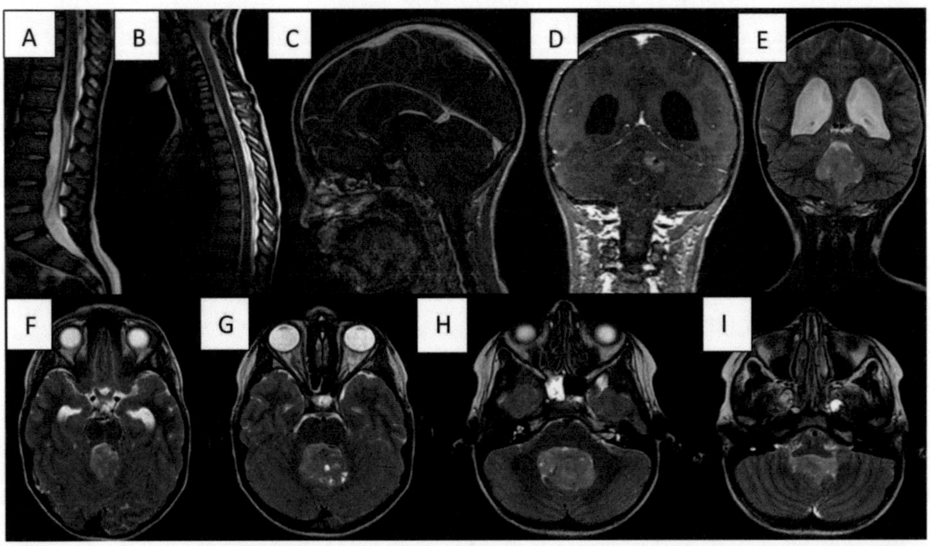

Figure 5.
A: Sagittal section of T2 MRI sequence of the lumbar spine, indicating no signs of CSF metastases of medulloblastoma; B: Sagittal section of T2 MRI sequence of the cervical and thoracic spine, also showing no evidence of CSF metastases of medulloblastoma; C: Sagittal section of T1C MRI sequence of the brain, demonstrating medulloblastoma filling the fourth cerebral ventricle; D: Coronal section of T1C MRI sequence of the brain, displaying medulloblastoma within the fourth cerebral ventricle alongside a dilated supratentorial ventricular system; E: Coronal section of T2 MRI sequence of the brain, featuring a medulloblastoma within the fourth cerebral ventricle with a dilated supratentorial ventricular system; F, G, H, and I: Axial section of T2-sequence MRI of the brain, revealing medulloblastoma of the posterior cranial fossa.

found. The tumor cells were positive for synaptophysin and NSE (**Figure 6B**). Ki67 was observed in the densest areas of positivity in over 75% of cells in the extranodal areas. p53 was seen in 15% of cells in the extranodular areas but was not found in the nodal areas. YaP1 and GAB1 were negative. Beta-catenin showed cytoplasmic peri-membranous positivity, while it was negative in the nuclei. Based on the histological

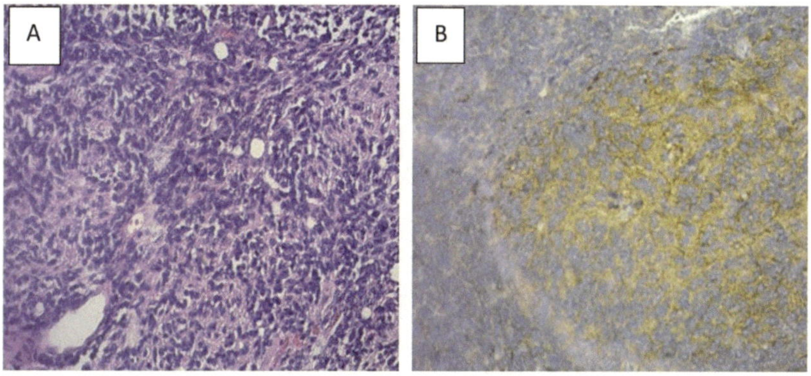

Figure 6.
A: Medulloblastoma—HE—microscope magnification ×400; B: Medulloblastoma—immunohistochemical staining for synaptophysin, microscope magnification ×400.

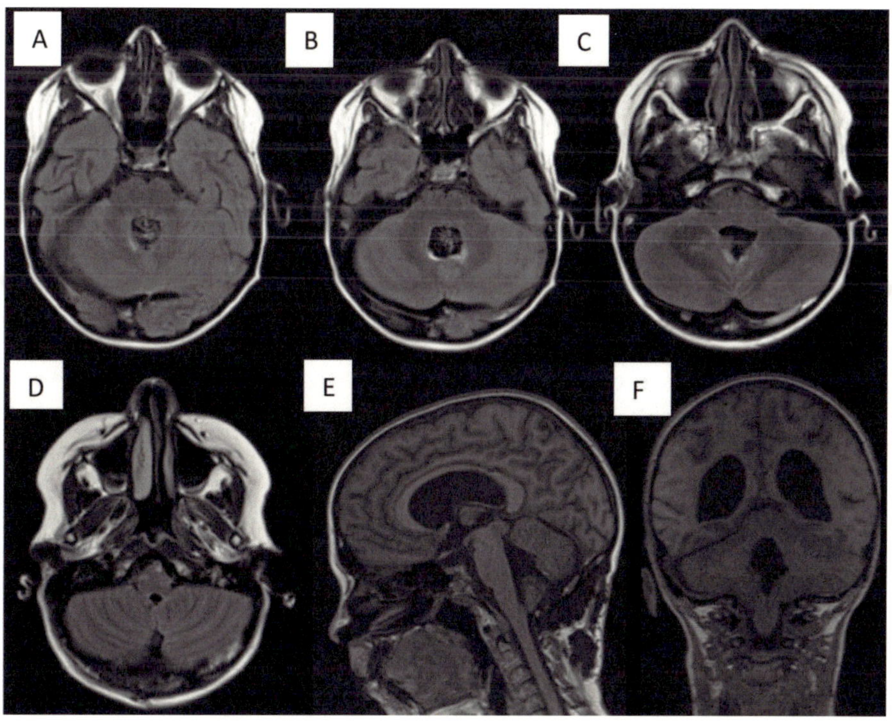

Figure 7.
A, B, C, and D: Axial sections of the T1 sequence through the posterior cranial fossa showing a completely removed tumor; E: Sagittal section T1 sequence shows a normal postoperative finding; F: Coronal section T1 sequence that also shows a regular finding, without signs of residual tumor.

picture, the tumor was determined as medulloblastoma. No amplification of the MYCN gene was found. Cerebrospinal fluid cytology showed no signs of leptomeningeal metastases. Three months after the operation, follow-up brain and spinal MRI were performed, which verified normal postoperative findings with no signs of residue, recurrence, or metastasis of the resected medulloblastoma (**Figure 7**). After the operation, 36 Gy craniospinal RT, tumor bed 54 Gy, and concomitant temozolomide were administered. Adjuvant chemotherapy was also performed according to the ACNS 0332 protocol, followed by six cycles vincristine d1, d8, cisplatin d1, and cyclophosphamide d2–3.

4. Ependymomas

4.1 Definition, WHO classification, and grading

Ependymomas are tumors that can appear in any part of the CNS and originate from ependymal cells lining the ventricular system and central canal [19]. With the development of knowledge, it has been realized that the group of tumors comprised by the term ependymoma includes various entities. Thus, both benign and extremely malignant tumors have been designated in this group. According to the new WHO 2021 classification, ependymomas are classified considering the location of appearance, histology, and molecular features [3]. Within the group of ependymal tumors the following entities can be distinguished: 1. SE—subependymoma; 2. ST-ZFTA—supratentorial, ZFTA-fusion-positive ependymoma; 3. ST-YAP1—supratentorial, YAP1-fusion-positive ependymoma; 4. PFA—group A posterior fossa ependymoma; 5. PFB—group B posterior fossa ependymoma; 6. SP-EPN—spinal ependymoma; 7. SP-MYCN—spinal ependymoma, MYCN-amplified; and 8. MPE—myxopapillary ependymoma [5]. Grading of ependymoma is based on the histological features of the tumor. Thus, the number of mitoses as well as the presence of microvascular proliferation and necrosis are observed [20]. Therefore, SE is a WHO grade 1 tumor, and MPE is a WHO grade 2 tumor [20]. No grades have been assigned to other molecular subtypes. If there is only a histological diagnosis without molecular analysis, grades 2 or 3 are assigned [20]. However, it should be pointed out that there are serious controversies in tumor grading, since not infrequently the gradation based on histological characteristics does not reflect the actual malignancy of the tumor and the poor prognosis [20]. Therefore, molecular stratification is extremely important [3, 5, 20].

4.2 Etiology

As with most tumors, the exact cause of ependymoma is still unknown [21]. However, it has been established that ependymomas occur somewhat more frequently in patients with neurofibromatosis type 2 (NF2) [21].

4.3 Epidemiology

Ependymomas can develop at any age of life; however, they most often occur in the pediatric population [22]. In terms of frequency, ependymomas are the third most common CNS tumors, following pilocytic astrocytomas and medulloblastomas [5, 22]. Ependymomas occur more often in males, and in children, they most often appear in the first 5 years of life [7, 23]. Ependymomas can occur within the entire neuroaxis. However, in 60% of cases, ependymomas develop in the region of the posterior cranial fossa, in 30% of cases in the supratentorial region, and in 10% of cases in the region of the spinal cord [21].

4.4 Pathology

Considering the fact that ependymomas can be benign as well as malignant, it is understandable that their histological characteristics differ [6, 22]. Benign ependymomas are tumors that are classified as WHO grade I tumors and include subependymomas [20, 22]. Subependymomas appear in the ventricular system of the brain and are histologically presented as hypocellular tumors with bland nuclei [6, 22]. WHO grade II and grade III ependymomas are not benign tumors; therefore, their histological presentation is different [6, 22]. The main histological feature of WHO grade II ependymoma is hypercellularity [6, 22]. WHO grade III ependymomas are anaplastic ependymomas that are histologically presented with numerous mitoses and necrosis [6, 22].

4.5 Clinical presentation

There are no symptoms that are pathognomonic for ependymomas. They may present like other CNS tumors and depend on the location of its occurrence as well as its degree of malignancy. Clearly, the clinical picture in benign tumors develops slowly, while in malignant tumors, it is much more dynamic. However, the clinical presentation mostly depends on the location of the ependymoma. Ependymomas that occur intracranially are different from those that occur intraspinally. Also, tumors that develop supratentorially differ from tumors that appear infratentorially, in the area of the posterior cranial fossa. Intracranial tumors commonly present with symptoms of increased intracranial pressure, most often with headache followed by nausea and vomiting. In young children, signs of elevated ICP can be a tense fontanelle and an increase in head circumference [21]. Supratentorial ependymomas can present with symptoms such as focal neurological deficits and epileptic seizures [19, 21]. Infratentorial ependymomas, in addition to the symptoms of elevated ICP, often present with ataxia, gait instability, diplopia, and facial palsies [19]. Children with diagnosed intraspinal ependymoma clinically present with back pain, weakness in the lower extremities, and impaired sphincter function [19].

4.6 Diagnostics

Diagnostics begins with a detailed patient history, which is usually provided by the accompanying parent [22]. After that, it is necessary to determine the clinical status of the patient, with special reference to the neurological status [22]. When it comes to intracranial tumors, including intracranial ependymomas, radiological diagnosis usually begins with MSCT or MRI of the brain [22]. Infratentorial ependymoma on MRI of the brain is shown as a solid tumor that spreads through the foramina of Luschka and Magendie [19]. Ependymoma presents as a heterogeneous signal in the T2 sequence [19]. In the T1 native sequence, it has a hypointense signal, and in the T1 postcontrast sequence, it shows heterogeneous enhancement [19]. When it comes to supratentorial ependymomas, on brain MR, they often show signs of calcification and bleeding and frequently contain a cystic component [19]. In the case of intraspinal ependymomas, it is necessary to perform an MRI of the affected part of the spine [22].

Intraspinal ependymomas are most often located in the lumbosacral spine [19]. The diagnosis of ependymoma is ultimately made on the basis of histological and molecular analysis of the tumor tissue [21].

4.7 Differential diagnosis

In the differential diagnosis of supratentorial ependymomas, other glial and embryonic tumors are considered; with infratentorial ependymomas, the following are most often considered: PA, medulloblastoma, and choroid plexus tumors [22].

4.8 Treatment

Currently, there are no guidelines for the treatment of individual molecular subgroups of ependymoma [22]. Surgical resection of the tumor has been proven the best option in the treatment of ependymoma [19, 21, 22]. Research has shown that gross total resection (GTR) significantly affects survival [19]. However, in some cases, it is not possible to completely remove the tumor due to its very sensitive location [21, 22]. In such patients, especially in the case of grade 2 or 3 ependymoma, further treatment is required, usually in the form of adjuvant RT [8, 11]. The use of chemotherapy in the treatment of ependymoma is limited [21, 22].

WHO grade 1 ependymoma does not require further treatment after neurosurgery in which complete resection of the tumor was achieved, although regular radiological monitoring of the patient is advisable [21]. On the other hand, even after successful surgical resection, WHO grade 2 and 3 ependymomas require further oncological treatment for residual tumor cells [21]. The type of adjuvant treatment is determined with regard to the results of surgery, the extent of the disease, and the age of the patient [21]. RT prevents local recurrence of the disease [21]. Chemotherapy is also given with the aim of preventing local recurrence of the disease, especially in very young children, and in order to avoid the use of RT [21].

According to the HIT-MED-Guidance, patients above the age of 18 months who after surgery have no signs of residual tumor or signs of ependymoma metastasis undergo RT of the tumor bed, while patients who are younger than the specified age receive chemotherapy [21]. Patients in whom postoperative follow-up brain MRI shows a residual ependymoma undergo adjuvant RT or chemotherapy, while patients with cerebrospinal fluid metastases undergo an individual approach to treatment [21].

However, the large multicenter COG ACNS021 study investigating treatment of ependymoma in children showed that even children as young as 1 year old can receive RT [19]. Accordingly, children aged between 12 and 18 months can receive adjuvant RT of 54 Gy, while children older than 18 months can receive RT of 59.4 Gy [19].

Since craniospinal radiation has not been shown to be superior to focal radiation when it comes to preventing distant relapses of the disease, and since most relapses are focal, focal radiation is still preferred [19].

Proton beam radiation is another form of adjuvant therapy after surgical resection of ependymoma [24]. With it, in addition to good disease control, the toxic effect of radiation on the surrounding healthy tissue can be avoided or reduced [24].

Treating infants, that is, children under 1 year of age, for ependymoma is very challenging. In such patients, surgery is followed by adjuvant chemotherapy, and after the child reaches 1 year of age, RT treatment is considered [19]. Although neoadjuvant chemotherapy has shown some success in the treatment of residual ependymomas in children after subtotal neurosurgical resection, its potential benefits have yet to be defined before considering repeated surgery or radiation [19]. Also, there is no evidence that chemotherapy is successful in the treatment of disseminated ependymomas [19].

4.9 Prognosis

The most important prognostic factor that affects the outcome of patients with intracranial ependymoma is the extent of the performed neurosurgery [22]. Therefore, the more radical the operation, the higher the degree of survival [22]. The location of intracranial ependymomas also plays an important role in survival. Thus, patients with supratentorial ependymoma have a worse prognosis [22]. According to the available information, the 5-year survival of a pediatric patient after complete surgical removal of an ependymoma with adjuvant RT is between 60% and 85% [21].

4.10 Case presentation

The patient, a 6-year-old girl, clinically presented with symptoms of instability and drifting while walking as well as increased irritability. Additionally, the parents noticed that 10 days before being admitted to the hospital, the girl had a slightly irregular head position due to the impossibility of straightening her neck. At the time of examination, symptoms of elevated ICP were also present, in the form of headaches accompanied by nausea and vomiting. The neurological status showed lowering of the right mouth corner, left-sided torticollis, and drifting while walking. Brain MRI performed as part of the diagnostic workup verified a tumor of the right cerebellar hemisphere, extending caudally to the level of the medulla oblongata, which it compressed, and cranially to the mesencephalon, where it also produced a compressive effect (**Figure 8**). Based on the above, a neurosurgical procedure was indicated, during which right-sided retrosigmoid osteoplastic craniotomy and resection of the tumor were performed. Following retraction of the petrous surface of the cerebellum and opening of the cistern of the right pontocerebellar angle, the tumor was accessed, and tumor tissue pervading the cranial nerve was found. The tumor tissue was grayish in color, sharply demarcated, and soft in consistency, with a compressive effect on the brain stem. With the help of an aspirator and bipolar tweezers, the tumor was completely removed and referred for histopathology analysis. During the operation, all neurovascular structures (the right trigeminus nerve, right facial nerve, and right vestibulocochlear nerve, as well as the basilar artery and right AICA) remained intact. The operation proceeded smoothly and without complications. The patient was then transferred to the pediatric intensive care unit for the duration of 24 hours. The early postoperative course was uneventful, and the patient was transferred to the Pediatric Department of the Clinic for Neurosurgery. Histopathology analysis of the resected tissue showed that the tumor consisted of gliovascular formations and smaller clusters of ependymal cells (**Figure 9**). In parts, the tumor created ependymal canals and rosettes. The tumor cells were oval, and mitosis was not found, neither were there signs of necrosis. Inside the tumor foci of cartilaginous, metaplasia and calcification were found. Immunohistochemically, the cells were GFAP-positive, S100-positive, and P54-negative, with EMA focal positivity. Proliferative activity measured with Ki67 was 2%, and 5% within the foci. The findings confirmed a grade 2 ependymoma with focal cartilaginous metaplasia. Oncological treatment with proton beam radiotherapy was performed postoperatively. The follow-up MRI of the neuroaxis

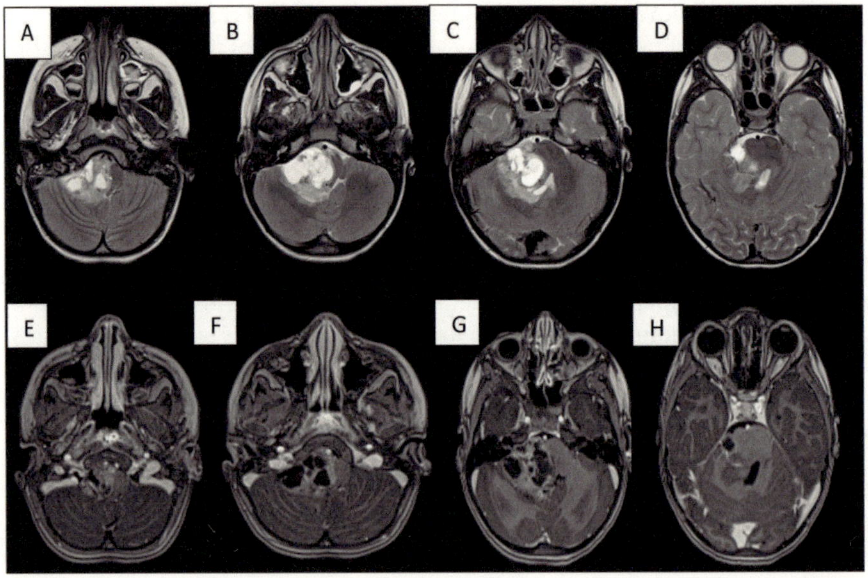

Figure 8.
A, B, C, and D: Axial T2 sequences of MRI of the brain showing an ependymoma in the posterior cranial fossa at the right pontocerebellar angle, causing significant compression on the brainstem; E, F, G, and H: Axial T1C sequences of MRI of the brain depict an ependymoma in the posterior cranial fossa at the right pontocerebellar angle, displaying heterogeneous contrast enhancement.

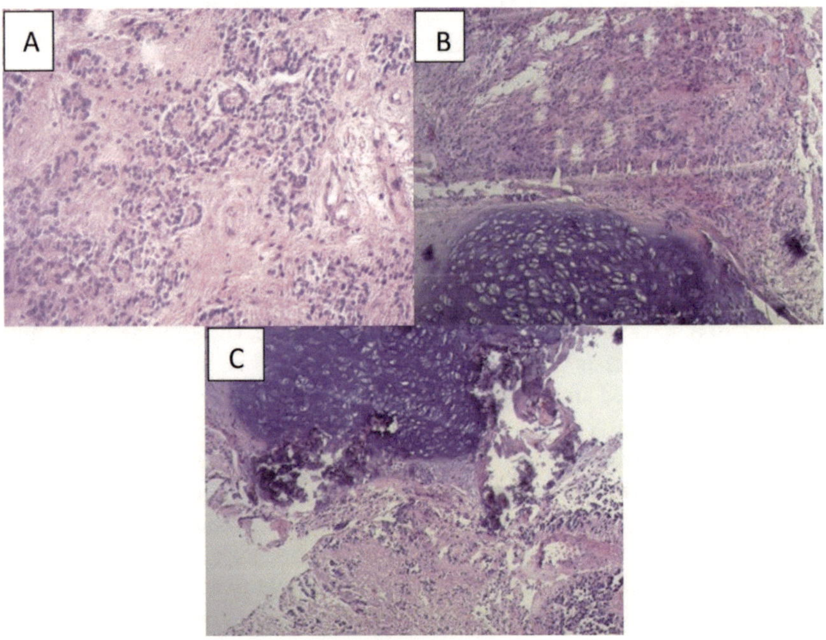

Figure 9.
A: Histological presentation of ependymoma with cartilaginous metaplasia—HE staining—microscope magnification ×200; B and C: Histological presentation of ependymoma with cartilaginous metaplasia—HE staining—microscope magnification ×100.

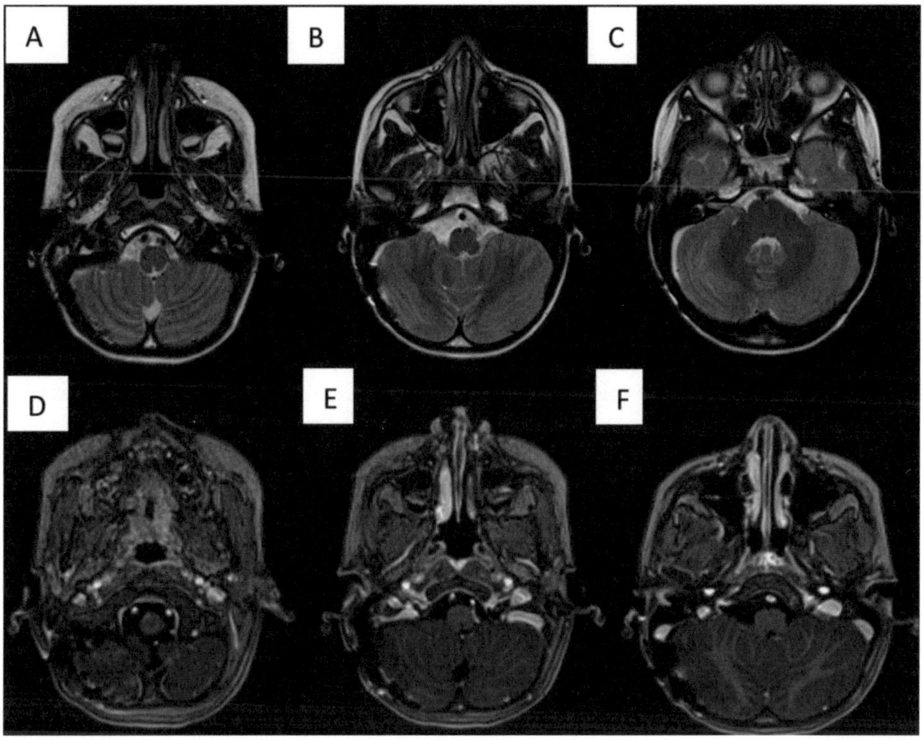

Figure 10.
A, B, and C show axial T2 sequences of MRI of the brain, confirming the complete removal of the ependymoma without any signs of remaining tumor or tumor recurrence. D, E, and F display axial T1C MRI sequences of the brain, also confirming the complete removal of the ependymoma with no signs of residual tumor or recurrence of tumor disease.

performed 1 year after the surgery confirmed a normal intracranial finding, with no signs of residual or recurrent tumor (**Figure 10**). There were no signs of hydrocephalus. MRI of the spine as well as CSF cytology showed no signs of CSF metastases.

5. Craniopharyngiomas

5.1 Definition, WHO classification, and grading

Craniopharyngiomas (CP) are benign brain tumors that typically occur in the sellar region [6]. According to the new CNS 5 tumor classification, adamantinomatous (ACP) and papillary craniopharyngiomas (PCP) are two separate entities and not subtypes of one tumor [25]. Both types of craniopharyngiomas are WHO grade 1 tumors [26].

5.2 Etiology

ACP is caused by a mutation of the CTNNB1 gene, which is an important factor in the regulation of the WNT β-catenin signaling pathway [25]. PCP is associated with the BRAF V600E mutation in 95% of cases [6]. Both of these tumors originate from ectoblastic remnants of the duct of Rathke [25].

5.3 Epidemiology

CPs are generally rare tumors that occur in the sellar region, a location where up to 10% of all CNS tumors in the pediatric population develop [25]. CP has two peaks of occurrence, one in the pediatric age and the other in the elderly [26]. In the pediatric population, these tumors most often appear in the first decade of life, equally in both genders [26]. ACP is a craniopharyngioma that occurs in the pediatric population, while PCP appears almost exclusively in adults [6].

5.4 Pathology

ACPs are mixed solid and cystic squamous epithelial tumors [6, 25]. They often contain calcifications and cholesterol-rich deposits [6]. An important characteristic by which ACP can be recognized macroscopically is the machine oil-like fluid that fills the cystic component of the tumor [25]. Typical microscopic features of ACP are nodules of wet keratin and large eosinophilic masses [26].

5.5 Clinical presentation

Clinically, patients with ACP most often present with symptoms of elevated ICP such as headache, nausea, and vomiting. Also, since ACP occurs in the sellar region, symptoms of compression on surrounding structures such as the optic apparatus and frontal lobe occur as a result of tumor growth [25]. Thus, as a result of tumor compression on the optical apparatus, 60–80% of patients develop symptoms of visual disturbances [25, 26]. The extension of the tumor into the area of the frontal lobe can result in behavioral changes [25]. A special group of symptoms that are pathognomonic for tumors in the sellar region are symptoms associated with hormonal imbalance that occurs due to affection of the pituitary gland and infundibulum [25, 26]. This type of symptom occurs in 40–80% of patients with APC [25, 26]. In childhood, hormonal imbalance is most often manifested by delayed puberty, amenorrhea, changes in body weight, and diabetes insipidus, which presents as polyuria and polydipsia [25].

5.6 Diagnostics

The diagnosis of craniopharyngioma, as with all other tumors, begins with taking the medical history and assessing the clinical status. This is followed by radiological diagnostics, which is often started with native and post-contrast MSCT of the brain, followed by MRI of the brain. Further diagnostics includes an eye examination and hormonal status assessment [6, 25, 26].

The radiological characteristics of ACP can best be explained with the help of the 90% rule: 90% are cystic, 90% have calcification, 90% enhance, and over 90% have a suprasellar component [25, 27]. On T1WI and T2WI, the cystic component of the tumor most often shows hyperintensity, while the solid component on T2WI has a mixed signal [25]. The solid component on the T1C sequence shows vivid enhancement [25]. Native MSCT has an important role in the detection of calcifications [25, 27].

5.7 Differential diagnosis

When it comes to the differential diagnosis of craniopharyngioma in children, the following come into consideration: arachnoid cyst, PCA, atypical teratoid/rhabdoid tumor (AT/RT), pituicytoma, pituitary adenoma, and Rathke cleft cyst [25].

5.8 Treatment

In the treatment of CP, an interdisciplinary approach is very important. Close cooperation of a pediatric neurologist, pediatric endocrinologist, ophthalmologist, radiologist, neurosurgeon, radiosurgery specialist, and oncologist is necessary. Of course, a clinical psychologist who provides psychological support to the patient also plays an important role in the treatment. Very often, the treatment of craniopharyngioma is not straightforward, but requires a combination of different forms of treatment, from open neurosurgery to radiosurgery and oncological treatment. One of the main reasons for the complexity of the treatment of these tumors is their unfavorable location, since they are surrounded by important neurovascular structures and in direct proximity to the pituitary gland. Another reason is the high rate of disease recurrence.

When it comes to surgical treatment of CPs, it is necessary to choose the best approach in order to achieve tumor resection and maximum safety during the resection. The possibilities include transcranial approach and endoscopic endonasal transsphenoidal approach (EETA). An additional surgical option in the treatment of craniopharyngioma is stereotactic or open biopsy [28]. Benefits of a biopsy can be multiple. Namely, in addition to obtaining a histopathology result, the compressive effect of the tumor on the surrounding structures is reduced by puncturing the cyst [26, 28]. The form of surgical treatment is most often based on the Kassam et al. classification system, which divides craniopharyngiomas depending on their relative position to the infundibulum of the pituitary gland [26]. Accordingly, four types of craniopharyngioma are distinguished: pre-infundibular, trans-infundibular, retro-infundibular, and, lastly, CP, which is located exclusively within the third cerebral ventricle [26]. Thus, in the first three types, the EETA approach is most often used in treatment, while in the last variant, a transcranial approach is strictly indicated, which includes transcallosal, transcortical, or transventricular approaches [26]. Frequently, in the early postoperative recovery after surgical treatment of craniopharyngioma, hormonal imbalance is verified, most often in the form of adrenal insufficiency, hypothyroidism, and diabetes insipidus [29]. All of the above must be anticipated and incorporated into the preoperative and postoperative management of patients [29].

Regarding surgical approaches in the treatment of CPs, the possibilities include the transsphenoidal, transcranial, and supraorbital approaches [30]. Research has shown that EETA has the best results [30, 31], since it is associated with a lower incidence rate of vision deterioration and a lower rate of recurrence of the tumor, as well as a higher rate of postoperative vision improvement [30, 31]. Research has also proved that EETA is an equally successful approach in both adult patients and children with craniopharyngiomas and does not depend on the size of the nasal cavity or the degree of pneumatization of the sphenoid sinus [31].

There is still no absolute consensus as to which form or combination of treatments is best in the treatment of CP. Surgical treatment is indicated in patients who present with symptoms of hormonal imbalance, that is, disorders in the functioning of the pituitary gland, and with symptoms of hydrocephalus [26]. In addition to the reduction of the tumor mass and thus the release of the compressed surrounding neurovascular structures, surgery is essential in order to obtain histopathology findings [26]. The more radical the surgical intervention, the higher the incidence of dysfunction of the hypothalamus and pituitary gland [29]. Currently, it is considered that surgical treatment in combination with adjuvant external beam irradiation is the best treatment combination in the first attempt to treat patients with CB [32]. Also, it is considered that limited resection, combined with RT that does not damage the hypothalamus and pituitary gland, is a better treatment option than radical surgery that removes the tumor and leads to damage to the hypothalamic-pituitary axis [32]. RT of cystic CP can lead to cyst enlargement [32].

In the early postoperative period, the main complication is hormonal imbalance, which is most often manifested as DI, hypothyroidism, and sexual dysfunction [29]. For this reason, during this period, it is very important to perform frequent hormone level checks as well as monitor sodium and urine osmolarity [26, 29].

Recurrence of CP occurs in an interval between 1 and 4 years [32]. The treatment of recurrent CP is more demanding than the treatment of initial CP, due to the presence of adhesions and post-radiation changes in the surgical field [32], which contributes to less successful results than with primary treatment [32].

RT plays an important role in the treatment of CP and is used in the prevention of tumor recurrence as well as in the treatment of recurrent CP growth [26]. RT has shown particularly good results as an adjuvant form of treatment to surgical treatment of CP [26, 32]. Different forms of RT are used in the treatment of CP, such as conventional external RT, proton beam therapy (PBT), stereotactic radiotherapy (SRS), RS, and brachytherapy [26]. The main complication of RT is impaired pituitary function [29]. Brachytherapy is used in the treatment of dominantly cystic forms of CP and involves intracystic irradiation [32]. In almost 90% of patients with the cystic form of CP, shrinkage of the cyst is seen, while the efficiency in mixed CP is lower, and tumor reduction is recorded in about 60% of patients [32].

SRS is also used in the treatment of CP. This form of treatment involves the delivery of fractionated radiation exclusively to the tumor surface while preserving the surrounding sensitive neural structures [32]. SRS has shown great success in the treatment of smaller-volume CPs as well as in the treatment of smaller residues and relapses of the tumor, while the success rate of this method drops significantly in larger-volume tumors [32]. The success rate of SRS treatment of smaller-volume CP is between 60% and 90% [32].

Experiences in the use of chemotherapy in the treatment of CP are quite limited. One of the therapeutic options is intracystic treatment with Bleomycin [26, 32]. This form of treatment can contribute to the successful reduction of the tumor volume. However, there are real risks of the toxic effect of the antineoplastic agent in the case of uncontrolled leakage into the surrounding neural tissue, which can even have a lethal outcome [26, 32].

5.9 Prognosis

Five-year survival in patients with CP is around 90%, with a very high tumor recurrence rate of up to 50% [26].

5.10 Case presentation

The patient, a 4-year-old girl, presented clinically with behavioral changes, poor appetite, fatigue, and headache. At the time of examination, the child was GCS 12, with no signs of lateralization. In the Emergency Department, MRI of the brain was performed, which verified an extensive neoplastic process in the sellar region with extensive suprasellar extension (**Figure 11**). In view of the above, an operation was indicated, during which right-sided frontoparietal osteoplastic parasagittal

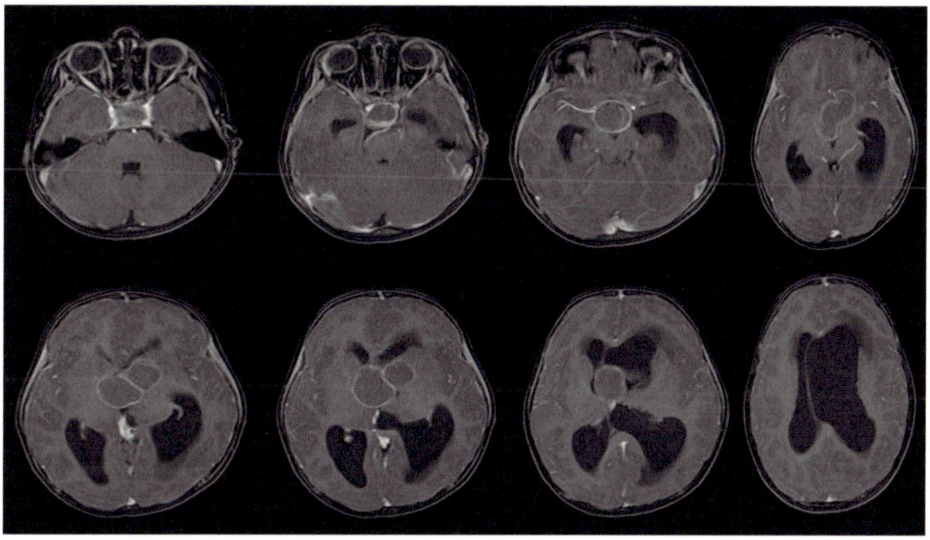

Figure 11.
This image displays axial T1C sequences of MRI images of the brain, confirming the presence of a craniopharyngioma with a large suprasellar extension and signs of accompanying hydrocephalus.

craniotomy and maximum reduction of the tumor were performed. Histopathological analysis confirmed a craniopharyngioma of the adamantinomatous type (**Figure 12**). Histologically, the tumor tissue consisted of clusters of well-differentiated epithelial cells palisading peripherally in places, with more abundant formation of cornified material. Calcifications were also present. Immunohistochemically, the tumor cells were cytoplasmically positive for beta-catenin. Postoperatively, the patient underwent multidisciplinary monitoring for dysfunction of the hypothalamic-pituitary axis and the consequent occurrence of central diabetes insipidus, secondary adrenal insufficiency, and secondary hypothyroidism. A follow-up MRI of the brain performed 3 months after the operation verified a significant reduction of the tumor with minimal residual tumor present. One year after the first operation, the girl presented again with headache and deterioration of vision. The control MRI of the brain verified an increase in the cystic component of the tumor, pressing into the area of the hypothalamus and pushing the chiasm anteriorly (**Figure 13**). Additional surgical

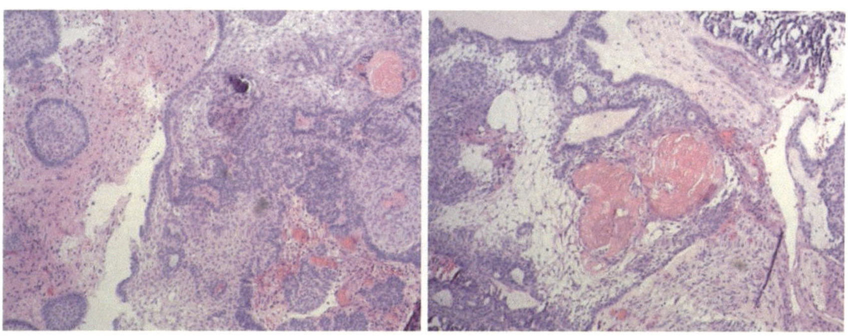

Figure 12.
Craniopharyngioma—histological HE staining, microscope magnification ×200.

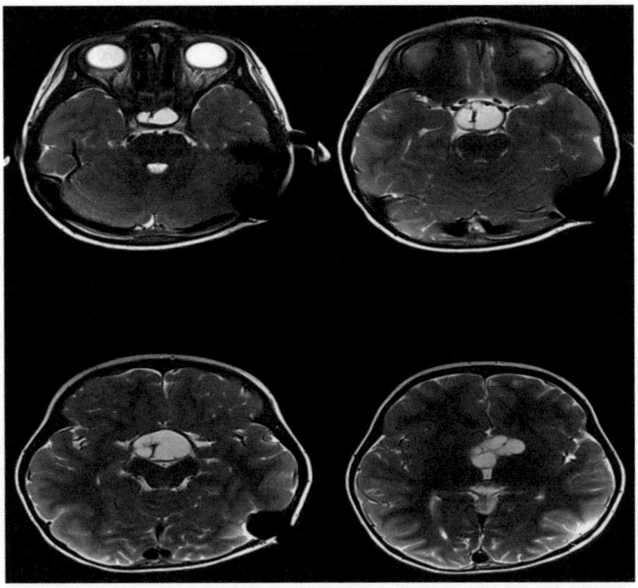

Figure 13.
This picture shows the second postoperative MRI of the brain, an axial section in T2 sequence, which verifies the recurrence of the cystic component of the tumor process, especially in the suprasellar area.

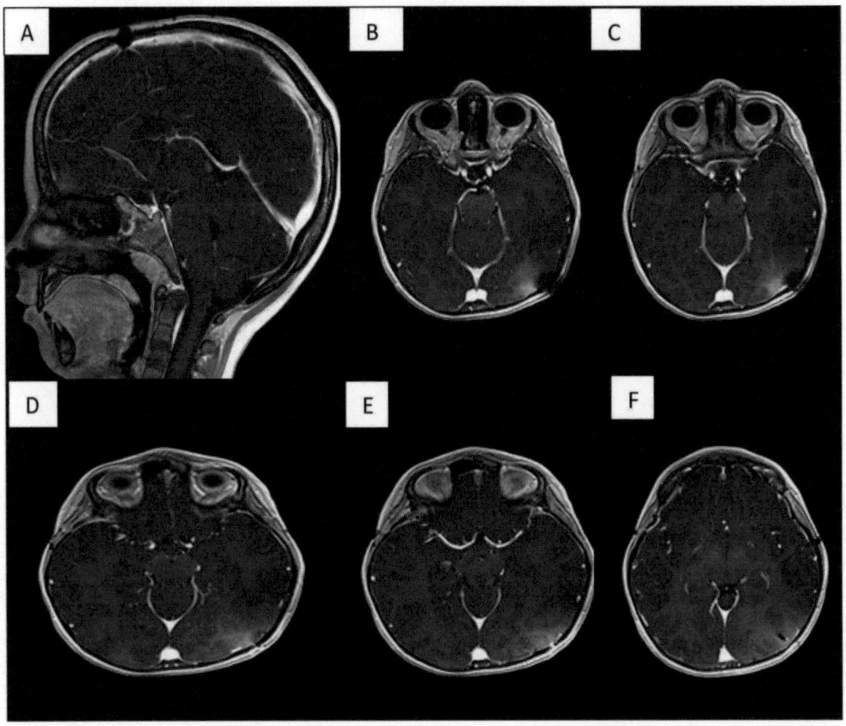

Figure 14.
A: Postoperative T1C sequence, sagittal section shows complete removal of a craniopharyngioma through two neurosurgical procedures. B, C, D, E, and F: T1C sequence, axial section showing complete removal of a craniopharyngioma through two neurosurgical procedures.

treatment was indicated. Left pterional osteoplastic craniotomy was performed, after which a subfrontal approach through the opto-carotid triangle was used to reach the area of the tumor, which was completely removed in this act. Follow-up MRI of the brain showed a normal postoperative finding (**Figure 14**).

6. Conclusions

Open neurosurgery of resection or reduction of the tumor process still has a large and important role in the treatment of CNS tumors, especially in the pediatric population. CNS tumors in children very often occur in the area of the posterior cranial fossa, and they can be benign or malignant. It is the surgical procedure that brings numerous benefits, such as reducing the volume of the tumor, removing the compressive effect, obtaining the histology of the tumor, and very often solving the issue of hydrocephalus.

Acknowledgements

The authors wish to thank Aleksandra Žmegač Horvat for language editing of the manuscript.

Conflict of interest

In writing this chapter, the authors declare that there was no conflict of interest of any kind.

Thanks

It is a great honor and privilege to participate in the writing of such a comprehensive textbook. The Republic of Croatia Ministry of Health Reference Center for Pediatric Neurosurgery, which operates as part of the Department of Neurosurgery at the UHC Zagreb, has extensive knowledge and experience in the treatment of pediatric patients with tumor diseases of the central nervous system. The authors would like to thank their colleagues from the aforementioned center for the medical documentation provided, which was used in the writing of the clinical case presentation section in this chapter.

Acronyms and abbreviations

ACP	adamantinomatous craniopharyngioma
AT/RT	atypical teratoid/rhabdoid tumor
CMB	classic medulloblastoma
CNS	central nervous system
CP	craniopharyngioma
CT	chemotherapy
DNMB	desmoplastic/nodular medulloblastoma

EETA	endoscopic endonasal transsphenoidal approach
D/ENMB	medulloblastoma with extensive nodularity
HT	hormonal therapy
LC/AMB	large cell/anaplastic medulloblastoma
MB	medulloblastoma
MPE	myxopapillary ependymoma
MRI	magnetic resonance imaging
MSCT	multislice computed tomography
PA	pilocytic astrocytoma
PBT	proton beam therapy
PCP	papillary craniopharyngioma
RS	radiosurgery
RT	radiotherapy
SE	subependymoma
SRS	stereotactic radiosurgery
WHO	World Health Organization

Author details

Miroslav Vukić* and Ivan Pašalić
University Hospital Center Zagreb, Zagreb, Croatia

*Address all correspondence to: vukicmd@gmail.com

IntechOpen

References

[1] Scheithauer BW. Development of the WHO classification of tumors of the central nervous system: A historical perspective. Brain Pathology. 2009;**19**(4):551-564. DOI: 10.1111/j.1750-3639.2008.00192.x. Epub 2009 Sep 2

[2] Torp SH, Solheim O, Skjulsvik AJ. The WHO 2021 classification of central nervous system tumours: A practical update on what neurosurgeons need to know—A minireview. Acta Neurochirurgica. 2022;**164**(9):2453-2464. DOI: 10.1007/s00701-022-05301-y. Epub 2022 Jul 26

[3] Louis DN, Perry A, Wesseling P, Brat DJ, Cree IA, Figarella-Branger D, et al. The 2021 WHO classification of tumors of the central nervous system: A summary. Neuro-Oncology. 2021;**23**(8):1231-1251. DOI: 10.1093/neuonc/noab106

[4] Knight J, De Jesus O. Pilocytic astrocytoma. In: In: StatPearls. Treasure Island (FL): StatPearls Publishing; 2024. Available from: https://www.ncbi.nlm.nih.gov/books/NBK560614/. [Updated 2023 Aug 23]

[5] Damodharan S, Puccetti D. Pediatric central nervous system tumor overview and emerging treatment considerations. Brain Sciences. 2023;**13**(7):1106. DOI: 10.3390/brainsci13071106

[6] Louis DN, Ohgaki H, Wiestler OD, Cavenee WK. WHO Classification of Tumours of the Central Nervous System. Revise 4th ed. Lyon: IARC Press; 2016

[7] Soon WC, Goacher E, Solanki S, Hayes J, Kapetanstrataki M, Picton S, et al. The role of sex genotype in paediatric CNS tumour incidence and survival. Child's Nervous System. 2021;**37**(7):2177-2186. DOI: 10.1007/s00381-021-05165-0. Epub 2021 May 5

[8] Collins VP, Jones DT, Giannini C. Pilocytic astrocytoma: Pathology, molecular mechanisms and markers. Acta Neuropathologica. 2015;**129**(6):775-788

[9] Kameda-Smith MM, Green K, Hutton DL, Jeelani NUO, Thompson DNP, Hargrave D, et al. The role of reoperation in pediatric cerebellar pilocytic astrocytoma. Journal of Neurosurgery. Pediatrics. 2024:1-7. DOI: 10.3171/2024.2.PEDS23236. Epub ahead of print

[10] Muthukumar N. Hydrocephalus associated with posterior fossa tumors: How to manage effectively? Neurology India. 2021;**69**(Supplement.):S342-S349. DOI: 10.4103/0028-3886.332260

[11] Brown MT, Friedman HS, Oakes WJ, Boyko OB, Hockenberger B, Schold SC Jr. Chemotherapy for pilocytic astrocytomas. Cancer. 1993;**71**(10):3165-3172. DOI: 10.1002/1097-0142(19930515)71:10<3165::aid-cncr28207 11044>3.0.co;2-n

[12] Ruella M, Giovannini S, Pirozzi Chiusa C, Perez Zabala J, Argañaraz R, Mantese B, et al. Retrospective cohort study assessing postoperative functional outcome, cerebellar mutism and hydrocephalus. World Neurosurgery: X. 2023;**19**:100180. DOI: 10.1016/j.wnsx.2023.100180

[13] Ellison DW, Korshunov A, Northcott PA, Taylor MD, Kaur K, Clifford SC. Medulloblastoma. In: WHO Classification of Tumours Editorial Board. Central Nervous System Tumours, WHO Classification of Tumours

Series. 5th ed. Vol. 6. Lyon (France): International Agency for Research on Cancer; 2021. Available from: https://publications.iarc.fr/601

[14] Jackson K, Packer RJ. Recent advances in pediatric medulloblastoma. Current Neurology and Neuroscience Reports. 2023;**23**(12):841-848. DOI: 10.1007/s11910-023-01316-9. Epub 2023 Nov 9

[15] Radiopaedia. Medulloblastoma [Internet]. Available from: https://radiopaedia.org/articles/medulloblastoma [Accessed: May 20, 2024]

[16] Mahapatra S, Amsbaugh MJ. Medulloblastoma. In: StatPearls. Treasure Island (FL): StatPearls Publishing; 2024. Available from: https://www.ncbi.nlm.nih.gov/books/NBK431069. [Updated 2023 Jun 26]

[17] Kijima N, Kanemura Y. Molecular classification of medulloblastoma. Neurologia Medico-Chirurgica (Tokyo). 2016;**56**(11):687-697. DOI: 10.2176/nmc.ra.2016-0016. Epub 2016 May 26

[18] Chang CH, Housepian EM, Herbert C Jr. An operative staging system and a megavoltage radiotherapeutic technic for cerebellar medulloblastomas. Radiology. 1969;**93**(6):1351-1359

[19] Korones DN. Pediatric ependymomas: Something old, something new. Pediatric Hematology Oncology Journal. 2023;**8**(2):114-120

[20] Kresbach C, Neyazi S, Schüller U. Updates in the classification of ependymal neoplasms: The 2021 WHO classification and beyond. Brain Pathology. 2022;**32**(4):e13068. DOI: 10.1111/bpa.13068. Epub 2022 Mar 21

[21] Riabowol G, Yiallouros M. Ependymoma—Brief Information [Internet]. 2024. Available from: https://dx.doi.org/10.1591/poh.patinfo.ependy.kurz.1.20070626

[22] Zamora EA, Alkherayf F. Ependymoma. In: StatPearls. Treasure Island (FL): StatPearls Publishing; 2024. Available from: https://www.ncbi.nlm.nih.gov/books/NBK538244. [Updated 2023 Jun 26]

[23] McGuire CS, Sainani KL, Fisher PG. Incidence patterns for ependymoma: A surveillance, epidemiology, and end results study. Journal of Neurosurgery. 2009;**110**(4):725-729

[24] Indelicato DJ, Ioakeim-Ioannidou M, Bradley JA, Mailhot-Vega RB, Morris CG, Tarbell NJ, et al. Proton therapy for pediatric ependymoma: Mature results from a bicentric study. International Journal of Radiation Oncology, Biology, Physics. 2021;**110**(3):815-820. DOI: 10.1016/j.ijrobp.2021.01.027. Epub 2021 Jan 27

[25] Maia R, Miranda A, Geraldo AF, Sampaio L, Ramaglia A, Tortora D, et al. Neuroimaging of pediatric tumors of the sellar region-a review in light of the 2021 WHO classification of tumors of the central nervous system. Frontiers in Pediatrics. 2023;**11**:1162654. DOI: 10.3389/fped.2023.1162654

[26] Ortiz, Torres M, Shafiq I, Mesfin FB. Craniopharyngioma. In: StatPearls. Treasure Island (FL): StatPearls Publishing; 2024. Available from: https://www.ncbi.nlm.nih.gov/books/NBK459371. [Updated 2023 Apr 24]

[27] Castillo M, Mukherji SK. Imaging of the Pediatric Head, Neck, and Spine. Philadelphia: Lippincott-Raven; 1996

[28] Trippel M, Nikkhah G. Stereotactic neurosurgical treatment options for craniopharyngioma. Frontiers in

Endocrinology. 2012;**3**:63. DOI: 10.3389/fendo.2012.00063

[29] Zhou Z, Zhang S, Hu F. Endocrine disorder in patients with craniopharyngioma. Frontiers in Neurology. 2021;**12**:737743. DOI: 10.3389/fneur.2021.737743

[30] Webb KL, Pruter WW, Hinkle ML, Walsh MT. Comparing surgical approaches for craniopharyngioma resection among adults and children: A meta-analysis and systematic review. World Neurosurgery. 2023;**175**:e876-e896. DOI: 10.1016/j.wneu.2023.04.037. Epub 2023 Apr 14

[31] Schelini JC, Cavalheiro S, Dastoli PA, Hirai ÉR, Atallah C, Costa M, et al. Endoscopic endonasal transsphenoidal approach for pediatric craniopharyngiomas: A case series. International Journal of Pediatric Otorhinolaryngology. 2020;**130**:109786. DOI: 10.1016/j.ijporl.2019.109786. Epub 2019 Nov 19

[32] Lithgow K, Hamblin R, Pohl U, et al. Craniopharyngiomas. In: Feingold KR, Anawalt B, Blackman MR, et al., editors. Endotext. South Dartmouth (MA): MDText.com, Inc.; 2000. Available from: https://www.ncbi.nlm.nih.gov/books/NBK538819. [Updated 2022 Feb 26]